NUTRITION AND DIET RESEARCH PROGRESS

AF769701

LINOLEIC ACIDS

SOURCES, BIOCHEMICAL PROPERTIES AND HEALTH EFFECTS

IGHO ONAKPOYA
EDITOR

NOVA BIOMEDICAL
New York

Copyright © 2012 by Nova Science Publishers, Inc.

All rights reserved. No part of this book may be reproduced, stored in a retrieval system or transmitted in any form or by any means: electronic, electrostatic, magnetic, tape, mechanical photocopying, recording or otherwise without the written permission of the Publisher.

For permission to use material from this book please contact us:
Telephone 631-231-7269; Fax 631-231-8175
Web Site: http://www.novapublishers.com

NOTICE TO THE READER

The Publisher has taken reasonable care in the preparation of this book, but makes no expressed or implied warranty of any kind and assumes no responsibility for any errors or omissions. No liability is assumed for incidental or consequential damages in connection with or arising out of information contained in this book. The Publisher shall not be liable for any special, consequential, or exemplary damages resulting, in whole or in part, from the readers' use of, or reliance upon, this material. Any parts of this book based on government reports are so indicated and copyright is claimed for those parts to the extent applicable to compilations of such works.

Independent verification should be sought for any data, advice or recommendations contained in this book. In addition, no responsibility is assumed by the publisher for any injury and/or damage to persons or property arising from any methods, products, instructions, ideas or otherwise contained in this publication.

This publication is designed to provide accurate and authoritative information with regard to the subject matter covered herein. It is sold with the clear understanding that the Publisher is not engaged in rendering legal or any other professional services. If legal or any other expert assistance is required, the services of a competent person should be sought. FROM A DECLARATION OF PARTICIPANTS JOINTLY ADOPTED BY A COMMITTEE OF THE AMERICAN BAR ASSOCIATION AND A COMMITTEE OF PUBLISHERS.

Additional color graphics may be available in the e-book version of this book.

Library of Congress Cataloging-in-Publication Data

ISBN: 978-1-62257-384-4
Library of Congress Control Number: 2012941597

Published by Nova Science Publishers, Inc. † New York

Contents

Preface

Nutritional science has grown over the past few years, and research into the relationship between nutrition and health is an ever expanding area. Linoleic acid (LA) is an omega-6 essential fatty acid which is involved in a number of physiologic and biologic processes. It is a component of natural diet, and also commonly available as an over-the-counter supplement.

This book, Linoleic Acids: Sources, Biochemical Properties and Health Effects, provides essential information about the basic and applied research relating to LA.

The opening two chapters give a thorough overview of the natural sources of LA, its antioxidant properties, and how LA and its derivatives influence the nutritional and health value of our diet.

The linoleic and fatty acid composition of meat is influenced by the type of diet through which animals are fed, and this thus has health implications for human health. A chapter in this book is devoted to examining the effect of the type of forage on the LA composition of agricultural animals in the Russian Siberia.

The oxidative stability of linoleic acid, as well as the processes involved in its extraction from natural sources affects the flavor and nutritional value of edible oils. The mechanism of oxidation and antioxidation of linoleic and unsaturated fatty acids is extensively described in this volume.

Chapters are also devoted to examining the procedures used for the extraction of linoleic and fatty acids in the nutrition industry, and describe the pros and cons of such processes. The influence of geographical location on the LA content of virgin olive oil, as well as the effect of the type of olive oil on consumer preferences is also investigated.

The use of nutritional supplements as anti-obesity agents is quite common, and a chapter is dedicated to evaluating the evidence relating to the role of LA isomers as weight loss aids. Chapters also discuss the effectiveness of LA derivatives in the management of atopic dermatitis as well as the prevention of ischemic stroke. The last two chapters are monographs which explore the potential relationships between dietary LA and the development of various types of cancers.

Food researchers and technologists, physicians, dieticians, nutritionists and biochemists will find the information in this book very useful.

In closing, I would like to thank the authors of each chapter for their valuable contributions, without which this volume wouldn't have been possible.

In: Linoleic Acids
Editor: Igho Onakpoya

ISBN: 978-1-62257-384-4
© 2012 Nova Science Publishers, Inc.

Chapter I

Linoleic and α-Linolenic Acid Content of Pork, Beef, and Lamb Lipids

***Pilar Teresa Garcia*[1] *and Jorge J. Casal*[2]**
[1]Area Bioquímica y Nutrición.Tecnología Alimentos, Centro de Investigación en Agroindustria, CIA Instituto Nacional de Tecnnología Agropecuaria, INTA, Argentina
[2]Universidad de Moron. Buenos Aires. Argentina

Abstract

Linoleic acid (LA) and α- linolenic acid (ALA) belong to the n-6 and n-3 series of polyunsaturated fatty acids (PUFA) respectively. They are defined as essential fatty acids (EFA) since they are not synthesized in the human body. Because LA is the metabolic precursor of arachidonic acid (AA) and bioactive eicosanoids derived from AA, there is concern that dietary LA could augment tissue AA content, eicosanoid formation and consequently enhance the risk of and/or exacerbate conditions associated with acute and chronic diseases such as cancers, cardiovascular disease, inflammation, neurological disorders, etc. The n-6/n-3 ratio is considered as a nutritional index for the healthiness of food for human consumption. The concentration of LA and ALA in pork, beef or lamb lipids is dependent on whether or not the species is a ruminant. In ruminant animals, the majority of the dietary unsaturated fatty acids are hydrogenated to saturated fatty acids in the rumen during digestion. Non- ruminant meat contains proportionally more unsaturated fatty acids. LA and ALA proportions in meat lipids are affected by several variables including breed, sex, type of muscle, anatomical location, feeding regimen, botanical composition, freshness of grass, supplementation, altitude, etc. All of these variables influence also the ratio LA/ALA. Dietary design will in the future be of great importance for improving the nutritional value of meats.

List of Abbreviations

AA	Arachidonic acid
ALA	α-linoleic acid
CHD	Cardiovascular heart disease
CLA	Conjugated linoleic acid
DHA	Docosapentaenoic acid
EFA	Essential fatty acids
EPA	Eicosapentaenoic acid
FA	Fatty acids
LA	Linoleic acid
LD	Longissimus dorsi
MUFA	Monounsaturated fatty acids
NL	Neutral lipids
PL	Phospholipids
PUFA	Polyunsaturated fatty acids
SFA	Saturated fatty acids

1. Introduction

Linoleic acid (LA) and α-linoleic acid (ALA) belong to the n-6 (omega 6) and n-3 (omega 3) series of polyunsaturated fatty acids (PUFA) respectively. They are defined as essential fatty acids (EFA) since they are not synthesized in the human body and are mostly obtained from the diet. Hence it is essential to provide these two acids in the diet, because they are precursors of long chain PUFA. In the absence of LA and ALA growth, learning and visual acuity are negatively influenced and the risk for cardiovascular disease is increased [1]. LA is the most prominent PUFA in the Western diet. It is practically found in every food that we eat. Because LA is the metabolic precursor of arachidonic acid (AA) and bioactive eicosanoids derived from AA, there is concern that dietary LA could augment tissue AA content, eicosanoid formation and subsequently enhance the risk of and/or exacerbate conditions associated with acute and chronic diseases such as cancers, cardiovascular diseases, inflammation, neurological disorders, etc. [2]. The recommended intake for humans of n-6 fatty acids (FA) is approximately 4 % of dietary energy with a minimum of 1.5%, and the intake of n-3 FA should be about 0.75% of dietary energy to avoid EFA deficiency. The n-6/n-3 ratio is considered as a nutritional index for the healthiness of food for human consumption and it should not exceed a value of 4 in the human diet to lower the risk of cardiovascular heart disease (CHD) [3]. To ensure balanced eicosanoid production, the ratio n-6/n-3 should be between 4:1 and 6:1 [4]. This is one of the main reasons why the meat obtained from animals raised on pasture is considered to have a higher value for human health, compared to the meat from animals fed concentrates. There is much evidence that increased consumption of n-3 FA protect from CHD and that excessive consumption of n-6 FA at the expense of n-3 promote CHD and other diseases. Analysis of n-3 PUFA intake, intake recommendations, and health claims are often limited to C18:3 (ALA), C20:5 (EPA) and C22:6 (DHA) and often omit C22:5 (DPA). DPA is an intermediate in the production of

DHA from EPA and its contribution in ruminant lipids is higher than EPA and DHA. The functional and nutritional attributes of DPA are largely unknown but some studies show that DPA appears to be a primary end point for the synthesis of n-3 PUFA from ALA [5].

Health related concerns about meat lipids is limited to its relatively high concentrations of hypercholesterolemic, saturated fatty acids (SFA), low concentration of hypo-cholesterolemic PUFA and the presence of cholesterol. The nutritional value depends on the amounts of SFA, monounsaturated fatty acids (MUFA), n-3 and n-6 PUFA, CLA, cholesterol and the ratio n-6/n-3. The FA composition of meat is dependent on whether or not the species is a ruminant. In ruminant animals (e.g. cattle, sheep) the majority (>90%) of dietary unsaturated FA are hydrogenated to SFAs in the rumen during digestion. Non- ruminant meat (e.g. pork, poultry) contains proportionally more unsaturated FA, but its composition is still dependent on the FA profile of the animal feed. The FA profile of meat will also vary depending on the proportion of lean meat and fat present. The proportions of LA and ALA from ruminant meats, beef and lamb, are affected by several factors, mainly the ruminal biohydrogenation of the LA and ALA from dietary grass and cereals lipids. The FA composition of adipose tissue and muscle in meat animals is affected by a number of factors including diet, total fat content, breed, genotype, age and gender. It also differs among adipose depot sites throughout the carcass [6]. Other factors are season, feeding regimen, botanical composition, freshness of grass, supplementation, altitude, etc. Dietary lipids may be supplied mainly as grasses, forages, seed oils, rich oil cereals, fish oils, etc. In most species, fat content of the meat shows higher variability, depending on the balance between dietary energy content and metabolic requirements, associated with the genetic characteristics of the animal. Sex and age differences in muscle FA composition can often be explained by the degree of fatness and associated changes in the triacylglycerol/phospholipid ratio. However, even after correction for fatness, differences in the carcass lipid FA composition were reported between steers and heifers, and between bulls and steers [7, 8]. Studies comparing FA composition between bulls and heifers without any confounding effects of diet and age are scarce. Sex and breed differences in beef FA composition are to a great extend associated with the content of intramuscular fat due to a higher proportion of membrane phospholipids (high in PUFA) and a lower proportion of triacylglycerol (high in SFA and MUFA) in leaner animals. Phopholipids (PL) are characterized by a high PUFA content and depends on the metabolic fibre type of the muscle. The phospholipid content is relatively constant and less influenced by species, breed, nutrition, and age. In contrast to PL, the content of triacylglycerols varies widely between 0.2 and 5 g /100g fresh tissue [9], and is mainly dependent of the fat level, breed, and the location of the muscle. Animal growth rate, through its effects on fat formation, can strongly influence muscle FA composition [10]. The discrepancy in results might be related to differences in type or quality of forage, or to the differences in breeds. Gender is also known to affect the fat deposition, e.g. castration is associated with increased fat deposition. Studies in humans have suggested that gender is also associated with the differences in the capacity for conversion of ALA to EPA, DPA and DHA. The conversion of ALA to EPA, DPA and DHA and LA to AA is dependent on the sequential activities of Δ6 and Δ5 desaturases and on elongation of the carbon chain [11].

Table 1. Influence of breed, sex and anatomical location on linoleic acid (LA), α-linolenic acid (ALA) and LA/ALA ratio in pork body lipids

Item	LA %	ALA%	LA/ALA	Reference
LD Sire Minimum	10.0	0.47a	21.28	[16]
LD Sire Maximum	11.7	0.71b	16.42	
SM LW x (LR x LW)	10.70b	0.61	17.54	[17]
SM D x (LR x LW)	9.39b	0.57	16.47	
SM P x (LR x LW)	11.52a	0.58	19.86	
Sub fat N Stress negative	10.21	0.39	26.18	[18]
Sub fat Nn Stress carrier	10.08	0.39	25.85	
Sub fat Nn Stress positive	10.97	0.43	25.51	
Sub fat inner layer Duroc Barrows	7.93b	0.52b	15.25	[19]
Sub fat inner layer Yorkshire Barrows	9.04a	0.62a	14.58	
Sub fat outer layer Duroc Barrows	10.3a	0.58a	17.76	[19]
Sub fat outer layer Yorkshire Barrows	9.88a	0.58a	17.21	
Sub fat inner layer Duroc Gilts	8.08b	0.51b	15.84	[19]
Sub fat inner layer Yorkshire Gilts	9.62a	0.63a	15.27	
Sub fat outer layer Duroc Gilt	9.22b	0.49b	18.82	[19]
Sub fat outer layer Yorkshire Gilts	12.04a	0.73a	16.49	
LD Castrated males	10.2b	0.54	18.89	[16]
LD Females	11.4a	0.58	19.66	
SM Castrated males	9.93b	0.56b	17.73	[17]
SM Females	11.12a	0.61a	18.23	
Sub fat Castrated males	11.56b	1.02b	11.33	[17]
Sub fat Females	12.73a	1.10a	11.57	
LT Barrow	9.27b	0.79b	11.73	[22]
LT Gilt	11.4a	0.89a	12.81	
Back fat Female 3% rapeseed oil	15.93a	3.45a	4.62	[24]
Back fat Castrated 3% rapeseed oil	13.93b	3.03b	4.60	
Back fat Female 3% palm oil	13.63a	1.25a	10.90	[24]
Back fat Castrated 3% palm oil	12.38b	1.17b	10.58	
LD Female 3% rapeseed oil NL	5.11	0.93a	5.49	[24]
LD Castrated 3% rapeseed oil NL	4.81	1.01a	4.76	
LD Female 3% palm oil NL	4.61	0.43b	10.72	[24]
LD Castrated 3% palm oil NL	4.19	0.39b	10.74	
LD Female 3% rapeseed oil PL	35.11	1.99a	17.64	[24]
LD Castrated 3% rapeseed oil PL	35.02	2.06a	17.00	
LD Female 3% palm oil PL	34.96	1.55b	22.55	[24]
LD Castrated 3% palm oil PL	36.45	1.59b	22.92	
BF Muscle Castrated NL	6.34	0.51	12.43	[25]

Item	LA %	ALA%	LA/ALA	Reference
BF Muscle Gilts NL	6.25	0.52	12.02	
BF Muscle Castrated PL	28.27a	0.79	35.78	[25]
BF Muscle Gilts PL	27.96b	0.78	35.85	
LD Entire males	7.58a	0.58a	13.07	[26]
LD Female	6.16b	0.47b	13.11	
Sub fat Barrows	9.48	0.37	25.62	[18]
Sub fat Gilts	11.36	0.44	25.82	
ST Duroc Barrows	6.7b	1.1a	6.09	[27]
ST Duroc Gilts	7.3a	1.2a	6.08	
SM Duroc Barrows	7.8b	1.0a	7.08	[27]
SM Duroc Gilts	8.4a	1.3a	6.46	
Sub fat Outer Layer Loin	13.66a	1.10a	12.42	[12]
Sub fat Inner Layer Loin	11.71b	0.99b	11.83	
Intermuscular fat Loin	12.01b	0.94b	12.78	

a,b,c indicate a significant difference ($p<0.05$) between breed, sex or anatomical location reported within each respective study. "na" indicates that the value was not reported in the original study.

Abbreviations: LW: Large White; D: Duroc; P: Pietrain; LR: Landrace; LD: *Longissimus dorsi*: SM: Semimembranosus; LT: *Longissimus thoracis*; BF: *Biceps femoris*; ST: *Semitendinosus*; Sub: subcutaneous; NL: Neutral lipids; PL: Phospholipids.

Table 1 a. Influence of production system on linoleic acid (LA), α-linolenic acid (ALA) and LA/ALA ratio in pork body lipids

Item	LA %	ALA%	LA/ALA	Reference
Total carcass No fat	6.62	0.47	14.09	[28]
Total carcass Tallow 10%	10.5d	0.93	11.29	
Total carcass High oleic SFO oil 10%	11.6c	0.72	16.11	
Total carcass Sunflower oil (SFO) 10%	27.5[a]	0.70	39.29	
Total carcass Linseed oil 10%	13.3d	14.18	0.94	
Total carcass Fat blend 10%	12.9	5.42	2.38	
Total carcass Oil blend 10%	11.7	8.86	1.32	
LD Control	11.65d	0.49d	23.77	[29]
LD Linseed (10%) 30 days	12.09c	2.46c	4.91	
LD Linseed (10%) 60 days	13.03b	3.32b	3.92	
LD Linseed (10%) 90 days	15.98a	4.15a	3.85	
Carcass fat No fat	6.62e	0.47b	14.09	[30]
Carcass fat Tallow (T)	10.5d	0.93c	11.29	
Carcass fat High oleic sunflower oil	11.6c	0.72d	16.11	
Carcass fat Sunflower oil (SFO)	27.5a	0.70db	39.29	
Carcass fat Linseed oil (LO)	13.3b	14.18a	0.94	
LD Palm kernel oil	0.92b	0.63b	1.46	[31]
LD Palm oil	11.13b	0.57b	19.53	
LD Soybean oil	13.24a	0.87a	15.22	
LT Basal	11.2	0.55b	20.36	[22]
LT Linseed 3%	10.4	1.24a	8.39	
LT Fish oil 10%	8.84	0.47b	18.81	
BF Muscle NL Indoors	6.09	0.47b	12.96	[25]
BF Muscle NL Free-range	6.51	0.56a	11.63	
BF Muscle PL Indoors	27.46b	0.77	35.66	

Table 1 a. (Continued)

Item	LA %	ALA%	LA/ALA	Reference
BF Muscle PL Free-range	28.77a	0.80	35.96	
LD Low fat	6.08a	0.46a	13.22	[26]
LD Low fat + 4.8g fish oil	6.09a	0.48ab	13.24	
LD 41.2 g palm kernel oil	7.31b	0.52ab	14.06	
LD 38.7g palm kernel oil + 2.5g fish oil	7.05ab	0.56ab	12.59	
LD 36.1g palm kernel oil +5.2g fish oil	7.39b	0.57ab	12.96	
LD 34g palm kernel oil +7.2g fish oil	7.29b	0.58b	12.57	
LD Sunflower diet LA/ALA 20.7	14.48a	0.42b	34.48	[32]
LD Linseed diet LA/ALA 1.5	12.88b	2.28a	5.65	
SM Sunflower diet LA/ALA 20.7	16.29a	0.50b	32.57	[32]
SM Linseed diet LA/ALA 1.5	13.62b	2.54a	5.36	
LD Control diet Total fatty acids	17.5a	0.8b	20.5a	[84]
LD Linseed- enriched diet	14.1b	1.3a	10.5b	
LD Control diet Phospholipids	30.2a	0.9b	33.3a	
LD Linseed-enriched diet Phospholipids	27.0b	1.8a	14.8b	
Sub fat Outer layer Diet rich SFA	12.4b	na		[21]
Sub fat Outer layer Diet rich PUFA	18.4a	na		
Sub fat Inner layer Diet rich SFA	10.9b	na		[21]
Sub fat Inner layer Diet rich PUFA	17.9a	na		
LD Duroc Diet SFA (35.7%) NL	4.7b	na		[21]
LD Duroc Diet PUFA (58.0%) NL	7.2a	na		
LD Duroc Diet SFA (35.7%) PL	25.5b	na		[21]
LD Duroc Diet PUFA (58.0%) PL	27.3a	na		
Subcutaneous fat 1.5 % Corn oil	17.0a	1.04	16.35	[33]
Subcutaneous fat 1.5 % Tallow	13.1b	1.35	9.70	
Subcutaneous fat 1.5% CLA	14.6ab	1.04	14.04	
LD Control + 0% fat blend high LA	11.1d	na		[34]
Control + 2% fat blend high LA	14.4c	na		
Control + 4% fat blend high LA	18.1b	na		
Control + 8% fat blend high LA	20.9a	na		
Backfat Control + 0% fat blend high LA	10.3d	na		[34]
Control + 2% fat blend high LA	13.4c	na		
Control + 4% fat blend high LA	16.8b	na		
Control + 8% fat blend high LA	21.0a	na		

a,b,c ,d indicate a significant difference ($p<0.05$) between production system reported within each respective study. "na" indicates that the value was not reported in the original study.

Abbreviations: LD: *Longissimus dorsi*: SM: *Semimembranosus*; LT: *Longissimus thoracis*; BF: *Biceps femoris*; Sub: subcutaneous fat; NL: Neutral lipids; PL: Phospholipids.

2. LA and ALA Proportions of Pig Body Lipids

Porcine carcass fat is deposited in four depots, with different anatomical locations: visceral, subcutaneous, intermuscular, or intramuscular. Considerable anatomical variations in FA composition in pigs have been reported. Recently some authors have suggested that not all adipose tissues are similar but each shows specific development and catabolism. There is a gradient of decreasing LA and ALA concentrations from the outer layer of subcutaneous, through the inner layer, to intermuscular adipose tissue [12]. There was a statistically positive correlation between the LA concentration of the different adipose tissue and the half carcass muscle content. Some results for LA and ALA proportions in different pork lipids samples are presented in Tables 1 and 1a. LA is an EFA derived entirely from the diet and is at much higher concentrations in pigs compared to beef and lamb. This is because this FA, an important constituent of grains and oilseeds, is not broken down during digestion in the pig stomach, but passes directly from the small intestine to the blood and thus to their tissues.

2.1. Breed Effects on LA and ALA Proportions of Pig Body Lipids

Evidence for breed differences in FA composition and in the activities of several enzymes involved in fat synthesis and FA metabolism has been cited in several studies [13]. Within-breed genetic variation in the proportion of major FA in back fat and intramuscular fat is also considerable. Average heritability higher than 0.5 have been reported for the proportion of LA and carcass leanness is positively associated to the content of most PUFA [14]. Heritabilities ranging between 0.24 and 0.73 were found for intramuscular fat content [13].

The interaction of genetic with dietary factors may further contribute to differences in intramuscular FA composition. An increased PUFA proportion was found in pigs when fat deposition was reduced by restricted feeding compared to *ad libitum* feed intake [15]. Intramuscular fat of Duroc contained less LA than halothane negative British Landrace pigs [13]. Sire affected the proportion of ALA but no changes were detected in LA. Sire had no effects on the total n-6 PUFA and the main constituent LA, but it affected the total and individual n-3 PUFA [16]. Alonso et al. reported that crossbreeding affected the proportions of LA in the intramuscular fat of Pietrain x (Landrace x Large White) compared with Duroc x (Landrace x Large White) but no differences were obtained for ALA. They concluded that the differences among crossbreeding are not very important in relation to the FA composition [17]. Differences in adipose tissue FA composition among stress genotypes were not significant and it seems that stress exerts no effects on LA or ALA concentrations [18]. Differences in both layers of back fat between Duroc and Yorkshire gilts in LA and ALA have been detected [19]. Significant breed differences in the proportions of LA between Duroc and Hampshire pigs have been observed; Hampshire lipids presented higher values of LA than Duroc [20]. The effect of diet on the on the FA composition is variable according to pig genotype. This was demonstrated in one study that investigated the effects of dietary fat saturation and dietary vitamin A on the FA composition of the offspring of two terminal sires: Duroc and Landrace x Large White [21].

2.2. Sex Effects on LA and ALA Proportions of Pigs' Body Lipids

Gender is also known to affect the fat deposition, e.g. castration is associated with increased fat deposition. The results of several studies reporting an effect of sex on the FA composition on pigs are shown in Table 1. Studies in humans have suggested that gender is also associated with the differences in the capacity for conversion of ALA to EPA, DPA and DHA. The conversion of ALA to EPA, DPA and DHA and LA to AA is dependent on the sequential activities of $^{\Delta}6$ and $^{\Delta}5$ desaturases and on elongation of the carbon chain [11].

The effects of sex in the FA composition of female and castrated pigs were studied in several studies. Sex had a significant effect on the LA proportions of *Semimembranosus* muscle and subcutaneous fat. The concentrations of LA and ALA were significantly higher in female than in castrated male pigs [16]. Similar results were reported for *Longissimus thoracis* muscles from crossbred pigs [22]. Significant sex differences were found in LA proportions: barrows 8.55% vs. 10.65% in gilts in *M. Longissimus lumborum*. Higher levels of LA and ALA were detected in female pigs, independent of feeding [23]. Feeding and gender gave rise to significant differences in PL and neutral lipids (NL) fractions of FA composition. Female pigs showed a higher content of LA in the NL fraction compared with castrates [24]. Sex was a significant factor in the variation in the FA profile of pig lipids [25]. Percentages of LA and ALA were higher in entire males than females [26]. Several muscles of Duroc barrows and gilts presented higher values of LA compared with barrows but no significant differences in ALA [27]. Gender influenced the proportion of LA ($p<0.01$) and ALA ($p<0.001$), gilts had more LA and ALA than barrows [18].

2.3. Production System Effects on LA and ALA Proportions of Pig Body Lipids

It is well known that FA composition can be manipulated by feeding strategies (Table 1a). The dietary FA can be either directly incorporated into animal tissues or they can be used as substrates for in vivo FA biosynthesis. The inclusion of tallow, high-oleic sunflower oil, sunflower oil, linseed oil, a fat blend and an oil blend in finishing diet vs. feeding a semi-synthetic diet with no added fat affected the carcass FA composition. Carcasses from gilts fed sunflower oil had the greatest proportion of LA, whereas carcasses of linseed-fed gilts had the greatest percentages of ALA [28]. The percentages of LA and ALA of pork intramuscular fat of muscle LD were affected by diet with the changes in the PL fraction being minor, while significant differences between feeding regimes were found in back fat and in the neutral fraction of *Longissimus dorsi* (LD) muscle [24]. The effect of duration of dietary linseed feeding on subcutaneous fat, intramuscular fat depot and muscle mass of growing-finishing barrows have also been researched. In all depots LA and ALA increased with increasing time on linseed regardless of tissue type [29]. Different dietary fat sources affected the FA composition of whole pigs (carcass + viscera). The highest LA content in total carcass fat was observed in animals fed with sunflower oil and the highest ALA content was observed in animals fed linseed oil [30].

Three dietary oils namely: palm kernel, palm and soybean, affected the LA and ALA proportions of pig body lipids, with LA and ALA being significantly higher on the soybean diet [31]. Feeding crossbred pigs with linseed oil or fish oil to a level of 1.2% affected LA and ALA proportions. In *Longissimus thoracis* muscle LA was lower in fish oil compared with linseed but ALA proportion was greatest in the meat of linseed group [22]. Free-range rearing produced in the neutral fraction of *M. Biceps femoris* of Hampshire crossbred pigs, more ALA with no differences in LA, when compared to indoor rearing. However, in the PL fraction, free-range contained more LA with no differences in ALA; sex effects were very small, and only in the phospholipid fraction [25]. Crossbred male and female pigs fed six different diets with increasing dietary fish oil levels showed differences in LA and ALA. Most palm kernel oil groups had higher percentages of LA than low fat groups, and a tendency to higher percentages of ALA, significant only for the group fed the highest proportion of fish oil [26]. A high ALA diet (linseed diet), and a high LA diet (sunflower diet) affected the FA composition of pigs adipose tissues and muscle. Feeding the linseed diet increased ALA proportion and decreased LA/ALA ratio in all tissues, while the sunflower diet led to an increase in LA content. LA/ALA ratio was reduced in pigs fed a linseed diet compared to pigs fed an enriched LA diet [32]. The dietary fat saturation affected the FA composition of the offspring of two terminal sires Duroc and Landrace x Large White. The pigs fed the saturated fat diet had less LA than those fed the polyunsaturated diet [21]. Differences in the supplemented diet, with corn oil or tallow, affected the percentages of LA without affecting the ALA concentrations in pig adipose tissues [33]. Landrace pigs showed a tendency towards increased LA levels, particularly in the loin and *Longissimus thoracis et lumborum*, whereas Duroc pigs seemed to be the most resistant to change the FA composition according to the diet [34].

3. LA and ALA Proportions of Beef Lipids

As a result of the FA imbalance in human diet, dietary strategies have been developed to improve the nutritional and health value of the intramuscular fat of cattle. Thus, manipulation of the FA composition of ruminant meat to reduce SFA content and the n-6/n-3 ratio, whilst simultaneously increasing PUFA and CLA content, is of major importance in beef research. There are three major factors that influence the FA composition of beef: age, diet and breed type (Tables 2 and 2a). Age and breed type specifically affect the concentration of MUFA in beef by affecting SDC gene expression and activity, whereas diet is the sole source of EFA, LA and ALA. Genetic and nutritional approaches have been widely studied in relation to FA composition of beef (Tables 2 and 2a) but it is acknowledged that genetic factors generally provide smaller differences than dietary factors. Although breed differences are generally small, they do reflect differences in gene expression or enzymes involved in FA synthesis.

Table 2. Influence of breed, sex and anatomical location on linoleic acid (LA), α-linolenic acid (ALA) and LA/ALA ratio in bovine body lipids

Item	LA %	ALA%	LA/ALA	Reference
LD Angus	4.07	0.85a	4.79	[40]
LD Charolais x Angus	4.38	0.84a	5.21	
LD Holando x Angus	4.41	0.73b	6.04	
LD German Holstein Grass	4.32b	1.67c	2.59	[41]
LD German Holstein Concentrate	4.11b	0.34b	12.09	
LD German Simental Grass	6.56a	2.22a	2.81	
LD German Simental Concentrate	5.22ab	0.46b	11.34	
LD grass Nguni	2.41	2.41	1.00	[42]
LD grass Bonsmara	2.49	2.48	1.00	
LD grass Angus	2.21	2.20	1.00	
Subcutaneous fat Brahman	4.3	0.9	4.77	[43]
Subcutaneous fat Hereford	1.7	0.7	2.42	
Subcutaneous fat Angus	1.9	0.1	19	
Subcutaneous fat Australian	1.6	0.5	3.2	
Subcutaneous fat J. Black	2.0	0.2	10	
Subcutaneous fat Hanwoo	4.2	0.4	11	
L. thoracis Simmental NL	3.91b	0.46a	8.5	[44]
L. thoracis Holstein NL	8.00a	0.53a	15.09	

Table 2. (Continued)

Item	LA %	ALA%	LA/ALA	Reference
L. thoracis Simmental PL	35.02a	1.42	24.66	[44]
L. thoracis Holstein PL	30.33b	1.36	22.30	
Steer Subcutaneous fat	2,6a	0.67b	3.88	[7]
Heifer Subcutaneous fat	1.9b	0.90a	2.11	
Steer Intramuscular fat NL	2.2	0.68	3.24	[7]
Heifer Intramuscular fat NL	2.0	0.92	2.17	
Steer Intramuscular fat PL	21.3	1.9	11.21	[7]
Heifer Intramuscular fat PL	22.2	2.1	10.57	
LT Simmental Heifers C	5.7b	0.21b	27.14	[45]
LT Simmental Bulls C	10.8a	0.34a	31.76	
Adipose tissue Heifers C	2.4b	0.18b	10.00	[45]
Adipose tissue Bulls C	3.5a	0.24a	14.58	
LD Autumn Male NL	2.83	0.68	4.16	[46]
LD Spring Male NL	2.74	0.56	4.89	
LD Autumn Female NL	2.74	0.58	4.72	[46]
LD Spring Female NL	2.55	0.63	4.04	
LD Autumn Male PL	16.58b	2.48	6.69	[46]
LD Spring Male PL	19.17a	2.25	8.52	
LD Autumn Female PL	15.73	2.15	7.32	[46]
LD Spring Female PL	16.45	2.58	6.37	
Raw steaks Muscle	3.5a	1.2a	2.92	[35]
Raw steaks Marbling	1.4b	0.7b	2.00	
Adipose tissue Brisket	1.63c	na		[6]
Adipose tissue Chuck	1.86ab	na		
Adipose tissue Flank	1.95ab	na		
Adipose tissue Loin	1.97ab	na		
Adipose tissue Plate	1.98a	na		
Rib	1.95ab	na		
Round	1.76bc	na		
Sirloin	1.87ab	na		
LD Bulls 14 months	6.31a	1.40a	4.51	[47]
LD Bulls 18 months	5.21b	1.10b	4.74	
LD Heifers 14 months	4.12c	0.89c	4.63	
LD Heifers 18 months	3.55d	0.78d	4.55	
L. lumborum	4.15a	0.93a	4.46	[61]
Subcutaneous fat	0.95b	0.44b	2.16	
L. lumborum steers	8.63b	1.69	5.11	[8]
L. lumborum bulls	10.44a	1.67	6.25	

a,b,c indicate a significant difference ($p<0.05$) between breed, sex or anatomical location reported within each respective study. "na" indicates that the value was not reported in the original study.

Abbreviations: LD: *Longissimus dorsi*; LT: *Longissimus thoracis*; NL: Neutral lipids; PL: Phospholipids.

Table 2a. Influence of production system on linoleic acid (LA), α-linolenic acid (ALA) and LA/ALA ratio in bovine body lipids

Item	LA%	ALA %	LA/ALA	Reference
LD Pasture (P) only	3.41b	1.30a	2.62	[40]
LD P + 0.7% grain	3.61b	0.89b	4.06	
LD P + 1% grain	3.93b	0.74b	5.31	
LD Grain	6.19a	0.28c	22.11	
LD Concentrate/ silage	2.98b	0.80b	3.73	[50]

Item	LA%	ALA %	LA/ALA	Reference
LD Grass	3.29b	1.76a	2.94	
LD Grass + Sunflower oil	4.74a	1.12b	4.23	
LD Grass + linseed oil	3.86b	1.81a	2.13	
Subcutaneous fat D1	0.88b	0.48a	1.83	[85]
Subcutaneous fat D2	0.86b	0.44a	1.95	
Subcutaneous fat D3	0.99b	0.47a	2.11	
Subcutaneous fat D4	0.92b	0.49a	1.88	
Subcutaneous fat YOTM	1.13b	0.42ab	2.69	
Subcutaneous fat YUTM	1.57a	0.24b	6.54	
LD Feedlot	11.95	0.48a	24.89	[51]
LD Pasture + 4 months C	10.07	0.84a	11.99	
LD Pasture + 2 months C	11.38	1.96b	5.81	
LD Pasture	12.55	5.53c	2.27	
LD Finishing Pasture	5.07b	2.39	2.12	[52]
LD Finishing Maiz silage	6.04a	1.58	3.82	
LT Autumn Carnalentejana –PDO beef	8.11c	0.31	26.16	[53]
ST Autumn	11.4b	0.37	30.81	
LT Spring	10.0b	0.32	31.25	
ST Spring	11.3b	0.39	37.66	
LT Intensively produced beef	11.0b	0.30	36.66	[53]
ST	17.7a	0.42	42.14	
LD Grass silage	3.52	1.88a	1.87	[54]
Grass silage + 4% soybean meal	2.50	0.83b	3.01	
Grass silage + 8% soybean meal	2.72	0.72b	6.46	
LD Cull cows Grass silage	1.87b	0.71b	2.63	[63]
LD Cull cows Red clover silage	2.64a	1.54a	1.71	
LD PL Simmental bulls LA	22.6	2.5	9.04	[55]
LD PL Simmental bulls ALA	23.7	4.3	5.51	
LD TRI Simmental bulls LA	1.8	0.5	3.60	
LD TRI Simmental Bulls ALA	2.3	0.9	2.55	
L.thoracis Linseed NL	8.20a	0.64a	12.81	[44]
L.thoracis Control NL	3.71b	0.35b	10.6	
L.thoracis Linseed PL	31.72a	1.62a	19.50	[44]
L.thoracis Control PL	33.62a	1.17b	28,74	
LD Forage: Concentrate 60 :40% NL	0.92	0.36	2.55	[56]
LD F:C + Linseed NL	0.79	0.59	1.33	
LD F:C + Fish oil NL	0.57	0.38	1.50	
LD F:C + Linseed-fish oil NL	0.72	0.41	1.76	
LD Forage:Concentrate 60 :40% PL	11.4	2.13	5.35	[56]
LD F:C + Linseed PL	10.1	4.34	2.33	
LD F:C + Fish oil PL	8.4	2.37	3.54	
LD F:C + Linseed-fish oil PL	9.2	3.49	2.64	
Ground beef Control	2.09	0.21b	9.95	[57]
Ground grass fed	1.71	0.67a	2.55	
Strip steak Control	2.38	0.13b	18.31	
Strip steack grass fed	2.01	0.71a	2.83	
LD Angus Concentrate NL	1.7a	0.1b	17.00	[70]
LD Angus Grass silage NL	0.6b	0.4a	1,5	
LD Angus Concentrate PL	18.6a	0.5b	37.2	
LD Angus Grass silage PL	5.9b	3.3a	1.78	
Control	2.67	0.36	7.42	[58]
Control + Vitamina E	2.83	0.35	8.08	
Control + Flaxseed	2.51	1.35	1.86	
LT Semi-intensive 12 months	14.2a	3.54a	4.01	[36]
LT Semintensive 14 months	10.5b	3.24a	2.97	
LT Intensive 12 months	9.95b	0.33b	30.15	

Table 2a. (Continued)

Item	LA%	ALA %	LA/ALA	Reference
LT Intenive 14 months	10.7b	0.37b	27,22	
Longissimus lumborum Spring	4.26b	0.81a	5.26	[37]
Longissimus lumborum Autumn	4.32b	0.44b	9.82	
Semitendinosus Spring	9.38a	1.32a	7.11	[37]
Semitendinosus Autumn	10.15a	0.91b	11.15	
LD Tall fescue	6.15	0.56	10.98	[59]
LD Alfalfa	6.75	0.80	8.44	
LD Red clover	5.91	0.60	9.85	
LM Grass Total lipid	2.35b	1.37a	1.72	[60]
LM Grass + sunflower oil Total lipid	3.17a	0.87b	3.64	
LM Grass-linseed oil Total lipid	2.59b	1.35a	1,92	
LM Grass NL	1.21b	0.84a	1.44	[60]
LM Grass + sunflower oil NL	1.45a	0.56b	2.59	
LM Grass-linseed oil NL	1.26b	0.83a	1.52	
LM Grass PL	12.05c	5.92a	2.04	
LM Grass + sunflower oil PL	17.93a	3.53b	5.08	
LM Grass-linseed oil PL	14.66b	5.92a	2.48	
LM Corn oil 0%	2.42	0.76a	3.18	[61]
LM Corn 0.75%	2.67	0.69b	3.87	
LM Corn 1.5%.	2.55	0.60b	4.25	

a,b,c indicate a significant difference ($p<0.05$) between production system reported within each respective study. "na" indicates that the value was not reported in the original study.

Abbreviations: LD: *Longissimus dorsi*: SM: *Semimembranosus*; LT: *Longissimus thoracis*; ST: *Semitendinosus*; NL: Neutral lipids; PL: Phospholipids.

Evidence from research has indicated that the levels of LA and ALA proportions were highest in lean beef muscle; about 2-4 times the levels in adipose tissues, with no differences in the levels of LA and ALA among subcutaneous, seam fat and marbling. There were no differences in n-6/n-3 ratio according to fat location [35]. There were significant differences in the concentrations of LA in external fat samples from eight different carcass locations, with the brisket containing significantly less amounts than the other sampling sites ($p<0.001$) except the round [6]. Two production systems (semi-intensive vs. intensive), and two slaughter ages (12 vs.14 months) affected LA and ALA proportions in meat FA composition. The slaughter age affected LA and ALA proportions. LA and ALA are strongly positively correlated to intramuscular fat of *Longissimus* muscle at the quantitative level (mg/100g fresh tissue), but there are negative correlation coefficients for the relative proportion of these FA to intramuscular fat. The relationships between intramuscular fat and the FA profile of triglycerides and PL fractions are weaker compared to total muscle fat [36]. Only small effects of slaughter season on LA and ALA proportions in intramuscular fat of Mirandesa PDO veal were detected, but significant changes by the muscle type were observed [37].

3.1. Breed Differences in LA and ALA Proportions of Beef Lipids

In cattle, there is evidence of genetic variation in the FA composition of adipose tissue triacylglycerols, with breed differences observed in studies comparing Jersey and Limousin. However, in the phospholipid fraction, the total amount of PUFA does not differ among crossbred groups, because certain amounts of unsaturated FA are required to maintain the physical properties of the cell at the body temperature of mammals [38]. Intramuscular fat had significant between-breed- differences in ALA content with no differences in LA, but in subcutaneous fat breed type it affected LA and ALA concentrations. Unfortunately, most bovine FA composition in the literature originates from breeds on diverse diets, ages, sexes, anatomical sites, etc. This makes it difficult to extrapolate the results and compare breeds because of the confounding effects of plane of nutrition, age, fatness, live-weight, developmental traits and other factors that affect lipid metabolism [39]. Significant differences in the percentages of ALA in LD muscles, with non-significant differences in LA percentages have been detected among Angus, Charolais x Angus and Holando breeds [40]. Feeding German Simmental and German Holstein bulls on either grass-based or indoor concentrate system affected LA and ALA percentages. The grass-based bulls had increased percentages of ALA in both breeds but the percentages of LA were only affected by the breed type, being higher in German Simmental intramuscular fat [41]. No breed differences in the proportions of LA and ALA were detected in Nguni, Bonsmara and Angus steers [42]. The LA and ALA data from a large number of studies that varied widely in age of cattle, breed type, and finishing diets, indicated that large variations in FA composition can occur across production systems [43]. Italian Simmental and Holstein bulls presented different diets had differences in *Longissimus thoracis* muscle percentages for ALA in PL and NL fractions, but with no differences in the NL for LA [44].

3.2. Sex Differences in the LA and ALA Proportions in Beef Lipids

Sex affects the FA composition of subcutaneous NL and intramuscular neutral and PL of *Longissimus lumborum* muscle. Steers presented higher values of LA in subcutaneous fat and heifers higher values of ALA in the NL of subcutaneous and intramuscular fats [7]. Important differences between heifers and bulls in intensively fed beef cattle have been reported. Bulls contained greater amounts of LA and ALA compared with heifers [45]. The influence of slaughter season and sex on the FA composition of intramuscular total lipids, NL and PL in several muscles of Barrosa-PDO calves has been studied. In LD muscle, only the LA content of the PL fraction was affected by sex and season. The proportions of LA and ALA in NL of LD muscle of Barrosa –PDO calves were not affected by season or sex. Small but significant differences were detected in LA proportions in the PL fraction. Males had higher LA content than females [46]. Differences in muscle FA between bulls and heifers raised under similar conditions have also been detected. Bulls presented higher levels of LA and ALA compared with heifers [47]. Similar differences were observed between intact males and females of Chinese native Quichuan cattle, and a possible effect of sex hormones on enzymatic systems affecting lipid metabolism was suggested [48]. Several studies demonstrated sex-dependent differences in the FA composition of muscle and subcutaneous adipose tissue of cattle slaughtered at different ages. The expression of the stearoyl –CoA desaturase gene was higher in the adipose tissue of heifers compared to bulls, and its variation partly contributed to sex and age differences in the FA composition of bovine adipose tissue [47]. Castration affected the FA composition of bull calves of Mertolenga breed. Entire males had significantly higher values of LA and ALA, indicating that castration has an effect on the FA composition of intramuscular fat of *Longissimus lumborum* [8].

Table 3. Influence of breed, sex and anatomical location on linoleic acid (LA), α-linolenic acid (ALA) and LA/ALA ratio in lamb body lipids

Item	LA %	ALA%	LA/ALA	Reference
LD Kivircik	7.3b	1.44b	5.07	[67]
LD Sakiz	8.0a	1.55a	5.16	
LL Texel x Polwarth	6.28b	1.78	3.53	[68]
LL Texel x Corriedale	8.39a	1.94	4.32	
Muscle LD	6.77	2.64b	2.56	[49]
Muscle ST	7.49	2.79b	2.68	
Muscle SM	8.48	3.17a	2.68	
Pasture LD	6.77	2.64a	2.56	[49]
Pasture leg muscles	7.37	2.89b	2.55	
Pasture LD Total lipids	6.77	2.64	2.56	[49]
Pasture LD Triacylglycerols	2.71	1.32	2.05	
Pasture LD Phospholipids	13.04	2.75	4.74	
LD muscle	9.62a	2.58a	3.73	[65]
SM muscle	10.77a	2.71a	3.97	

a,b indicate a significant difference ($p<0.05$) between breed, sex or anatomical location reported within each respective study. "na" indicates that the value was not reported in the original study.

Abbreviations:

LD: *Longissimus dorsi*: ST: *Semitendinosus*; LL: *Longissimus lumborus*; NL: Neutral lipids; PL: Phospholipids.

Table 3 a. Influence of production system on linoleic acid (LA), α-linolenic acid (ALA) and LA/ALA ratio in lamb body lipids

Item	LA %	ALA %	LA/ALA	Reference
Subcutaneous fat Grass pellets	2.23b	2.43a	0.92	[76]
Subcutaneous fat Concentrate	3.47a	0.44b	7.89	
LD Grass Hay	4.65b	2.27a	2.00	[67]
LD Grass + concentrate	10.7a	0.72b	14.86	
LD Soy oil	9.36a	0.93b	10.06	[73]
LD Soy oil + 33 % linseed oil	7.52d	1.57c	4.79	
LD Soy oil + 66 % linseed oil	6.74c	2.62d	2.57	
LD Linseed oil	5.0b	3.05a	1.64	
LD Soy oil NL	4.56a	0.70b	6.50	[73]
LD Soy oil + 33 % linseed oil NL	3.54d	1.08d	3.28	
LD Soy oil + 66 % linseed oil NL	2.99c	1.77c	1.69	
LD Linseed oil NL	2.26b	1.87a	1.21	
LD Soy oil PL	23.9a	1.29b	18.53	[73]
LD Soy oil + 33 % linseed oil PL	19.6d	2.55c	7.69	
LD Soy oil + 66 % linseed oil PL	17.8c	4.73d	3.76	
LD Linseed oil PL	13.5b	5.93a	2.28	
LD Sucking-lamb Average	9.33	1.88	4.96	[74]
Rearing in Autumn	9.82	2.57a	3.82	
Rearing in Winter	8.86	1.21b	7.32	
LD Grazing subterraneous clover	5.13a	1.97a	2.60	[75]
LD Grazing Italian ryegrass	4.10b	1.52b	2.69	
LD 30 days age	8.67b	2.04b	4.25	[65]
LD 50 days age	8.23b	2.70a	3.05	
LD 70 days age	11.05a	2.52ab	4.38	
LD muscle	9.62a	2.58a	3.73	[65]
SM muscle	10.77a	2.71a	3.97	
Leg Control	8.6a	1.1b	7.82	[86]

Item	LA %	ALA %	LA/ALA	Reference
Leg CLA	8.6a	1.3b	6.61	
Leg Saflower oil	12.4b	1.7a	10.33	
Adipose tissue Control	5.8c	1.2a	4.83	[86]
Adipose tissue CLA	3.3b	0.5b	6.60	
Adipose tissue Safflower oil	8.4a	0.7c	12.00	
LD Grass pellets	4.04b	2.91a	1.39	[76]
LD Concentrate diet	5.99a	0.57b	10.51	
LD Concentrate diet *Ad libitum*	5.46ab	0.48b	11.38	
LT Grass low growth rate NL	0.6b	1.3a	0.46	[10]
LT Grass high growth rate NL	1.4c	1.1a	1.27	
LT Grain low growth rate NL	2.7a	0.7b	3.86	
LT Grain high growth rate NL	2.7a	0.7b	3.86	[10]
LT Grass low growth rate PL	11.0b	3.2a	3.44	[10]
LT Grass high growth rate PL	9.7b	2.9a	3.34	
LT Grain low growth rate PL	14.3c	0.9b	15.88	
LT Grain high growth rate PL	14.6a	0.9c	16.22	
LD Control	5.49b	0.82a	6.70	[77]
LD Control + 5% sunflower oil	8.11a	0.56b	22.52	
Fat Control	3.43b	0.57a	6.02	[77]
Fat Control + 5% sunflower oil	6.08a	0.47b	12.94	
LT Control (C)	9.44b	0.82b	11.52	[78]
LT Control + Lucerne + 10% soybean	13.3a	1.01c	13.17	
LT Lucerne	13.9a	1.17a	11.88	
LT Lucerne + Lucerne + 10% soybean	14.8a	1.14a	12.98	
Muscle Control no fat	9.61a	0.56b	17.16	[64]
Muscle Control + wheat + linseed	10.61a	2.47a	4.30	
Muscle Control + corn- linseed	9.31a	2.21 a	4.21	
LL Control	1.77a	0.86a	2.06	[79]
LL Linseed	1.86a	0.85a	2.19	
LL Rapeseed	1.57b	0.62ab	2.53	
LL Safflower seed	1.75a	0.66a	2.65	
LL Sunflower seed	1.80a	0.52b	3.46	
LD Grassed 9 am to 5pm	8.68ab	2.77a	3.13	[80]
LD Grassed 9 am to 1 pm	8.33a	2.32b	3.59	
LD Grassed 1 pm to 5 pm	9.09a	2.80a	3.25	
LD Ewe control	1.84a	0.87a	2.11	[81]
LD Ewe linseed oil	1.71b	0.70b	2.44	
LD Lamb control	1.56	1.28	1.22	
LD Lamb Linseed oil	1.52	1.27	1.19	
Muscle Concentrate + concentrate	3.17	1.34d	2.37	[82]
Muscle Silage + concentrate	3.55	1.84c	1.93	
Muscle Concentrate + silage	3.08	2.17b	1.42	
Muscle Silage + silage	3.27	2.87a	1.14	
LT Prep-partum Hay	5.30	1.85	2.86	[83]
LT Pre-partum Grazing	5.04	1.85	2.72	
LT Post-partum Hay	4.89	1.65a	2.96	
LT Post-partum Grazing	5.45	2.07b	2.63	

a,b,c,d indicate a significant difference ($p<0.05$) between production system reported within each respective study. "na" indicates that the value was not reported in the original study.

Abbreviations: LD: *Longissimus dorsi*: SM: *Semimembranosus*; LT: *Longissimus thoracis*; LL: *Longissimus lumborums*; NL: Neutral lipids; PL: Phospholipids.

3.3. Production Systems Differences in LA and ALA Proportions in Beef Lipids

Diets based on pasture, pasture supplemented with 0.75% and 1% corn, or concentrate affects LA and ALA percentages on the FA of LD muscle. As the corn in the diet increases, LA increases and ALA decreases [49]. Similar results were observed in crossbred heifers offered a control diet of grass silage and concentrate or rations designed to enhance the concentration of conjugated linoleic acid (CLA) [50]. Alentejano bulls were used to investigate the effect of four feeding systems (pasture only, pasture feeding followed by 2 or 4 months of finishing on concentrate, and concentrate only) on the FA composition of muscle LD. No significant differences were observed for LA among all treatments. In contrast meat from the pasture diet had the highest percentages of ALA [51]. A pasture finishing system and an indoor finishing system (maize, silage and concentrate) affected the intramuscular FA profile of Rubia Gallega steers. Intramuscular fat of finished steers contained higher concentrations of LA but no differences were detected for ALA [52]. Differences in LA content of meat between bullocks reared in a semi-intensive system and bullocks produced in a conventional intensive concentrate–based system have been investigated. Seasonal differences were only detected in LA proportions [53]. Feeding of high concentrate diets significantly decreased the proportion of ALA in LD muscle lipids of cattle [54]. Two diets, one rich in LA and the other rich in ALA, affected the FA composition of the classes of lipids in the intramuscular fat of German Simmental bulls. The bulls fed ALA had higher concentrations of ALA in PL and triglycerides [55]. Long-term addition of linseed to the diet of young bulls increased ALA in neutral and phospholipid fractions of *Longissimus thoracis* lipids [44]. The effects of different sources of dietary n-3 PUFA on the FA composition of steers *Longissimus thoracis* muscle have been investigated. The proportions of LA in neutral and phospholipid fractions were significantly lowered by fish oil feeding ($p<0.05$), with a smaller non-significant effect by linseed [56]. The nutrient composition of grass-fed beef in the USA study for inclusion in the USDA National Database for Standard Reference compared the FA composition of grass-fed beef and conventionally fed (control) beef [57]. Dietary vitamin E with or without flaxseed affected beef FA composition. Feeding flaxseed increased ALA and this response was further accentuated by the inclusion of high levels of vitamin E in the diet [58]. Two production systems, semi-intensive vs. intensive affected the LA and ALA concentrations of meat FA. Pasture fed bulls presented higher percentages of ALA and lower percentages of LA than intensive ones [36].

Slaughter season affected the FA composition of Mirandesa purebred calves raised in a semi-extensive production system, and slaughtered in spring or autumn. LA was higher in *Semitendinosus* and *Semimembranosus* muscles in autumn and ALA in spring [37]. The FA composition of the distinctive pasture types did not influence the intramuscular fat composition in beef steers [59]. The FA composition of muscle fat and adipose tissue of grazing heifers supplemented with plant oil- enriched concentrates has been studied. Sunflower oil increased LA and linseed oil ALA in total lipids, NL and PL of *Longissimus lumborom* muscle [60]. Supplemental corn oil fed to steers grazing endophyte-free tall fescue affected the FA composition of *Longissimus lumborum* muscle. Corn oil supplementation linearly increased LA, whereas ALA was linearly decreased [61]. The contribution of LA and ALA in subcutaneous adipose tissue of steers and cows produced in the USA, Australian crossbred cattle, Japanese Black steers and Hanwoo steers fed under different production conditions varies. The values detected for LA were from 1.6 to 4.2% and for ALA from 0.1 to 0.9% [62]. The effect of feeding dairy cull cows with grass or red clover silage, on the proportions of LA and ALA in muscle LD has also been reported. Red clover silage increased had increased percentages of LA and ALA [63].

4. LA and ALA Proportions in Lamb Body Lipids

Fatty acid composition is an important factor in the classification of lamb meat quality due to its relationship to meat odor and flavor and the relationship of FA to the nutritional value of fat for human consumption. Several strategies have been tested in recent years to improve the nutritional value of meat of intensively-reared lambs, kept indoors and fed high-concentrate diets rich in LA and poor in ALA. Incorporating linseed rich in lipid and ALA induced a high ALA muscle content in the range of 1.5-3% [64]. In lamb production, more than in other species, each country or region has its own specific weight age and type of carcass criteria, depending on its own production system as well as the culture and the customs of the people [65].

4.1. Breed Differences in LA and ALA Proportions of Lamb Body Lipids

It is generally assumed that breed differences in intramuscular fat are largely due to variability in maturity stage, such that, when compared at the same weight, breeds with larger mature size tend to be leaner than breeds with similar mature size [66]. Breed effect on LA and ALA were reported when lambs from two Turkish breeds, Kivircik and Sakiz, were fed a commercial concentrate and hay in the ratios of either 75:25 or 25:75. Breed significantly affected LA and ALA proportions. Sakiz lambs contained higher percentages of ALA and LA compared with Kivircik [67]. The lipid profile of Texel x Polwarth and Texel x Corriedale ram lambs finished on pastures rich in white clover has been studied. LA was higher in the *Longissimus lumborum* samples of Texel x Corriedale lambs but ALA was similar in both crossbreed lambs. The ratio LA/ALA was higher for Texel x Corriedale [68].

4.2. Effect of Production System on LA and ALA Proportion on Lamb Body Lipids

Lambs finished on pasture tend to show higher amounts of PUFA than those finished with grain based diets [67, 69] due to a higher ingestion of C18 PUFA in the diet. The muscles of herbage-feed lambs had higher levels of ALA when compared with concentrate-fed lambs. This finding is consistent with the results of dietary trials in cattle [41, 70]. The ratio n-6/n-3 was lower in the muscle of the lamb fed herbage when compared to the animals fed concentrate. This is in agreement with other studies on lamb and cattle [10]. Some reports describe a higher content of LA and ALA in meat of ruminants grazing red or white clover legumes, when compared to meat of animals fed with grasses and other legumes. It is believed that in red clover-rich diets, the fermentation and biohydrogenation in the rumen are different from those obtained with perennial ryegrass due to the inhibition of proteolysis and lipolysis by the plant enzyme polyphenol oxidase, which is present in clover [71]. Differences in the FA composition of forage crops due the influence of cutting and season were reported [72]. Replacement of sunflower oil with linseed oil increased the content of ALA and decreased the LA content in meat lipids. In PL, LA decreased from 23.9% in the lamb fed sunflower to 13.5% in the lambs fed linseed [73]. The FA profile of lambs reared in autumn and slaughtered at Christmas were different from those reared in winter and slaughtered at Easter. The lambs reared in autumn had similar levels of LA but greater levels of ALA [74]. Grazed forage species influenced the LA and ALA percentages in lamb meat lipids. The differences could be related to the chemical composition of the forage species grazed by lambs that influence the rumen conditions and the growth and activities of ruminal bacteria and the acidic composition of the forage species that influenced the biohydrogenation steps. The grazing on *T.subterraneum* as monoculture and associated with *multiflorum* increased the LA and ALA of the LD of the lambs [75].

Significant differences on LA and ALA proportions were observed the FA composition of lambs slaughtered at three different ages (30, 50 and 70 days) [64]. Forage and concentrate diets affected the FA composition of sheep tissues. Forage presented less LA and more ALA than concentrate in LD muscle lipids [76]. The significant decrease of LA/ALA ratio in grass fed lambs is another feature important for human nutrition, because it reaches a level of 3.4/3.6 in PL and 0.5/1.4 in NL [10]. The effects of feeding lambs with diets high in LA have also been reported. Lambs were fed either safflower supplemented diet containing 6% oil from safflower seeds or a control diet containing no added oil. Safflower supplemented lambs had higher percentages of LA and lower of ALA than concentrate lambs [77]. Initial diet and duration of supplementation with soybean oil affected the FA composition of intramuscular fat of Merino Branco ram lambs [78]. Feeding lambs with a control or extruded linseed diet and with either wheat or corn affected ALA concentration in lamb lipids. In agreement with published results, feeding extruded linseed increased the proportion of ALA in muscle and adipose tissue of intensively- reared lambs fed high–starch concentrates. The type of cereal grain was not a major factor for transfer of ALA in carcasses [63]. Supplemental oilseeds in the diet (sunflower seed, safflower seeds, rapeseed, and linseed) affected the FA composition of different tissues of mature ewes with significant differences in LA and ALA due to the different dietary oils [79]. Morning vs. afternoon grazing affected LA and ALA proportions in intramuscular FA composition. The restriction of time at pasture, either in the morning or in the afternoon, affected the content of LA and ALA of lamb meat lipids [80]. The effect of maternal linseed supplementation and/or lamb linseed supplementation on muscle and subcutaneous adipose tissue FA composition of indoor lambs has been determined. Feeding linseed to ewes increased ALA proportion in milk. However, the proportion of ALA in lamb tissues was not affected [81]. The FA profile of lamb muscle was strongly influenced by the ewe diet and milk FA profile. The diet with only silage produced meat with a higher proportion of ALA [82]. The feeding source exerted a greater effect on milk FA during the post- partum period, than during the pre-partum period. Feeding strategy also influences the ALA content of lamb meat [83]. Dietary CLA supplementation (0.33 g/day) or feeding LA rich oil (safflower oil 6%) produced differences in LA and ALA concentrations in lamb tissues [84].

Conclusion

The concentration of LA and ALA in pork, cattle or lamb lipids is dependent on whether or not the species is a ruminant. In ruminant animals (e.g. cattle, sheep) the majority of the dietary unsaturated FA are hydrogenated to SFAs in the rumen during digestion. Non-ruminant meat (e.g. pork, poultry) contains proportionally more unsaturated FA, but its composition is still dependent on the FA profile of the animal feed.

LA and ALA proportions on lipids of pork, beef or lamb are affected by several variables such as breed, sex, type of muscle, anatomical location, feeding regimen, botanical composition, freshness of grass, supplementation, altitude, etc. Dietary lipids may be supplied as grasses, forages, oil seeds, oil rich cereals, oils fish, etc. In most species, fat content of the meat is variable, depending on the balance between dietary energy intake and metabolic requirements, as well as with the genetic characteristics of the animal. All of these variables influence the ratio of LA to ALA. Dietary design will in the future be of great importance for improving the nutritional value of meats.

References

[1] Williams, C.M. (2000). Dietary fatty acids and human health. *Annales de Zootecnie*, 49: 165-180.

[2] Whelan, J. (2008). The health implications of changing linoleic acid intakes. *Prostaglandins, Leukotrienes and Essential Fatty Acids*, 79:165-168).

[3] Enser, M., Hallett, K., Hewitt, B.J., Fursey, G.A. & Woods, J.D. (1996). Fatty acid content and composition of English beef, lamb and pork at retail. *Meat Science*, 42:443-456.

[4] Gester, H. (1998). Can adults adequately convert alpha-linolenic acid to eicos-apentaenoic acid and docosahexanoic? *International Journal for Vitamin and Nutritional Research*, 68, 159-173.

[5] Howe, P., Meyer, B., Record, S. & Baghurst, K. (2006). Dietary intake of long-chain omega 3 polyunsaturated fatty acids: contribution of meat sources. *Nutrition*, 22:47-53.

[6] Turk, S. N. & Smith, S .B. (2009). Carcass fatty acid mapping. *Meat Science,* 81, 658-663.

[7] Zembayashy, M., Nishimura, K., Lunt, D.K. & Smith, S.B. (1995). Effect of breed and sex on the fatty acid composition of subcutaneous and intramuscular lipids of finishing steers and heifers. *Journal of Animal Science*, 73: 3325-3332.

[8] Monteiro, A.C.G., Santos-Silva, J., Bessa, R.J.B., Navas, D.R. & Lemos, J.P.C. (2005). Fatty acid composition of intramuscular fat of bulls and steers. *Livestock Production Science*, 99:13-19.

[9] Sinclair, A.J. & O`Dea, K. (1990). Fats in human diets through history: Is the Western diet out of step? In: J.D. Wood and A. V. Fisher (Ed.). Reducing Fat in Meat Animals. 1. Elservier Applied Science, Nueva York.

[10] Aurousseau, B., Bauchart, D., Calichon, E., Micol, D. & Priolo, A. (2004). Effect of grass concentrate feeding systems and rate of growth on the triglyceride and phos-

pholipids and their fatty acids in the M. *Longissimus thoracis* of lambs. *Meat Science*, 66:531-541.

[11] Sprecher, H. (2000). Metabolism of highly unsaturated n-3 and n-6 fatty acids. *Biochim Biophys Acta,* 1486:219-231.

[12] Monziols, M., Bonneau, M., Davenel, A. & Kouba, M. (2007). Comparison of the lipid content and fatty acid composition of intermuscular and subcutaneous adipose tissues in pig carcasses. *Meat Science*, 76: 54-60.

[13] Cameron, N.D. & Enser, M. (1991). Fatty acid composition of lipid in *Longissimus dorsi* muscle of Duroc and British Landrace pigs and its relationship with eating quality. *Meat Science*, 29:295-307.

[14] Selliers, P. (1998). Genetic of meat and carcass traits. In: Rothschild, M.F., Ruvinsky, A. (Eds.). The Genetic CBA International, New York pp. 463-510.

[15] Cameron, N.D., Wood, J.D., Enser, M., Wihittington, F.M., Penman J.C.& Robinson, A.M. (2000). Sensitivity of pig genotypes to short-term manipulation of plasma fatty acids by feeding linseed. *Meat Science,* 56:379-386.

[16] Ntawibizi, M., Raes, K., Buys, N. & De Smet, S. (2009). Effect of sire and sex on the intramuscular fatty acid profile and índices for enzyme activities in pigs. *Livestock Science*, 122:264-270.

[17] Alonso,V., Campo, M.C., Español, S., Roncales, P. & Beltran, J.A. (2009). Effects of crossbreeding and gender on meat quality and fatty acid composition in pork. *Meat Science*, 81:209-217.

[18] Piedrafita, J., Christian, L.L. & Lonergan, S.M. (2001). Fatty acid profile in three stress genotypes of swine and relationships with performance, carcass and meat quality traits. *Meat Science*, 57:71-77.

[19] Garcia, P.T., Andrada, V., Lloveras, M.R., Sancho, A.M. & Casal, J.J. (2009). Sire and sex on pork subcutaneous fatty acid profile and enzyme activities. *Proceedings of the 55th International Congress Meat Science & Technology* .Copenhagen, Denmark PI.9.12.

[20] Garcia, P.T., Casal, Olsen, C. & Berra, G. (1986) A comparison of distribution and composition of intramuscular fat in Duroc Jersey and Hampshire pigs at 100 kg live-weight. *Meat Science*, 16:283-295.

[21] Olivares, A., Daza, A., Rey, A.I. & Lopez-Bote, C.J. (2009). Interactions between genotype, dietary fat saturation and vitamin A. concentration on intramuscular fat content and fatty acid composition in pigs. *Meat Science*, 82:6-12.

[22] Haak, L., De Smet, S., Fremaut, D., Van Walleghem, K. & Raes, K. (2008). Fatty acid profile and oxidative stability of pork as influenced by duration and time of dietary linseed or fish oil supplementation. *Journal Animal Science,* 86:1418-1425.

[23] Zhang, S., Knight, T.J., Stalder, K.J., Goodwin, R.N., Lonergan, S.M. & Beitz, D.C. (2007). Effects of breed, sex, and halothane genotype on fatty acid composition of pork *Longissimus* muscle. *Journal Animal Science, 85*:583-591.

[24] Tikk, K., Tikk, M., Aaslyng, M.D., Karlsson, A.H., Lindahl, G.& Andersen, A.H. (2007). Significancie of fat supplemented diets on pork quality- Connections between specific fatty acids and sensory attributes of pork. *Meat Science* 77:275-286.

[25] Hogberg, A., Pickova, J., Dutta, P.C., Babol, J. & Bylund, A. C. (2001). Effect of rearing system on muscle lipids of gilts and castrated male pigs. *Meat Science*, 58: 223-229.

[26] Hallenstvedt, , E., Kjos, N.P., Rehnberg, A. C., Overland, M.& Thomassen, M. (2010). Fish oil in feeds for entire male and female pigs: changes in muscle fatty acid composition and stability of sensory quality. *Meat Science,* 85:182-190.

[27] Garcia, P.T. & Casal, J.J. (1993). Effects of sex and carcass fatness on pork intramuscular lipids. *Revista de Investigaciones Agropecuarias*, 24:59-70.

[28] Realini, C.E., Duran-Montge, P., Lizardo, R., Gispert, M., Oliver, M.A. & Esteve-Garcia, E. (2010). Effect of source of dietary fat on pig performance, carcass characteristics and carcass fat content, distribution and fatty acid composition. *Meat Science*, 85: 606-612.

[29] Huang, F.R., Zhan, Z.P., Luo, J. & Peng, J. (2008). Duration of dietary linseed feeding affects the intramuscular fat, muscle mass and fatty acid composition in pig muscle. *Livestock Science,* 118:132-139.

[30] Duran-Montge,P., Realini,C.E., Barroeta,A.C., Lizardo, R.G.& Esteve-Garcia, E. (2010). *De novo* fatty acid synthesis and balance of fatty acids of pigs fed different fat sources. *Livestock Science,* 132: 157-164.

[31] Teye, G.A., Sheard, P.R., Whittington, F.M., Nute, G.R., Stewart, A. & Wood, J.D. (2006). Influence of dietary oil and protein level on pork quality. 1. Effects on muscle fatty acid composition, carcass, meat and eating quality. *Meat Science*, 73:157-165.

[32] Guillevic, M., Kouba, M. & Mourot, J. (2009). Effect of a linseed or a sunflower diet on performances, fatty acid composition, lipogenic enzyme activities and stearoyl-CoA-desaturase activity in the pig. *Livestock Science,* 124: 288-294.

[33] Smith, S. B., Hively, T.S., Cortese, G.M., Han, J.J., Chung, K.Y., Castañeda, P. et al. (2002). Conjugated linoleic acid depresses the Δ9 desaturase index and stearoyl coenzyme A desaturese enzyme activity in porcine subcutaneous adipose tissue. *Journal Animal Science*, 80: 2110-2115.

[34] Pascual, J.V., Rafecas, M., Canela, M.A., Boatella, J., Bou, R., Barroeta, A. C. & Codony, R. (2007). Effect of increasing amounts of linoleic-rich dietary fat on the fat composition of four pig breeds. *Meat Science*, 100: 1639-1648.

[35] Jiang, T., Busboom, J.R., Nelson, M.L., O`Fallon, J., Ringkob, T.P., Joos, D. & Piper, K. (2010). Effectof sampling fat location and cooking on fatty acid composition of beef steaks. *Meat Science*, 84:86-92.

[36] Humada, M.L. Serrano, E., Sañudo, C.,Rolland, D.C. & Dugan, M.E.R. (2012). Production system and slaughter age effects on intramuscular fatty acids from Young Tudanca bulls. *Meat Science*, 678-685J

[37] Pestana, J.M, Costa, A.S.H., Alves, S.P., Martins, S.V. & Alfaia, C.M. (2012) Seasonal changes and muscle type effect on the nutritional quality of intramuscular fat in Mirandesa-PDO veal. *Meat Science*, 90:819-827.

[38] Malau,-Aduli, A.E.O.Siebert, B.D., Bottema, C.D.K.& Pitchford, W.S. (1998). Breed comparison of the fatty acids composition of muscle phospholipids in Jersey and Limousin cattle. *Journal of Animal Science*, 76:766-773.

[39] Dance, I.J.E., Matthews, K.R. & Doran, G. (2009). Effect of breed on fatty acid composition and stearoyl-CoA desaturase protein expression in the S*emimembranosus* muscle and subcutaneous adipose tissue of cattle. *Livestock Science*, 125:291-297.

[40] Garcia, P.T., Pensel, N.A., Sancho, A.M., Latimori, N.J., Kloster, A. M., Amigone, M.A. & Casal, J.J. (2008). Beef lipids in relation to animal breed and nutrition in Argentina. *Meat Science,* 79:500-508.

[41] Nuernberg, K., Dannenbrger, D., Nuernberg, G., Ender, K., Voigt, J., Scollan, N.D., Wood, J.D., Nute, G.R. & Richardson, R.I. (2005). Effect of grass-based and a concentrate feeding system on meat quality characteristics and fatty acid composition of *Longissimus* muscle in different cattle breeds. *Livestock Production Science,* 94:137-147.

[42] Muchenje, v., Hugo, A., Dzama, K, Chimonyo, M., Strydom, P.E. & Raats, J.G. (2009). Cholesterol levels and fatty acid profiles of beef from three cattle breeds raised on natural pasture. *Journal of Food Composition and Analysis,* 22:354-358.

[43] De Smet, S., Raes, K. & Demeyer, D. (2004). Meat fatty composition as affected by fatness and genetic factors: A review. *Anim. Res*., 53: 81-98.

[44] Corazzin, M., Bovolenta, S., Sepulcri, A.& Piasentier, E. (2012). Effect of whole linseed addition on meat production and quality of Italian Simmental and Holstein young bulls. *Meat Science*, 90:99-105.

[45] Karolyi, D., Dikic, M., Salajpal, K. & Juric, I. (2009). Fatty acid composition of muscle adipose tissue of beef cattle. *Italian Journal of Animal Science*, 8:264-266. .

[46] Costa, P., Roseiro, L.C:, Partidario, A., Alves, V., Bessa, R.J.B., Calkins, C.R., Santos, C. (2006). Influence of slaughter season and sex on fatty acid composition, cholesterol and alfa-tocopherol contents on different muscles of Barrosa-PDO veal. *Meat Science*, 72: 130-139.

[47] Barton, L., Bures, D., Kott, T. & Rehak, D. (2011). Effects of sex and age on bovine muscle and adipose tissue fatty acid composition and stearoyl-CoA desaturase mRNA expression. *Meat Science,* 89:444-450.

[48] Zhang, Y. Y., Zan, L.S., Wang, H.B., Xing, Y.P., Adoligbe, C.M. & Ujan, J.A. (2010). Effect of sex on meat quality characteristics of Qinchuan cattle. *African Journal of Biotechnology*, 9: 4504-4509.

[49] Garcia, P.T., Casal, J.J., Fianuchi, S., Magaldi, J.J., Rodriguez, F.J. & Nancucheo, J.A. (2008). Conjugated linolenic acid (CLA) and polyunsaturated fatty acids in muscle lipids of lamb from the Patagonian area of Argentina. *Meat Science,* 79: 541-548.

[50] Sarries, M.V., Murray, B.E., Moloney, A.P., Troy, D. & Berian, M.J. (2009). The effect of cooking on the fatty acid composition of *Longissimus dorsi* muscle from beef steers fed rations designed to increase the concentration of conjugated linoleic acid in tissue. *Meat Science*, 81:307-312.

[51] Alfaia, C.P.M., Alves, S.P., Martins, S.I.V., Costa, A.S.H., Fontes, C.M.G.A., Lemos, J.P.C., Bessa, R.J.B. & Prates, J. A. M. (2009). Effect of the feeding system on intramuscular fatty acids and conjugated linoleic acid isomers of beef cattle, with emphasis on their nutritional value and discriminatory ability. *Food Chemistry*, 114:939-946.

[52] Varela, A., Oliete, B., Moreno, T., Portela, C., Monserrat, L. & Caballo, J. et al. (2004). Effect of pasture finishing on the meat characteristics and intramuscular fatty acid profile of steers of the Rubia Gallega breed. *Meat Science*, 67:515-522.

[53] Alfaia, C.M.M., Ribeiro, V.S.S., Lourenco, M.R.A., Quaresma, M.A.G., Martins, S.I.V., Portugal, A.P.V. et al. (2006). Fatty acid composition, conjugated linoleic acid isomers and cholesterol in beef from crossbred bullocks intensively produced and from Alentejana purebred bullocks reared according to Carnalentejana-PDO specifications. *Meat Science*, 72: 425-436.

[54] Faucitano, L., Chouinard, P.Y., Fortin, J.J., Mandell, I.B., Lafreniere, C.& Girard, C.L., Berthiaume, R. (2008). Comparison of alternative beef production systems based on forrage finishing or grain-forage diets with or without growth promotans: 2. Meat quality, fatty acid composition, and overall palatability. *Journal Animal Science*, 86:1678-1689.

[55] Herdmann, A., Martin, J., Nuernberg, G., Wegner, J., Dannenberger, D. & Nuernberg, K. (2010). How do n-3 fatty acid(short-time restricted vs. unrestricted) and n-6 fatty acid enriched diets affect the fatty acid profile in different tissues of German Simmental bulls ?. *Meat Science*, 86:712-719.

[56] Scollan, D.E., Choi, N.J., Kurt, E., Fisher, A.V., Enser, M. & Wood, J.D. (2001). Manipulating the fatty acid composition of muscle and adipose tissue in beef cattle. *British Journal of Nutrition*, 85:115-124.

[57] Leheska, J.M, Thompson, L.D., Howe, J. C., Hentges, E., Boyce, J., Brooks, J. C.et al. (2008). Effects of conventional and grass –feeding systems on the nutrient composition of beef. *Journal Animal Science*, 86: 3575-3585.

[58] Juarez, M., Dugan, M.E.R., Aldai, N., Aalhus, J.L., Patience, J.F., Zijlstra, R.T.& Beaulieu, A.D.(2011). Increasing omega-3 levels through dietary co-extruded flaxseed supplementation negatively affects pork palatability. *Food Chemistry,* 126:1716-1723.

[59] Dierking, R.M., Kallenbach, R.L. & Grun, I.U. (2010). Effect of forage species on fatty acid content and performance of pasture-finished steers. *Meat Science*, 85: 597-605.

[60] Noci, F., French, P., Monahan, F.J.& Moloney, A.P., (2007). The fatty acid composition of muscle fat and subcutaneous adipose tissue of grazing heifers supplemented with plant oil-enriched concentrates. *Journal Animal Science,* 85:1062-1073.

[61] Pavan, E. & Duckett, S.K. (2007). Corn oil supplementation to steers grazing endophyte-free tall fescue. II Effects on Longissimus muscle and subcutaneous adipose fatty acid composition and stearoyl-CoA desaturase activity and expression. *Journal Animal Science*, 85.1731-1740.

[62] Smith, S.B., Gill, C.A., Lunt, D.K. & Brooks, M.A. (2009). Regulation of fat and fatty acid composition in beef cattle. *Asian –Australasian Journal of Animal Science*, 22:1225-1233.

[63] Lee, M.R. F., Evans, P.R., Nute, G.R., Richardson, R.I. & Scollan, N.D. (2009). A comparison between red clover silage and grass silage feeding on fatty acid composition, meat stability and sensory quality of the M. *Longissimus* muscle of dairy cull cows. *Meat Science*, 81:738-744.

[64] Berthelot, V., Bas, P. & Schmidely, P.(2010). Utilization of extruded linseed to modify fatty acid composition of intensively-reared lamb meat: Effect of associated cereals (wheat vs. corn) and linoleic acid content of the diet. *Meat Science,* 84: 114-124.

[65] Oriani, G., Maiorano, G., Filetti, F., Di Cesare, C., Manchisi, A. & Salvatori, G. (2005) effect of age on fatty acid composition of Italian Merino suckling lambs. *Meat Science*, 71: 557-562.

[66] Kyame, T., Brenoe, U.T. & Vangen, O. (2006). Body tissue development in lambs of two genetic lines analysed by X-ray computer tomography. *Small Ruminant Research*. 65: 242-250.

[67] Demirel, G., Ozpinar, H., Nazli, B. & Keser, O. (2006). Fatty acid of lamb meat from to breeds fed different forage: concentrate ratio. *Meat Science*, 72:229-235.

[68] Faria, P.B., Bressan, M.C., Vieira, J.O., Vicente- Neto, J., Ferrao, S.P.B., Rosa, F.C., Monteiro, M., et al. (2012). Meat quality and lipid profiles in crossbreed lambs finished on clover-rich pastures. *Meat Science*, 90:733-738.

[69] Bressan, M.C., Rossato, L.V., Rodrigues, E.C., Alves, S.P., Bessa, R.J.B. Ramos, E. M. et al. (2011). Genotype x environment interactions for fatty acid profiles in *Bos indicus* and *Bos taurus* finished on either pasture or grain. *Journal of Animal Science*, 89:221-232.

[70] Warren, H.E., Scollan, N.D., Nute, G.R., Hughes, S.I., Wood, J.D. & Richardson, R.I. (2008). Effects of breed and a concentrate or grass silage diet on beef quality in cattle of 3 ages. II Meat stability and flavor. *Meat Science,* 78: 270-278.

[71] Lourenco, M., Van Ranst, G., Vlaeminck, B., De Smet, S. & Fievez, V. (2008). Influence of different dietary forages on the fatty acid composition of rumen digests as well as ruminant meat and milk. *Animal Feed Science and Technology*, 145:418-437.

[72] García, P. T., Pordomingo, A., Perez, C. A., Rios, M.D. & Casal, J.J. (2007). Influence of cutting and season on the fatty acid composition of forage crops for grazing forage beef production. *Proceedings 53nd International Congress Meat Science & Technology,* 97-98-

[73] Jeronimo, E., Alves, S.P., Prates, J.A.M., Santos-Silva, J.& Bessa, R.J.B. (2009). Effect of dietary replacement of sunflower oil with linseed oil on intramuscular fatty acids of lamb meat. *Meat Science*, 84: 499-505.

[74] Mazzone, G., Giammarco, M., Vignola, G., Sardi, L. & Lambertini, L. (2010). Effects of rearing season on carcass and meat quality of suckling Apennine light lambs. *Meat Science*, 86:474-478.

[75] Chiofalo, B., Simonella, S., Di Grigoli, A., Liotta, L.,Frenda, A.S., Lo Presti, V., Bonanno, A. & Chiofalo, V.(2010). Chemical and acidic compostion of *Longissimus dorsi* of Comisana lambs fed with *Trifolium subterraneum* and *Lolium multiflorum. Small Ruminant Research,* 88:89-96.

[76] Daniel, Z.C.T.R., Wynn, R.J., Salter, A.M. & Buttery, P.J. (2004). Differing effects of forage and concentrate diets on the oleic acid and the conjugated linoleic acid content of sheep tissues. *Journal of Animal Science*, 82:747-758.

[77] Kott, R.W., Hatfield, P.G., Bergman, J.W., Flyn, C.R., Van Wagoner, H. & Boles, J.A. (2003). Feedlot performance, carcass composition, and muscle and fat CLA concentrations of lambs fed diets supplemented with safflower seeds. *Meat Science*, 49: 11-17.

[78] Bessa, R.J.B., Lourenco, M., Portugal, P.V. & Santos-Silva, J. (2008). Effects of previous diet and duration of soybean oil supplementation on light lamb carcass composition, meat quality and fatty acid composition. *Meat Science,* 80:1100-1105.

[79] Peng, Y.S., Brown, M.A., Wu, J.P. & Liu, Z. (2010). Different oilseed supplements alter fatty acid composition of different adipose tissues of adult ewes. *Meat Science*, 85:542-549.

[80] Vasta, V., Pagano, R.I., Luciano, g., Scerra, M., Caparra, P., Foti, F. et al. (2012). Effect of morning vs. afternoon on intramuscular fatty acid composition in lamb. *Meat Science*, 90:93-98.

[81] Berthelot, V., Bas, P., Pottier, E. & Normand, J. (2012). The effect of maternal linseed supplementation on muscle and subcutaneous adipose tissue fatty acid composition of indoor lams. *Meat Science*, 90: 548-557.

[82] Bernes, G., Turner, T. & Pickova, J. (2012). Sheep fed only silage supplement with concentrates. 2. Effects on lamb performance and fatty acid profile of ewe milk and lamb meat. *Small Ruminant Research*, 102: 114-124.
[83] Joy, M., Ripoll, G., Molino, F., Dervishi, E. & Alvarez Rodriguez, J. (2012). Influence of the type of forage supplied to ewes in pre- and post-partum periods on the meat fatty acid of suckling lambs. *Meat Science*, 90:775-782.
[84] Enser, M., Richardson, R. I., Wood, J.D., Gill, B.P. & Sheard, P.R. (2000). Feeding linseed to increase the n-3 PUFA of pork: Fatty acid composition of muscle, adipose tissue, liver and sausages. *Meat Science,* 55: 201-212.
[85] Dugan, M.E.R., Rollan, D.C., Aalhus, J.L., Aldai, N. & Kramer, J.K.G (2008). Subcutaneous fat composition of youthful and mature Canadian beef. *Canadian Journal of Animal Science,* 88:591-599.
[86] Mir, Z., Rushfeldt, M.I., Paterson, L.J. & Weselake, P. (2000). Effects of dietary supplementation with CLA or linoleic rich oil in the lamb content of lamb tissues. *Small Ruminant Research,* 36:25-31.

In: Linoleic Acids
Editor: Igho Onakpoya
ISBN: 978-1-62257-384-4
© 2012 Nova Science Publishers, Inc.

Chapter II

Linoleic Acid Content and Antioxidant Properties of Different Tree Nuts: A Review

A. Beltrán, M. Ramos, A. Valdés and M.C. Garrigós
Analytical Chemistry, Nutrition & Food Sciences Department,
University of Alicante, Alicante, Spain

ABSTRACT

Tree nuts are characterized by high total lipid content, ranging from 45 to 75% depending on the nut type. Their lipid profile is composed mainly of heart-protective monounsaturated fatty acids (MUFAs) and polyunsaturated fatty acids (PUFAs). In this sense, it is possible to distinguish a group of nuts rich in MUFAs (mainly oleic acid) such as hazelnuts, almonds and pistachios from another rich in PUFAs (mainly linoleic acid) such as sunflower seeds. Despite their high fat content, nuts contain many valuable nutritional components which have been associated with several health benefits such as their influence on the serum lipid profile and reduction of cardiovascular disease risk in humans. These effects have been linked to their fatty acid composition and the presence of some minor compounds presenting antioxidant activity (i.e. polyphenols and tocopherols) and to the cholesterol lowering effects of phytosterols. Linoleic acid (LA) is one of the essential fatty acids in humans that must be supplied into the diet (nuts being one of the main sources of LA) and it is the starting point for the synthesis of a variety of other unsaturated fatty acids. After ingestion, LA is converted into arachidonic acid, 20:4 (n-6), which, together with eicosapentanoic acid, is the starting point for the synthesis of eicosanoids and prostaglandins that are important mediators in many inflammatory and cardiovascular diseases. In this chapter, the linoleic acid content of different tree nuts, their antioxidant properties and potential use as natural dietary antioxidants, as well as other applications are discussed.

List of Abbreviations

CHD	Coronary heart disease
FAMEs	Fatty acids methyl esters
FAOSTAT	Food and Agriculture Organization Statistical Database and Data-sets
FID	Flame ionization detector
GC	Gas chromatography
HPLC	High performance liquid chromatography
LA	Linoleic acid
MUFA	Monounsaturated fatty acid
NMR	Nuclear magnetic resonance
PFE	Pressurized fluid extraction
PUFA	Polyunsaturated fatty acid
RAE	Retinol activity equivalent
SFA	Saturated fatty acid
SFE	Supercritical fluid extraction
TP	Tocopherols
TT	Tocotrienols
USDA	United States Department of Agriculture

Introduction

Extensive research has been carried out on nuts and health outcomes during the last two decades due to the publication of a report from the pioneering Adventist Health Study showing association of nut consumption with a lower risk of coronary heart disease (CHD) [1], demonstrating that a diet enriched with nuts reduced serum cholesterol levels compared to a standard healthy diet. This interest is reflected in a considerable increase in the total world production of nuts in the last decade from 7.407.465 tonnes in 2000 to 13.392.753 tonnes in 2010 (Figure 1).

By definition, tree nuts are dry fruits with a seed in which the ovary wall becomes hard at maturity [1]. The most popular edible tree nuts are almonds (*Prunus amigdalus*), hazelnuts (*Corylus avellana*), walnuts (*Juglans regia*), and pistachios (*Pistachia vera*). Other common edible nuts are pine nuts (*Pinus pinea*), cashews (*Anacardium occidentale*), pecans (*Carya illinoiensis*), macadamias (*Macadamia integrifolia*), and Brazil nuts (*Bertholletia excelsa*). The consumer definition also includes peanuts (*Arachis hypogea*), which botanically are groundnuts or legumes but are widely identified as part of the nuts food group. Although chestnuts (*Castanea sativa*) are tree nuts as well, they are different from all other common nuts because of being starchier and having a different nutritional profile [1]. For the purpose of this review, the term "nuts" will include all common tree nuts and also chestnuts and peanuts.

According to the FAOSTAT database [2], cashew is the world's most popular nut which ranks first with a global production of 3.585.807 tonnes (29%), followed by walnut with 2.545.388 (20%), almond with 2.531.722 tonnes (20%), chestnut accounting for 1.958.547 tonnes (16%), peanut with 912,179 (7%), hazelnut reaching a value of 888.328 tonnes (7%) and Brazil nut presenting a value of 91.107 (0.2%) tonnes in 2010.

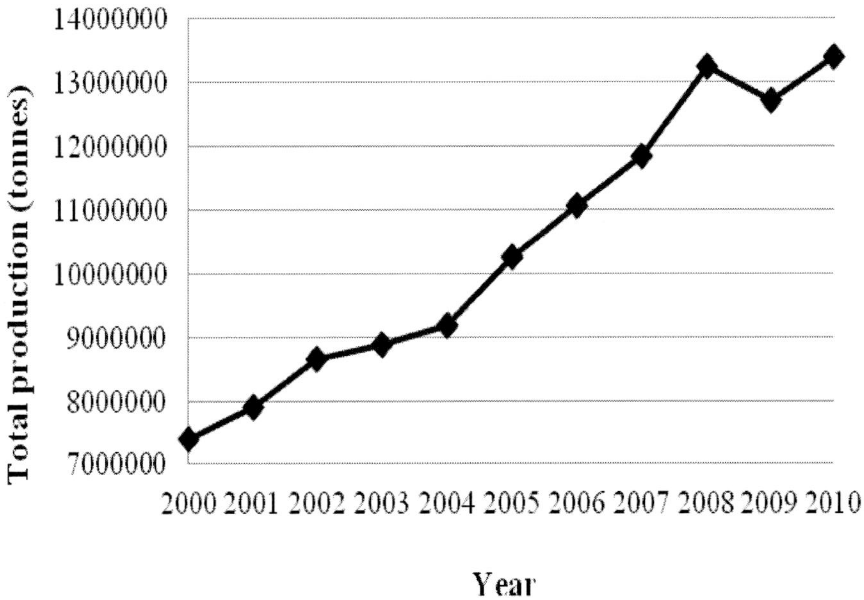

Figure 1.Total world production (tonnes) of nuts between the years 2000 and 2010 [2].

The nut crops swept through the countries with high tolerance to extreme weather conditions characterized by wet winters and hot summers. As it can be seen in Figure 2, China (40%), Vietnam (16%) and Turkey (14%) were the main nut production countries in the world in 2010, with 2.906.440, 1.171.100 and 1.022.911 tonnes of nuts, respectively; followed by Nigeria (601.000 tonnes), Côte d'Ivoire (390.950 tonnes), Spain (258.700 tonnes), Italy (238.100 tonnes) and Mexico (163.099 tonnes). Also, Syrian Arab Republic, Brazil, Philippines and Morocco are other countries with partial production of nuts in the world reaching a value of 161.500, 146.223, 141.318 and 113.422 tonnes, respectively [2].

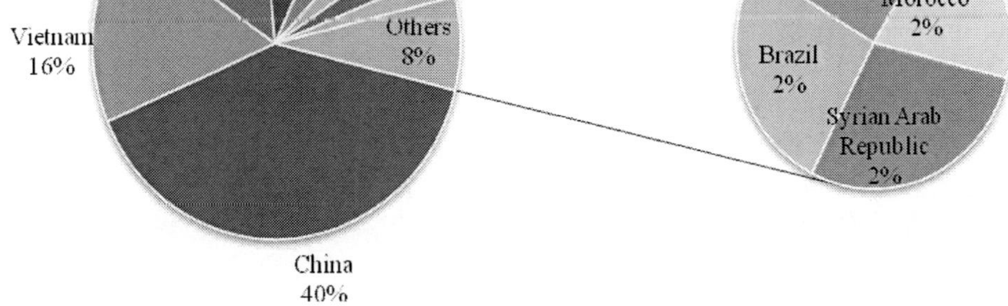

Figure 2. Geographic distribution of the total world production of nuts in 2010 [2].

From the point of view of the current situation in the food industry, nuts are consumed regularly as snacks, desserts or part of a meal; and are eaten whole (fresh, salted, roasted or fried) [3], in spreads (peanut butter, almond paste), as oils or hidden in commercial products, mixed dishes, sauces, pastries, ice creams and baked foods [1].

Composition and Nutrient Values of Nuts: Macro and Micronutrients

As it can be seen in Table 1, tree nuts (almonds, hazelnuts, chestnuts, cashew nuts, Brazil nuts, macadamia nuts, walnuts and pistachios) and edible seeds (peanuts and sunflowers) are good sources of lipids and proteins. The lipid fraction is composed especially of oleic (C18:1) and linoleic (C18:2) fatty acids; with emphasis on the ω-6 to ω-3 relation in macadamia, walnut and chestnut whose profiles favour the reduction of cardiovascular disease risk. Their proteins present an amino acid profile that meets the requirements of school children and contain more sulfur-containing amino acids than legumes such as beans. These nuts and edible seeds are also good sources of phytosterols, mainly β-sitosterol; minerals, particularly calcium, iron, zinc, selenium and potassium; tocopherols (TP), especially α-TP; and insoluble fiber. These nutrient-dense foods contain bioactive substances that maximize their beneficial health effects and, for this reason, their study and consumption should be encouraged [4].

Table 1. Average value of macronutrients of 13 different nuts per 100 g of food sample [5]

Nut	Energy (Kcal)	Water (g)	Protein (g)	Fat (g)	Ash (g)	Carbohydrate (g)	Fiber (g)	Sugars (g)	Starch (g)
Black walnut	618	4.56	24.06	59.0	2.47	9.91	6.8	1.10	0.24
English walnut	654	4.07	15.23	65.2	1.78	13.71	6.7	2.61	0.06
Pine nut	673	2.28	13.69	68.4	2.59	13.08	3.7	3.59	1.43
Pistachio	562	3.91	20.27	45.4	2.91	27.51	10.3	7.66	1.67
Pecan	691	3.52	9.17	71.9	1.49	13.86	9.6	3.97	0.46
Peanut	570	6.39	26.15	49.6	2.03	15.82	9.5	na	na
Macadamia	718	1.36	7.91	75.8	1.14	13.82	8.6	4.57	1.05
Hazelnut	628	5.31	14.95	60.8	2.29	16.70	9.7	4.34	0.48
Cashew	553	5.20	18.22	43.9	2.54	30.19	3.3	5.91	23.49
Brazil nut	656	3.48	14.32	66.4	3.51	12.27	7.5	2.33	0.25
Almond	575	4.70	21.22	49.4	2.99	21.67	12.2	3.89	0.74
Chestnut	213	48.65	2.42	2.3	1.13	45.54	8.1	na	na
Sunflower seed	584	4.73	20.78	51.4	3.02	20.00	8.6	2.62	na

na = not available in the USDA Nutrient Database 2011.

Despite their similarities in water content (less than 6.4 % except in the case of chestnuts) and protein (13-26%) fractions, nuts have wide range of chemical composition. The majority of nuts present a content of 9-22% related to carbohydrate fraction, less than 3.5% of ash, between 1.10-3.97% of sugars and 0.06-1.67% related to starch content. Nuts are also a good source of dietary fiber, which ranges from 7-12 g per 100 g, and in standard servings provide 5–10% of daily fiber requirements [1]. Nevertheless, pistachio and cashew nuts differ from the rest in its high content in carbohydrates (27.51% for pistachio and 30.19% for cashews) and sugars (7.66 and 5.91%, respectively). Also, cashews present in their composition the lowest fiber content (3.7%) followed by pine nuts (3.3%). As has been previously mentioned, chestnuts are different from all other common nuts presenting a different nutritional profile. Although nuts present a very high sensory appeal and numerous health benefits, their consumption should be moderate due to their high caloric value, about 500–700 kcal per 100 g of portion, which is due to the fat content. In this respect, the majority of nuts have a high fat content ranging from 44-76 % by dry weight depending on the nut type, being good sources of unsaturated fatty acids including monounsaturated (MUFA) and polyunsaturated fatty acids (PUFA). Finally, smaller amounts of saturated fatty acids (SFA) are also present. Figure 3 shows the proportions of SFA, MUFA, and PUFA for different nuts. Regarding macadamias, hazelnuts, cashews, pecans, pistachios, peanuts and Brazil nuts, MUFA is the predominant fatty acid fraction. However, PUFA fraction is predominant for English walnuts (78%), Black walnuts (66%), pine nuts (60%) and sunflower seeds (50%).

In the case of chestnuts, a similar content of MUFA (37%) and PUFA (43%) is observed. Most of the tree nuts had a relatively low percentage of SFAs (less than 7%). Only Brazil nuts (15%), macadamias (12%) and cashew nuts (8%) present higher values of SFA. This fact has been crucial for these nuts to be excluded from the USDA qualified health claim for tree nuts [6].

In general, palmitic (C 16:0), stearic (C 18:0) and arachidic fatty acids (C 20:0) are the major SFAs present in nuts, with oleic (C 18:1), eicosenoic (C 20:1) and palmitoleic (C 16:1) acids being the dominant MUFAs. The most abundant PUFA present in the 13 nuts is linoleic acid (C 18:2) followed by α-linolenic acid. Table 2 shows the fatty acid composition of different nuts according to the USDA National Nutrient Database for Standard Reference 2011.

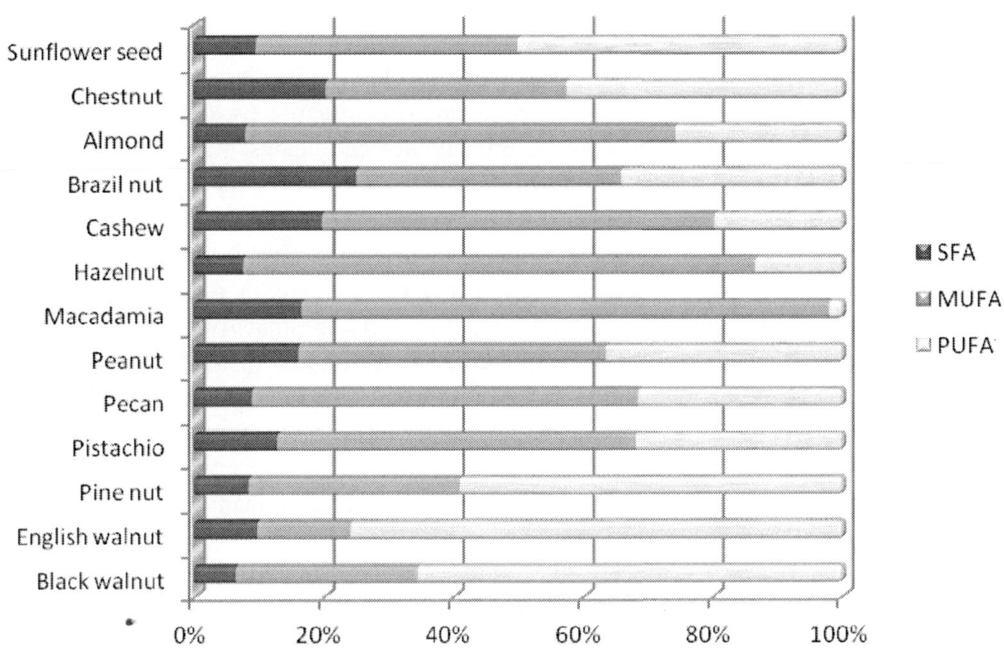

Figure 3. Fatty acids profile of nuts based on data from USDA Nutrient Database 2011 [4].

Table 2. Fatty acid composition of 13 different nuts expressed as g of fatty acid per 100 g of food sample [4]

Nuts	SFAs			MUFAs			PUFAs	
	C 16:0	C 18:0	C 20:0	C 16:1	C 18:1	C 20:1	C 18:2	C 18:3
Black walnut	1.923	1.445	0	0.063	14.533	0.408	33.072	2.006
English walnut	4.404	1.659	0.063	0	8.799	0.134	38.093	9.080
Pine nut	3.212	1.390	0.229	0.017	17.947	0.801	33.150	0.164
Pistachio	4.994	0.476	0.043	0.473	23.174	0.174	13.485	0.259
Pecan	4.366	1.745	0.069	0	40.594	0.207	20.628	0.986
Peanut	5.674	1.288	0	0.045	21.757	0.523	17.192	0.010
Macadamia	6.036	2.329	1.940	12.981	43.755	1.890	1.296	0.206
Hazelnut	3.097	1.265	0.102	0.116	45.405	0.131	7.833	0.087
Cashew	3.916	3.223	0.266	0.136	23.523	0.138	7.782	0.062
Brazil nut	9.085	5.794	0.160	0.226	24.223	0.052	20.543	0.035
Almond	3.044	0.013	0.658	0.243	30.611	0.010	12.061	0.006
Chestnut	0.384	0.021	0	0.021	0.749	0.010	0.798	0.095
Sunflower seed	2.210	1.690	0.115	0.020	18.380	0.085	23.050	0.060

Generally, C 18:1, 18:2, 16:0, and 18:0 are the dominant fatty acids in nuts, in descending order. In addition, English and Black walnuts are good sources of 18:3 (9.080 and 2.006 g per 100 g of portion, respectively). Among the 13 nuts, 8 contain higher oleic fatty acid content as follows: Hazelnut > Macadamia > Pecan > Almond > Brazil nut > Cashew > Pistachio > Peanut. However, Macadamia has markedly higher palmitoleic fatty acid content (13%) than the rest. The major linoleic fatty acid content is present in English walnut composition (38.093 g per 100 g) followed by Pine nut (33.15g), Black walnut (33.072g) and sunflower seed (23.05g). As it can be observed in Table 1, chestnuts contain the least amount of fat (2.26g of fat per 100 g of portion). For this reason, only 0.749 g of C 18:1 per 100 g of portion and 0.798 g for C 18:2 are present in their composition.

Nuts are also high in trace micronutrients including vitamins and minerals with antioxidant properties (Tables 3 and 4). Among antioxidant vitamins (A, C, and E), vitamin E is the most abundant in nuts and it is the primary defence against lipid peroxidation by protecting the human cells from free radical damage [7].Sunflower seeds have the highest amounts of vitamin E reaching values of 35.17 mg per 100 g of food sample; followed by almonds and hazelnuts with values of 26.22 and 15.03 mg, respectively. Vitamin A expressed as retinol activity equivalents (RAE) is present in great amounts in pine nuts (29 RAE), pistachios (21 RAE) and English walnuts (20 RAE); while chestnuts (43 mg) followed by hazelnuts (6.3 mg) and pistachios (5.6 mg) are rich in vitamin C. Thus, these nuts are potentially beneficial to human health. On the other hand, pine nuts, cashews and hazelnuts are good sources of vitamin K which acts as a regulator in the blood clotting mechanism and is required for bone maturation in the human body [8]. The vitamin B1 or thiamine is required by the organism because its phosphate derivatives are involved in many cellular processes. Macadamia and sunflower seeds are a good source of this vitamin since they contain thiamine amounts of 1195 and 1480 mg respectively. Another B group vitamin, Niacin or B3, has been used for over 50 years to increase levels of high-density lipoprotein (HDL) in blood; and has also been found to modestly decrease the risk of cardiovascular events in a number of controlled human trials. Niacin deficiency commonly results in pellagra [9]. Thus, the intake of all kinds of nuts provides significant amounts of this vitamin, except black walnut and Brazil nut with less than 0.295 mg of B3 per 100 g of food samples. Peanut followed by black walnut and sunflower are rich in pantothenic acid or vitamin B5; while peanut, sunflower and hazelnut provide significant amounts of Folate or vitamin B12. It is important to note the high content of Riboflavin or B2 vitamin in almonds presenting 1014 mg per 100 g of food sample in contrast of the rest with less than 0.4 mg. In general, the B group of vitamins are essential for energy production in the human body, as well as the synthesis and metabolism of proteins, carbohydrates, and fats. Vitamin E availability in nuts is noteworthy because aside the tree nuts being a good source of the vitamin, the nutrient is present in a more bioavailable form compared to other food matrices. Two different classes of the vitamin exist: TP and tocotrienols (TT). There are four isomers (α, β, γ, and δ) of each class, and the two classes differ in that the TT contain unsaturated side chains [5]. Table 4 shows the TP content of different nuts as they are the main source of vitamin E in contrast to TT.

In general, the major TP isomers present in nuts are α- and γ-TP, with the amounts present being dependent upon the nut type. In this sense, almonds and hazelnuts have dominant α-TP contents, whereas γ-TP levels are found in black walnuts, Brazil nuts, English walnuts, pecans, and pistachios. Pine nut is the only tree nut that contains fairly equal amounts of both α- and γ-TP.

Table 3. Average vitamin content of 13 different nuts per 100 g food sample [4]

Nut	Vitamin C[a]	Thiamine	Riboflavin	Niacin	Pantothenic acid	Folate. total	Vitamin A	Vitamin E[c]	Vitamin K
	mg	mg	mg	mg	mg	µg	RAE[b]	mg	µg
Black walnut	1.7	0.057	0.130	0.470	1660	31	2	1.8	2.7
English walnut	1.3	0.341	0.150	1125	0.570	98	20	0.7	2.7
Pine nut	0.8	0.364	0.227	4387	0.313	34	29	9.33	53.9
Pistachio	5.6	0.870	0.160	1300	0.520	51	21	2.3	na
Pecan	1.1	0.660	0.130	1167	0.863	0	3	1.4	3.5
Peanut	0.0	0.675	0.135	15925	1769	240	0	na	na
Macadamia	1.2	1195	0.162	2473	0.758	0	0	0.54	na
Hazelnut	6.3	0.643	0.113	1800	0.918	113	1	15.03	14.2
Cashew	0.5	0.423	0.058	1062	0.864	25	0	0.9	34.1
Brazil nut	0.7	0.617	0.035	0.295	0.184	22	0	5.73	0
Almond	0.0	0.211	1014	3385	0.469	50	0	26.22	0
Chestnut	43.0	0.238	0.168	1179	0.509	62	1	0	0
Sunflower seed	1.4	1480	0.355	8335	1130	227	3	35.17	0

[a]Vitamin C expressed as total ascorbic acid.
[b]Vitamin A expressed as RAE or retinol activity equivalents.
[c]Vitamin E as α-tocopherol.
na means "not available in the USDA Nutrient Database 2011".

To have a better knowledge of the composition of nuts, Table 5 shows the main mineral contents of the 13 different nuts. Compared to other common foods, nuts have an optimal nutritional density with respect to healthy minerals, such as copper, manganese, calcium, magnesium, phosphorus and potassium.

Table 4. Tocopherol isomer content in nuts expressed as milligrams per 100 g of kernels, n = 3 [5]

Nuts	α-Tocopherol	β-Tocopherol	γ-Tocopherol	δ-Tocopherol
Almond	23±1	0.16±0.03	0.57±0.04	nd
Black walnut	2.4±0.3	0.01±0.01	20.1±0.6	1.57±0.06
Brazil nut	5±2	0.03±0.02	14±4	0.21±0.10
Cashew	1.5±0.3	nd	5.6±0.6	0.37±0.03
English walnut	1.1±0.3	0.06±0.02	20±2	1.7±0.3
Hazelnut	26±2	0.9±0.2	4.1±0.6	0.20±0.02
Macadamia	nd	nd	0.01±0.02	nd
Pecan	1.2±0.3	0.8±0.3	22±2	0.60±0.22
Pine nut	12.5±0.9	nd	11.6±0.3	0.03±0.03
Pistachio	1.5±0.2	0.05±0.01	23±1	0.57±0.06

nd: non detected

Table 5. Average mineral content of 13 different nuts per 100 g of food sample [4]

Nut	Ca	Fe	Mg	P	K	Na	Zn	Cu	Mn	Se
	mg	mg	mg	mg	mg	mg	mg	mg	mg	μg
Black walnut	61	3.12	201	513	523	2	3.37	1360	3896	17
English walnut	98	2.91	158	346	441	2	3.09	1586	3414	4.9
Pine nut	16	5.53	251	575	597	2	6.45	1324	8802	0.7
Pistachio	105	3.92	121	490	1025	1	2.20	1300	1200	7.0
Pecan	70	2.53	121	277	410	0	4.53	1200	4500	3.8
Peanut	106	3.91	188	388	744	22	2.12	0.900	2640	7.2
Macadamia	85	3.69	130	188	368	5	1.30	0.756	4131	3.6
Hazelnut	114	4.70	163	290	680	0	2.45	1725	6175	2.4
Cashew	37	6.68	292	593	660	12	5.78	2195	1655	19.9
Brazil nut	160	2.43	376	725	659	3	4.06	1743	1223	1917
Almond	264	3.72	268	484	705	1	3.08	0.996	2285	2.5
Chestnut	27	1.01	32	93	518	3	0.52	0.447	0.952	0
Sunflower seed	78	5.25	325	660	645	9	5.00	1800	1950	53

In terms of the mineral content, it is important to note that all studied nuts contain high amounts of manganese (> 1000 mg per 100 g of food sample), except for chestnuts that contain only 0.952 mg. Pistachios contain the greatest amounts of potassium, with values reaching 1025 mg. Copper mineral is also abundant, being present in amounts more than 1000 mg in nuts except for peanuts, macadamias, almonds and chestnuts which contain under 1 mg per 100 g of portion. Almonds and Brazil nuts are rich in calcium, containing 264 and 160 mg respectively. Also, Brazil nuts and sunflower seeds contain higher amounts of magnesium and phosphorus. Comparing the majority of nuts, selenium is found particularly in Brazil nuts in greater concentrations (1917 μg). A high intake of calcium, magnesium and potassium, together with a low sodium intake, is associated with protection against bone demineralization, arterial hypertension, insulin resistance, and overall cardiovascular risk [1]. In this sense, numerous health benefits attributed to the consumption of tree nuts in daily diet have been reported [10, 11]. In the 2010 U.S. Dietary Guidelines, these benefits were documented since moderate evidence indicates that eating 1.5 ounces per day of peanuts and certain tree nuts (i.e., walnuts, almonds, and pistachios) reduces the risk of cardiovascular disease when consumed as part of diet. These health claims have been partially attributed to the lipid constituents in nuts, including unsaturated fatty acids, most of which are rich in MUFA (primarily oleic acid) and PUFA (primarily linoleic acid), the isomers of TP along with TT (vitamin E), and phytosterols [5]. In fact, nuts contain numerous types of antioxidants with different properties such as sterol esters, TP, TT, phytosterols, phytostanols, squalene, terpenoids, sphingolipids, and essential oils, among others, and phytochemicals such as phenolic acids, flavonoids (flavonols, flavones, flavanols or catechins, flavanones, anthocyanidins, isoflavanoids), stilbenes, lignans, hyrolyzable tannins, condensed tannins or proanthocyanidins, carotenoids, alkaloids, coumestan, phytates, terpenes, and phytoestrogens, among others. The actions of antioxidants have been attributed to their ability to scavenge free radicals, thereby reducing oxidative damage of cellular biomolecules such as lipids, proteins, and DNA [12].

Regarding the phytochemical composition, the term 'phytochemical' broadly refers to all plant derived chemicals. Hence, macronutrients such as plant carbohydrates (including dietary fibre), lipids and proteins could be categorised as phytochemicals. However, for the purposes of the present review, we will use the term 'phytochemical' to refer to micronutrients with health-promoting actions. A previous study categorised phytochemicals into six broad classes: alkaloids, organosulfurs, phenolics, carbohydrates, non-nutritive proteins and lipids [6]. Nuts contain the majority of phytochemical classes (Table 6).

Table 6. Phytochemical composition of nuts per 100 g of portion [13]

		Phenols		
	Phytosterols	Proanthocyanidins	Flavonoids	Carotenoids
Nuts	mg	mg	mg	μg
Almond	141	184.02	15.24	2
Cashew	na	8,68	1.98	22
Hazelnut	96	500.66	11.74	106
Peanut	220	15.62	0.66	0
Chestnut	22	0.05	0.02	na
Walnut	72	67.25	2.71	21
Brazil nut	na	0	0	0
Macadamia	116	0	0	na
Pecan	102	494.05	34.01	55
Pine nut	na	0	0.49	na
Pistachio	214	237.34	14.37	332

na = not available in the literature.

As it can be seen in Table 6, almonds contain great amounts of phytosterols, proanthocyanidins and flavonoids such as catechins, flavonols, and flavonones in their aglycone and glycoside form, while pistachios has the highest concentration of carotenoids in comparison with the other nuts.

Peanut contains a wide range of phytosterols while high amounts of proanthocyanidins are present in hazelnut followed by pecans, pistachios and almonds. Nevertheless, micro and macronutrient contents can be quite variable depending upon horticultural aspects such as cultivar type, growing region, climatic conditions, and harvest year or interactions of these factors, as well as the storage, processing, and assay conditions employed [14].

In this sense, the nutrient composition of almonds is dependent on the genotype since evaluations of local almond genotype selections from breeding trials have shown a wider range in total lipid content; for example, such as 25-61% lipids for Turkish and 40-67% for Spanish selections. Moreover, Spanish samples showed 67% of lipids in the 2002 harvest samples, but 59 and 61% lipids in the two subsequent harvest year samples [15].

Lipid Oxidation of Nuts: Mechanism and Factors

Linoleic acid (LA) is one of the essential fatty acids present in humans that must be supplied through the diet (nuts being one of the main sources of LA) and it is the starting point for the synthesis of a variety of other unsaturated fatty acids. After ingestion, LA is converted into arachidonic acid, 20:4 (n-6), which, together with eicosapentanoic acid, is the starting point for the synthesis of eicosanoids and prostaglandins that are important mediators in many inflammatory and cardiovascular diseases.

However, the high LA content of some nuts makes them quite susceptible to oxidative degradation resulting in a reduction in their shelf life. In this sense, oxidised lipids can accelerate deterioration of sensory quality in nuts and decrease consumer acceptance, the lipid oxidation of dried foods being influenced by a number of factors including antioxidants [16] metals, photosensitisers and oxygen content, heat intensity and light energy and the number of double bonds in fatty acids [17].

Regarding nut samples, lipid oxidation is the main cause of off-flavour development, with high temperatures and oxygen concentration being the most important factors affecting these processes [18].

The mechanism of the oxidation processes of nuts largely depends on the oxidative conditions. In this sense, the nature of the different compounds produced in the oxidation of nuts at room temperature in closed receptacles [19], could be different from those produced at higher temperatures [20]. Oxidative stability is an important indicator to determine oil quality and shelf life because low-molecular-weight off-flavour compounds are produced during oxidation, which can make oil unacceptable to consumers or for industrial use as a food ingredient [21].

In the oxidation process, the triglyceride structure undergoes changes with the consequence of the formation of a great number of compounds. It has been postulated that first of all, primary oxidation compounds, such as hydroperoxides, are generated. Among the secondary oxidation products, it is possible to find alkanals, (E)-2-alkenals and (E,E)-2,4-alkadienals, and also γ-oxygenated α,β-unsaturated aldehydes [22]. The mechanism of free radical autoxidation can be understood by a chain process consisting of initiation, propagation, and termination steps. When the compound undergoing reaction is a lipid or other compound of biological importance (protein, carbohydrate, nucleic acid), the process is normally referred to as peroxidation.

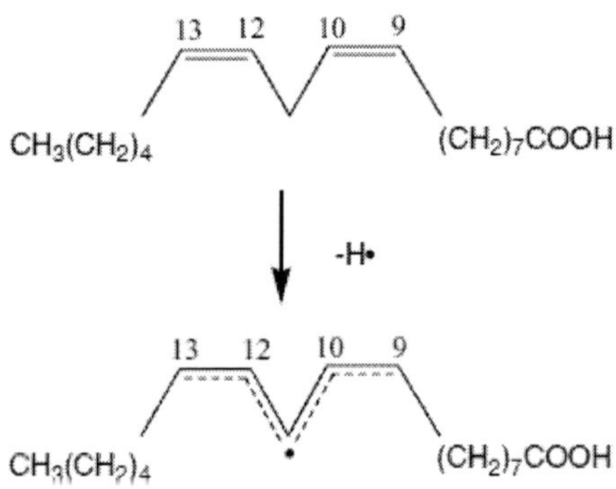

Scheme 1.

As it can be seen in Scheme 1, in the presence of initiators, oxidation of linoleic acid begins with the abstraction of a hydrogen atom of an allylic carbon generating an alkyl radical to be combined later with molecular oxygen.

The direct oxidation of unsaturated lipids by triplet oxygen is prevented by spin as the ground state of the lipid is of multiplicity singlet while the oxygen is triplet. This spin barrier can be overcome by the presence of initiators, which can produce radicals by different mechanisms which are described below:

a) Thermal dissociation of hydroperoxides (LOOH) present as impurities leading to the formation of alcoxyl radicals (LO•)

$LOOH \rightarrow LO\bullet + HO\bullet$

b) Exposure to light in the presence of a sensitizer as a ketone (LCOL):

$LCOL + h\nu \rightarrow LCO\bullet + L\bullet$

c) Decomposition of hydroperoxides catalyzed by metals (M) of variable oxidation state:

$LOOH + M^{2+} \rightarrow LO\bullet + OH^- + M^{3+}$

$LOOH + M^{3+} \rightarrow LOO\bullet + H^+ + M^{2+}$

Thermal oxidation of unsaturated lipids generally comprises initiation of autocatalytic decomposition of hydroperoxides which is normally catalyzed by metals in trace amounts because its presence is very difficult to remove. Since the reaction of singlet oxygen ($^1O_2$) with unsaturated lipids is highly favored because of the multiplicity singlet of the lipid and also occurs at speeds higher than those attained in the case of reactions with triplet oxygen, hydroperoxides formed enzymatically or photoxidativelly serve as free radical initiators, as shown in the above reactions [22]. At the stage of propagation, the alkyl radicals formed in the initiation step (L•), combine with molecular oxygen (O_2) to produce peroxyl radicals (LOO•). LOO • radicals have half-lives (7s) significantly higher than the radicals L• (10^{-8}s), allowing them to propagate the oxidation reaction by abstraction of hydrogen from selective unsaturated fatty acids to produce hydroperoxides as primary products and alkyl radicals:

$L\bullet + O_2 \rightarrow LOO\bullet$

$LOO\bullet + LH \rightarrow L\bullet + LOOH$

The first reaction of the propagation step is quite rapid, while abstraction of hydrogen from another unsaturated lipid is slower and, therefore, is the rate determining step of the reaction. Unsaturated fatty acids have different susceptibilities to the abstraction of hydrogen depending on the energies of dissociation of the labile CH bonds. Adjacent bonds to a double bond or a tertiary carbon atom are weak and easily broken. For the series of fatty acid-CH_2-

$(CH = CH\text{-}CH_2)_n\text{-}CH_2\text{-}(n = 1\text{-}3)$, the relative oxidation rate increases in proportion 1:40:80 respectively, the oxidation of monounsaturated fatty acids being much slower than those of polyunsaturated fatty acids [23].

After reaching a maximum value, the oxidation rate decreases in the final stage when the peroxyl radicals react with each other to form self-destructing non-radical through the termination reaction:

LOO• + LOO• → non radical product

At low temperatures, the peroxyl radicals can combine to produce peroxyl bond dimers (LOOL) with the formation of molecular oxygen:

LOO• + LOO• → LOOL + O_2

At low oxygen pressures and elevated temperatures, alkyl and alkoxyl radicals (LO •) may be combined to form dimers containing the ether group (LOL):

L• + LO• → LOL

Furthermore, the alkyl radicals can combine with each other giving rise to dimers with CC bonds:

2 L• → L-L

One of the most important reactions in the finishing stage involves the presence of an antioxidant (AH). The presence of antioxidants in nuts inhibits oxidation since they react with peroxyl radicals according to reaction:

LOO• + AH → A• + LOOH

A• + LOO• → non radical product

The radical antioxidant (A•) is stabilized by resonance and can not spread the oxidation reaction. Because of its lipophilicity, TP are considered the antioxidants responsible for lipid stabilization. However, although nuts generally contain suitable amounts of TP, fatty acid composition is more important for oxidative stability than TP content. Given the same concentration of antioxidants, the oxidative stability of a nut decreases with the increase of unsaturated fatty acids content [24].

The relative differences between the oxidative stability of nuts with different degrees of unsaturation are minimized as the oxidation temperature increases. The increase in the rate of oxidation induced by high temperatures prevails over the influence in the oxidative process of fatty acid composition in terms of mono and polyunsaturated fatty acids present in each of the different nuts. The importance of temperature on the rate of oxidation of fatty acids is explained by the quantitative relationship between the rate constant of reaction (K) and temperature (T) described by the Arrhenius equation [25]:

$$K = A \cdot e^{(-Ea/RT)}$$

where A is the preexponential factor which is a constant related to the geometry of the reaction medium, Ea is activation energy, R is the universal gas constant (8.314 JK^{-1} mol^{-1}) and T is the absolute temperature in Kelvin. The activation energy is correlated with the dissociation energy of the CH bonds (EDCH) using the equation given by Koreck et al. [26]:

$$E_a = 0{,}55\ [EDCH - 62{,}5]$$

Since EDCH presents an approximate value of 83 kcal mol^{-1} for bis-allylic hydrogens of linoleate and linolenate and it is approximately 10 kcal mol^{-1} greater for the hydrogens in the oleate, values of activation energy of 11 and 17 kcal mol^{-1} are obtained for linoleate and oleate, respectively. Furthermore, as the oxidation temperature increases, the contribution of the activation energy in the Arrhenius equation is less significant.

It is not easy to differentiate the individual effects of temperature and oxygen concentration in the oxidative process due to the strong interactions between them. At low or moderate temperatures and atmospheric pressure, the solubility of oxygen is higher and the peroxyl radical species are more common. Once the oxidation reaction with oxygen is initiated, the hydroperoxides are the major products generated. Under these conditions, the rate of formation of hydroperoxides is greater than the rate of decomposition. Compounds formed by the termination reactions are major products only in advanced stages of the oxidative process, i.e. at the end of the induction period when the initial substrate concentration susceptible to oxidation begins to decrease considerably.

At elevated temperatures, oxygen solubility decreases drastically although all the oxidation reactions are accelerated. The chemistry of oxidation at these temperatures is more complex, since the thermal and oxidative reactions occur simultaneously. As the oxygen pressure is reduced, the initiation reaction becomes more important because the concentration of alkyl radicals relative to peroxyl radicals increases, forming polymeric compounds through reactions that involve mainly the alkyl and alkoxy radicals. Under these conditions, the formation of new compounds is very rapid. Hydroperoxides practically disappear above 150 °C, indicating that the decomposition rate is greater than the rate of formation resulting in the synthesis of polymeric compounds in the early stages of heat treatment. Light is the third factor that exerts a major influence on the oxidative process. Minor compounds can be electronically excited due to absorption of light. After excitation, the molecule is capable of transferring their excess energy to a molecule of oxygen enabling it attain singlet spin multiplicity, which then reacts with the olefinic double bonds. However, as the temperature increases, the influence of light in the oxidation decreases, reaching a negligible effect at elevated temperatures.

Determination of Linoleic Acid Content in Different Nuts

The development of advanced analytical techniques (such as gas chromatography (GC), high performance liquid chromatography (HPLC), mass spectrometry (MS), nuclear magnetic resonance (NMR), capillary electrophoresis (CE), HPLC-NMR, HPLC-MS, GC-MS and CE-

MS) are an important and indispensable tools in food research; since the characterization, quantification and identification of macronutrients (lipids, proteins, carbohydrates and water fractions) and micronutrients such as vitamins, minerals, phenolic compounds, etc, present in nuts must be studied [27]. These techniques are used for quality control of natural products for human consumption, confirming their composition and ensuring the safety of the final product. However, the choice of an analytical technique depends on the physicochemical properties of the matrix and/or the target compound to be analyzed. For example, the preparation procedure, separation mechanism and technique and the type of detector to be employed depend on the polarity, size or volatility of the target compound.

Regarding the fatty acid profile determination, fatty acids present in nuts may be found in free form but generally they are combined forming complex molecules through amide or ester bonds. The free fatty acid concentration and fatty acid enrichment are measured with common procedures involving multiple steps, based on extraction from the nut and analysis [28]. Over the years, a broad range of extraction techniques have been performed. Folch et al. in 1957 developed one of the first simple methods for the isolation and purification of total lipids from animal tissues based on two steps. This method was based on mixing the sample with organic solvents such as chroloform/methanol in cells or tissue homogenates [29]. Nowadays, traditional or modified Folch procedure, or the commonly called Bligh and Dyer method [30], in which a chloroform/ methanol/water mixture is used to separate the lipids from all the non-lipids in samples containing 80% water, are generally employed in laboratories to quantitatively extract lipids. Total lipids of runner peanuts were extracted according to the classical Bligh-Dyer method with slight modifications with the aim of determining the fatty acid composition [31]. Due to increased interest in the new methods for the cultivation of new pistachio varieties, Tsantili et al. developed a technique based on some physical and compositional differences in nuts among varieties of different origin. The analysis of fatty acid profile was carried out with a lipid extraction by homogenizing of the samples with 20 mL chloroform/methanol in accordance with the Folch method [32].

However, these extraction techniques are time and resource consuming, potentially causing sample loss and contamination, and generating organic wastes. Therefore, these problems become more apparent when the number of samples to be extracted and analyzed is large and/or the specimen size is small. For this reason, the processes of extraction in nut samples have led to the search for transformation models that increase yields, preserve quality, reduce costs, and improve productivity. Among the extraction processes, the most commonly used one for several oleaginous seeds in industrial scale is cold or hot extraction using hydraulic or mechanic press with prior heating of the nuts [33]. Regarding laboratory scale, more tedious processes have been employed, such as solid–liquid extraction using petroleum ether, hexane, ethanol, methanol, and chloroform amongst other reagents isolated or combined, and also extraction using supercritical carbon dioxide (CO_2). Santos et al. carried out a chemical evaluation and thermal behavior study of Brazil nut oils obtained by different extraction processes using Soxhlet, hydraulic pressing, and supercritical carbon dioxide methods. The identification and quantification of the linoleic acid in oils obtained through the different extraction techniques showed values between 37.53 g/ 100 g oil for the extractions carried out by hydraulic pressing and 45.17 g /100 g oil using Soxhlet with hexane as solvent. Therefore, the results confirmed that with the solid-liquid extraction, the highest composition values for the Brazil nut oil were achieved [32]. The Soxhlet extraction technique was developed for the fat determination in milk [34]. This extraction technique is considered one of the most relevant techniques for isolating species and it has been the standard and reference method for solid-liquid extraction in many fields. Regarding the research studies on tree nuts, important commercially edible nuts as almonds, cashews, Brazil nuts, hazelnuts, macadamias, pecans, pine nuts, pistachios and walnuts have been characterized employing Soxhlet as extraction method [35, 36].

In recent years, many studies have been developed to improve Soxhlet extraction, because of some disadvantages such as long operation time (several hours), large solvent volumes, evaporation and concentration steps needed at the end of the extraction process, and inadequacy for thermolabile analytes [37]. For these reasons, improved methods based on Soxhlet extraction have been performed such as microwave-assisted Soxhlet extraction (MASE) [38]. This technique is based on the same principles as conventional Soxhlet extraction but uses microwaves as auxiliary energy to accelerate the process. This system has been used for the study of the oil content and the fatty acid composition of olive seeds, sunflower seeds, peanuts, croissants and beef steaks [39].

More recently, other alternatives to improve the extraction process have been proposed; such as supercritical fluid extraction (SFE), microwave-assisted extraction (MAE), pressurized fluid extraction (PFE), ultrasound-assisted extraction, etc. Supercritical fluid extraction is an alternative to conventional extraction methods due to several advantages over conventional techniques, among which are enhancing the use of low temperatures, efficiency in solvent use, prevention of oxidation reactions and the maintenance of the high product quality due to the absence of solvent in solute phase [40]. In theory, each compound possesses a unique extractability under different conditions of supercritical fluid related to factors such as extraction temperature, pressure, and analysis time. Thus, components in a sample are extracted in an ordered manner from a sample matrix under optimized conditions of SFE, allowing for convenient fractionation of the extract [41]. Supercritical fluid extraction using carbon dioxide as solvent was successfully used for fast and effective extraction of a wide variety of dyes and food compounds, due to carbon dioxide being not only cheap and readily available at high purity, but also safe to handle and environmentally friendly. It is easily removed by simple expansion to common environmental pressure values. Other supercritical fluids, such as ethane and propane, have also been evaluated as potential extraction solvents for fats and oils samples due to the higher solubility of lipids. However, the major drawback of these fluids is their flammability [42]. Consequently, SFE using carbon dioxide is approved for food processing without declaration [43]and it was successfully used for oil extraction from seeds like almond [44], pistachio [45], walnut [46], hazelnut [47] and Macadamia nut [48].

On the other hand, PFE is one of the so-called green technologies and it operates at high pressures and temperatures above the boiling point of the organic solvent. The use of higher temperatures increases the ability of solvent to solubilize the analytes and decreases the viscosity of liquid solvents allowing a better penetration of the solvent into the matrix. The use of a higher pressure facilitates the extraction of the analytes from samples by improving the solvent accessibility to the analytes that is trapped in the matrix pores [49].

The ultrasound assisted method as an alternative to improve the oil extraction of food samples has been recognized for application in the edible oil industry because of its capacity for improving the extraction efficiency and shortening the time required for this step since the implosion of bubbles formed during ultrasound application produces a highly efficient temperature and pressure due to the rapid adiabatic compression of gases and vapors within the bubbles or cavities [50]. This increase of temperature favors the solubility of the analytes and facilitates their diffusion from the sample matrix to the solvent. In addition, the increase of pressure facilitates the penetration of the solvent into the sample matrix and the transfer from the matrix to the liquid phase [51]. For these reasons, the methods based on ultrasound have been applied for extracting oil from different matrices. Qing-An Zhang et al. optimized the ultrasound assisted extraction parameters such as extraction time, extraction temperature, and solvent/sample ratio to obtain high extraction efficiency for different almond cultivars. The fatty acid composition analyzed by GC-MS was compared with the results obtained with Soxhlet extraction. The different procedures demonstrated that the amount of linoleic acid was the same when using both methods [52].

Once the extraction of the oil fraction is optimized, the determination of the fatty acid profile of a wide variety of biological samples is carried out by different analytical techniques, particularly by GC, which is considered a routine technique [53]. However, by employing the GC technique, separating carboxylated compounds becomes complicated due to their relatively high polarity. For this reason and with the purpose to analyze free fatty acids present in the sample, it is necessary to form non-polar derivatives with the aid of a derivatization method transforming the free fatty acids to fatty acid methyl esters (FAMEs); that are also more volatile compounds than the free fatty acid components [54]. The chromatographic determination of FAMEs and the separation into individual compounds is less frequently by high performance liquid chromatography (HPLC) [55]. Nowadays, there are many derivatization methods to obtain FAMEs that are adequate techniques. Initially, the Association of Official Analytical Chemists [56] and American Oil Chemists Society [55]. recommended the use of sulphuric acid–methanol reagent for preparing FAMEs. However, both organizations later accepted the use of the boron trifluoride (BF_3)–methanol reagent. Other methods for methylation of fatty acids that led to good results involve the use of hydrochloric acid–methanol, and diazomethane solutions, whereas the methods that employ silylating agents are less used [57]. Under acidic conditions, the most common derivatives of fatty acids are the methyl esters obtained by heating the oil extracted with excess of anhydrous methanol and BF_3 as catalyst. The use of this catalyst has found wide application as a good direct transesterification reagent (methylating the fatty acids directly from the acylglycerol parent lipid), and esterification reagent (converting free fatty acids to their methyl ester derivatives). The Official method UNE-EN ISO 5509-2000 suggests the BF_3 as catalyst in the preparation of FAMEs [58]. Other alternatives have been described using hydrochloric acid in methanol or sulphuric acid in methanol solutions. These methods are described as acid-catalysed methanolysis or transesterification techniques, and through their application it is possible to convert both acylglycerols and free fatty acids into methyl esters. However, these methods present the same disadvantages as other acid-catalysts in changing the isomeric distribution of conjugated fatty acids [59].

The derivatization carried out under the presence of basic catalysts has the aim to convert the fatty acids in esters. The reagents potassium hydroxide, sodium hydroxide and sodium methoxide are the most common catalysts used. Basic catalysis is faster than acid catalysis; however, alkali catalyst reactions require strict anhydrous conditions [56]. Another possibility is to combine potassium hydroxide and BF_3, both in methanol. Although the basic catalysis is faster than acid catalysis, the former will transform free fatty acids into their carboxylic salt and prevent their determination by GC analysis. A second acid catalysis avoids this problem but increases sample preparation time. In this sense, Milinsk et al. have studied different transesterification methods, which have been known for over 15 years and are currently used worldwide. The results showed that among all testing methods, those which used a basic catalysis for transesterification of unsaturated fatty acids were more effective [60].

Regarding the determination of fatty acids profile in nut samples, Gecgel et al. determined the free fatty acids content from hazelnuts, walnuts, almonds, and pistachio nuts using gas chromatography with flame ionization detector (FID) [61]. Fatty acids were identified by comparison of their retention times (Rt) with those of standards. In addition, Robbins et al. designed a study to quantify the healthful lipid constituents of 10 different types of commercially important tree nuts (almonds, black walnuts, Brazil nuts, cashews, English walnuts, hazelnuts, macadamias, pecans, pine nuts, and pistachios). The analysis of fatty acids was carried out by GC, the column employed was a (50%-cyanopropyl)-methylpolysiloxane J&W fused silica DB-23 capillary column and the detection of the compounds was performed by using a FID. The results indicated that higher amounts of linoleic acid were obtained in samples of Black walnuts followed by English walnuts and pine nuts [62]. The analysis by GC has also been used in a study based on compositional differences in pistachio among cultivars of different origin. Maskan et al. found that pistachio has high levels of linoleic acids, but the fatty acid contents were significantly affected by cultivar, with the exception of gondoic acid [63]. These studies are important because linoleic and linolenic acids present in nuts are essential for the human diet, provided their oxidation is prevented, whereas the high amount of oleic acid contributes to its oxidation stability. Although FID is the most widely used detection system in standard analytical methods, the employment of mass spectrometry (MS) as system of detection provides higher amounts of data and a better molecular mass structural information facilitating the identification of these compounds. Miraliakbari et al. used the GC-MS to confirm the identity of each FAME peak [64].

Although the HPLC technique is comparable with GC one regarding the rate of the analyses, its efficiency and resolution make it a more versatile determination method. This technique is not limited to volatile and thermally stable samples. The choice of the stationary phase will determine the selectivity of the process and the mode of operation, such as adsorption chromatography, partition, ion exchange or size gel filtration. The composition of fatty acids can be determined in extracted oils from nuts using reverse phase by using HPLC. In addition, triacylglycerides can be separated according to the number of carbon atoms and the instaurations. Another option is a combination of high resolution liquid chromatography with silver ion (SI-HPLC) [65]. This procedure has been used to describe and identify the source of oils and to detect certain adulterations [66].

An alternative technique which avoids problems present in GC determinations such as time-constraints, expensive cost and potential hazards to human health and environment because of the use of organic solvents, is infrared spectroscopy (IR). This technique has demonstrated to be fast, non-destructive, and a relatively inexpensive technology and regarded as an ideal method for fatty acid determination in different samples [67]. The infrared spectra obtained contain information about the degree of instauration, the total instauration, the number of carbons and the unsaturated fraction composition. Wu et al. studied the simultaneous evaluation of essential fatty acids in edible oils, such as α-linolenic and linoleic acids, by means of a fast and clean methodology based on near infrared spectroscopy (NIR) combined with chemometric analysis [68].

Finally, the analysis of fatty acids in nut samples can be carried out by using NMR equipments. This technique is based in a physical phenomenon in which a magnetic nuclei enclosed in a magnetic field absorb and re-emit electromagnetic radiation. The active nuclei most commonly used in NMR are H^1, C^{13}, P^{31} and F^{19}, all of them presenting the spin equal to ½. The NMR has been recognized as a viable technique for analyzing the fatty acid composition in oils, adulterations or instauration grade studies due to it is a simple and fast method, despite its low sensitivity [69].

Conclusion

Tree nuts are a rich source of unsaturated fatty acids, proteins and vitamins; compounds that may slow the ageing process, stimulate the immune system and protect against heart disease. In this regard, including nuts in a healthy dietary pattern will extend the cardioprotective effects beyond those attributable to the components of any diet excluding them.

Nuts undergo autoxidation and photosensitized oxidation reactions during processing and storage, producing off-flavor compounds and decreasing their quality. The antioxidant compounds found in nuts are good radical scavengers, conferring the ability to inhibit LA oxidation. A variety of sample preparation methods (extraction and derivatization) are available, and new methodologies for fatty acid profiles determination in samples of different nuts have been developed. Presently, the most commonly employed method for the oil extraction is the improved shoxlet technique. GC is the most common technique employed for the quantification of these compounds.

References

[1] Ros E. Health benefits of nut consumption. *Nutrients*, 2010, 2(7), 652-682.

[2] *http://faostat.fao.org/* Last accessed: February 2012.

[3] Zajdenwerg C, Branco G, Alamed, J, Decker E, Castro I. Correlation between sensory and chemical markers in the evaluation of Brazil nut oxidative shelf-life. *European Food Research and Technology*, 2011, 233(1), 109-116.

[4] Borges J, Veloso M. Chemical composition of nuts and edible seeds and their relation to nutrition and health. *Revista de Nutriciao*, 2010, 23 (2), 269-279.

[5] USDA National Nutrient Database for Standard Reference, Release 24 (2011). U. S. Department of Agriculture, Agricultural Research Service. *http://www.nal.usda.gov/fnic/foodcomp/search/*. Last accessed: February 2012.

[6] Robbins KS, Shi, EC, Shewfelt RL, Eitenmiller RR, Pegg R B. Update on the Healthful Lipid Constituents of Commercially Important Tree Nuts. *Journal of Agricultural and Food Chemistry,* 2011, 59(22), 12083-12092.

[7] Bolling BW, Oliver Chen CY, McKay DL, Blumberg JB. Tree nut phytochemicals: composition, antioxidant capacity, bioactivity, impact factors. A systematic review of almonds, Brazils, cashews, hazelnuts, macadamias, pecans, pine nuts, pistachios and walnuts. *Nutrition Research Reviews*, 2011, 24, 244–275.

[8] Verheugt FWA. Anticoagulant management in the cardiovascular setting. *Fundamental & Clinical Pharmacology*, 2012, 26(1), 11-15.

[9] Prousky J, Millman CG, Kirkland JB. Pharmacologic use of Niacin. *Journal of Evidence-Based Complementary and Alternative Medicine,* 2011, 16(1), 91-101.

[10] Kendall CW, Esfahani A, Truan J, Srichaikul K, Jenkins DJ. Health benefits of nuts in prevention and management of diabetes. *Asia Pacific journal of clinical nutrition*, 2010, 19(1), 110-116.

[11] Berryman CE, Preston AG, Karmally W, Deckelbaum RJ, Kris-Etherton PM. Effects of almond consumption on the reduction of LDL-cholesterol: a discussion of potential mechanisms and future research directions. *Nutrition Reviews,* 2011, 69(4), 171-185.

[12] Alasalvar C, Shahidi F. Natural antioxidants in tree nuts. European *Journal of Lipid Science and Technology*, 2009, 111(11), 1056-1062.

[13] López PU, Bulló M, Casas PA, Babio N, Salas JS. Nuts and oxidation: a systematic review. *Nutrition Reviews,* 2009, 67(9), 497-508.

[14] Jahanban AE, Jamei R, Jahanban RE. The importance of almond (Prunus amygdalus L.) and its by-products. *Food Chemistry*, 2010, 120(2), 349-360.

[15] Yada S, Lapsley K, Huang G. A review of composition studies of cultivated almonds: Macronutrients and micronutrients. *Journal of Food Composition and Analysis,* 2011, 24(4-5), 469-480.

[16] López C, Prats S, Berenguer V. Free radical lipid peroxidation: Mechanism and analysis. *Chem. Rev*, 2011, 5944-5972.

[17] Merrill L, Pike O, Ogden L, Dunn M. Oxidative Stability of Conventional and High-Oleic Vegetable Oils with Added Antioxidants. *Journal of the American Oil Chemists' Society*, 2008, 85, 771-776.

[18] Mexis SF, Badeka AV, Kontominas MG. Quality evaluation of raw ground almond kernels (*Prunus dulcis*): Effect of active and modified atmosphere packaging, container oxygen barrier and storage conditions. *Innovative Food Science and Emerging Technologies*, 2009, 10, 580-589.

[19] Guillén M, Goicoechea E. Formation of oxygenated α,β-unsaturated aldehydes and other toxic compounds in sunflower oil oxidation at room temperature in closed receptacles. *Food Chemistry*, 2008, 1, 157-164.

[20] Sanchez Prado L, Risticevic S, Pawliszyn J, Psillakis E. Low temperature SPME device: A convenient and effective tool for investigating photodegradation of volatile analytes. *Journal of Photochemistry and Photobiology A: Chemistry,* 2009, 206, 227-230.

[21] Choe E, Min D. Mechanisms and Factors for Edible Oil Oxidation. *Comprehensive reviews in food science and food safety*, 2006, 5, 169-186.

[22] Guillen MD, Goicoechea E. Oxidation of corn oil at room temperature: Primary and secondary oxidation products and determination of their concentration in the oil liquid matrix from ^1H nuclear magnetic resonance data. *Food Chemistry*, 2009,116, 183-192.

[23] Afaf KE. Effect of fatty acids and tocopherols on the oxidative stability of vegetable oils. *European Journal of Lipid Science and Technology*, 2006, 58, 1051-1061.

[24] Mateos R., Trujillo M., Pérez-Camino C., Moreda W., Cert A. Relationships between oxidative stability, triacylglycerol composition and antioxidant content in olive oil matrices. *Journal of Agricultural and Food Chemistry,* 2005, 53, 5766-5771.

[25] Labuza TP. Application of chemical kinetics to deterioration of foods. *Journal of Chemical Education*, 1984, 61(4), 348-358.

[26] Koreck S., Cheiner J., Howard JA., Ingold KU. Absolute rate constants for hidrocarbon autoxidation. *Canadian Journal of Chemistry*, 1972, 50, 2285-2288.

[27] Bernal J, Mendiola JA, Ibáñez E, Cifuentes A. Advanced analysis of nutraceuticals. *Journal of Pharmaceutical and Biomedical Analysis*, 2011, 55(4),758-774.

[28] Ruiz Rodriguez A, Reglero G, Ibañez E. Recent trends in the advanced analysis of bioactive fatty acids. *Journal of Pharmaceutical and Biomedical Analysis*, 2010, 51(2), 305-326.

[29] Folch J, Lees M, Stanley A. A simple method for the isolation and purification of total lipids from animal tissues. *Journal of Biology and Chemistry,* 1957, 226, 497.–509.

[30] Bligh EG, Dyer WJ. A rapid method of total lipid extraction and purification. *Canadian journal of biochemistry and physiology*, 1959, 37, 911– 917.

[31] Shin EC, Pegg RB, Phillips RD, Eitenmiller RR. Commercial Runner peanut cultivars in the USA: Fatty acid composition. *European Journal of Lipid Science and Technology,* 2010, 112(2), 195-207.

[32] Tsantili E, Takidelli C, Christopoulos MV, Lambrinea E, Rouskas D, Roussos PA. Physical, compositional and sensory differences in nuts among pistachio (Pistachia *vera L.*) varieties. *Scientia Horticulturae*, 2010, 125(4), 562-568.

[33] Santos OV, Correa NCF, Soares FASM, Gioielli LA, Costa CEF, Lannes SCS. Chemical evaluation and thermal behavior of Brazil nut oil obtained by different extraction processes. *Food Research International.* Available online 5 July 2011, In Press. 10.1016/j.foodres.2011.06.038.

[34] Virot M, Tomao V, Colnagui G, Visinoni F, Chemat F. New microwave-integrated Soxhlet extraction: An advantageous tool for the extraction of lipids from food products. *Journal of Chromatography A*, 2007, 1174(1–2), 138-144.

[35] Venkatachalam M, Sathe SK. Chemical Composition of selected edible nut seeds. *Journal of Agricultural and Food Chemistry*, 2006, 54 (13), 4705–4714.

[36] Bail S, Stuebiger G, Unterweger H, Buchbauer G, Krist S. Characterization of volatile compounds and triacylglycerol profiles of nut oils using SPME-GC-MS and MALDI-TOF-MS. *European Journal of Lipid Science and Technology*, 2009, 111(2), 170–182.

[37] Luque de Castro MD, García-Ayuso LE. Soxhlet extraction of solid materials: an outdated technique with a promising innovative future. *Analytica Chimica Acta*, 1998, 369 (1–2), 1-10.

[38] Luque-García JL,Luque de Castro MD. Focused microwave-assisted Soxhlet extraction: devices and applications. *Talanta*, 2004, 64(3), 571-577.

[39] Virot M, Tomao V, Ginies Ch, Visinoni F, Chemat F. Microwave-integrated extraction of total fats and oils. Journal of Chromatography A, 2008, 1196–1197, 57-64.

[40] Mezzomo N, Mileo BR, Friedrich MT, Martínez J, Ferreira SRS. Supercritical fluid extraction of peach (Prunus persica) almond oil: Process yield and extract composition. *Bioresource Technology*, 2010, 101(14), 5622-5632

[41] Sahena F, Zaidul ISM, Jinap S, Karim AA, Abbas KA, Norulaini NAN, Omar AKM. Application of supercritical CO_2 in lipid extraction – A review. *Journal of Food Engineering*, 2009, 95(2), 240-253.

[42] Temelli F. Perspectives on supercritical fluid processing of fats and oils. *The Journal of Supercritical Fluids*, 2009, 47(3), 583-590.

[43] Brunner G. Supercritical fluids: technology and application to food processing, *Journal of Food Engineering*, 2005, 67(1–2), 21-33.

[44] Marrone C, Poletto M, Reverchon E, Stassi A. Almond oil extraction by supercritical CO_2: experiments and modeling. *Chemical Engineering Science,* 1998, 53(21), 3711–3718

[45] Sheibani A, Ghaziaskar HS. Pressurized fluid extraction of pistachio oil using a modified supercritical fluid extractor and factorial design for optimization. LWT - *Food Science and Technology*, 2008, 41(8), 1472-1477.

[46] Martínez ML, Mattea MA, Maestri DM. Pressing and supercritical carbon dioxide extraction of walnut oil. *Journal of Food Engineering*, 2008, 88(3), 399-404.

[47] Özkal SG, Salgın U, Yener ME. Supercritical carbon dioxide extraction of hazelnut oil. *Journal of Food Engineering*, 2005, 69(2), 217-223.

[48] Silva CF, Mendes MF, Pessoa FLP, Queiroz EM. Supercritical carbon dioxide extraction of macadamia (*Macadamia integrifolia*) nut oil: experiments and modeling. *Brazilian Journal of Chemical Engineering,* 2008, 25(1), 175-181.

[49] Flores V, Saffi J, Melecchi MIS, Abad FC, Jacques RA, Martinez MM, Oliveira EC, Caramão EB. Comparison of soxhlet, ultrasound-assisted and pressurized liquid extraction of terpenes, fatty acids and Vitamin E from *Piper gaudichaudianum* Kunth. *Journal of Chromatography A*, 2005, 1105(1–2), 115-118.

[50] Luque de Castro MD, Priego Capote F. *Analytical Applications of Ultrasound.* Elsevier: Amsterdam; 2006, 393.

[51] Mijangos OF, Ruiz J, Lagunez L, Luque de Castro MD. Fast Ultrasound-assisted extraction of polar (phenols) and nonpolar (lipids) Fractions in *heterotheca inuloides* Cass. *Phytochemical Analysis*, 2011, 22(6), 484–491.

[52] Zhang QA, Zhang ZQ, Yue XF, Fan XU, Li T, Chen SF. Response surface optimization of ultrasound-assisted oil extraction from autoclaved almond powder, *Food Chemistry*, 2009, 116(2), 513-518.

[53] Janssen HG., Steenbergen H., Koning S. The role of comprehensive chromatography in the characterization of edible oils and fats. European *Journal of Lipid Science and Technology*, 2009, 111, 1171–1184.

[54] Aberoumand A. Identification of fatty acids in edible wild plants by gas chromatography. *Food Analytical Methods*, 2009, 2, 208–211.

[55] Ruiz-Rodriguez A, Reglero G, Ibañez E. Recent trends in the advanced analysis of bioactive fatty acids. *Journal of Pharmaceutical and Biomedical Analysis*, 2010, 51(2), 305-326.

[56] *www.aoac.org. Last access March 2012*

[57] Méndez E, Marrero D, González V. Evaluation of five methods for derivatization and GC determination of a mixture of very long chain fatty acids ($C_{24:0}$–$C_{36:0}$). *Journal of Pharmaceutical and Biomedical Analysis,* 2008, 46(1), 194-199.

[58] *Animal and vegetable fats and oils - Preparation of methyl esters of fatty acids.* (ISO 5509:2000)

[59] Aldai N, Murray BE, Nájera AI, Troy DJ, Osoro K. Derivatization of fatty acids and its application for conjugated linoleic acid studies in ruminant meat lipids. *Journal of the Science of Food and Agriculture*, 2005, 85(7), 1073-1083.

[60] Milinsk MC; Matsushita M, Visentainer JV, de Oliveira C,de Souza N. Comparative analysis of eight esterification methods in the quantitative determination of vegetable oil fatty acid methyl esters (FAME). *Journal of the Brazilian Chemical Society*, 2008, 19(8), 1475-1483.

[61] Gecgel U, Gumus T, Tasan M, Daglioglu O, Arici M. Determination of fatty acid composition of γ-irradiated hazelnuts, walnuts, almonds, and pistachios. *Radiation Physics and Chemistry*, 2011, 80(4), 578-581.

[62] Robbins KS, Shin ECh, Shewfelt RL, Eitenmiller RR, Pegg RP. Update on the Healthful Lipid Constituents of Commercially Important Tree Nuts. Journal of Agricultural and Food Chemistry, 2011, 59 (22), 12083–12092.

[63] Maskan M, Karataş S. Storage stability of whole-split pistachio nuts (*Pistachia vera L.*) at various conditions. *Food Chemistry,* 1999, 66(2), 227-233.

[64] Miraliakbari H, Shahidi F. Lipid class compositions, tocopherols and sterols of tree nut oils extracted with different solvents. *Journal of Food Lipids,* 2008, 15(1), 81-96.

[65] Neff WE, Adlof RO, List GR, El-Agaimy M. Analyses of Vegetable Oil Triacylglycerols by Silver Ion High Performance Liquid Chromatography with Flame Ionization Detection. *Journal of Liquid Chromatography*, 1994, 17(18), 3951-3968.

[66] Macher MB, Holmqvist A. Triacylglycerol analysis of partially hydrogenated vegetable oils by silver ion HPLC. *Journal of Separation Scienc*e, 2001, 24(3), 179-185.

[67] Zhou LJ, Wu H, Li JT, Wang ZY, Zhang LY. Determination of fatty acids in broiler breast meat by near-infrared reflectance spectroscopy. *Meat Science*, 2012, 90(3), 658-664.

[68] Wu D, Chen X, Shi P, Wang S, Feng F, He Y. Determination of α-linolenic acid and linoleic acid in edible oils using near-infrared spectroscopy improved by wavelet transform and uninformative variable elimination. *Analytica Chimica Acta*, 2009, 634(2), 166-171.

[69] Agiomyrgianaki A, Petrakis PV, Dais P. Detection of refined olive oil adulteration with refined hazelnut oil by employing NMR spectroscopy and multivariate statistical analysis. *Talanta*, 2010, 80(5), 2165–2171.

In: Linoleic Acids
Editor: Igho Onakpoya

ISBN: 978-1-62257-384-4
© 2012 Nova Science Publishers, Inc.

Chapter III

Oxidation of Linoleic Acid in Bulk, Micelle, Emulsion, and Microcapsule Systems

***Yoshiyuki Watanabe*[1], *Yasumasa Minemoto*[2] *and Shuji Adachi*[3]**

[1]Department of Biotechnology and Chemistry, Faculty of Engineering, Kinki University, Takaya, Higashi-Hiroshima, Japan

[2]Department of Applied Chemistry and Chemical Engineering, Toyama National College of Technology, Toyama, Japan

[3]Division of Food Science and Biotechnology, Graduate School of Agriculture, Kyoto University, Sakyo-ku, Kyoto, Japan

Abstract

Lipid oxidation is recognized to be very important from the viewpoint of its involvement in food spoilage and the relevance of lipid peroxidation *in vivo* to membrane damage, aging, heart disease and cancer. Linoleic acid and its acylglycerols are major constituents of lipids in foods. The oxidation kinetics for n-3 and n-6 polyunsaturated fatty acids (PUFAs) and their esters were investigated. Changes in the amounts of unreacted PUFA during the entire period could be expressed by the rate equation of the autocatalytic type. For n-3 PUFA, oxidation had to be separated into two parts. The respective oxidation processes of linoleoyl or oleoyl residue esterified with a variety of hydrophobic substances were measured at 80°C. The relationship between the molecular weight of the hydrophobic substance and the rate of oxidation of aliphatic residue was investigated. It was observed that as the molecular weight of the hydrophobic substance becomes lager, the rate constant for the oxidation tends to become smaller. However, for molecular weights exceeding 150, the values of the rate constants were found to be similar. The rate constant for the oxidation processes of linoleic acid mixed with a saturated fatty acid or its methyl ester was proportional to the molar fraction of the linoleic acid. The oxidation of methyl linoleate with an unsaturated fatty acid was promoted by the fatty acid. The antioxidative abilities of various antioxidants, such as acyl ascorbates, and alkyl ferulate, on the oxidation of linoleic acid were also kinetically analyzed. L-Ascorbic acid and PUFA were condensed by the immobilized lipase in acetone to produce the unsaturated acyl ascorbates. The PUFA moieties of the products were much more resistant to oxidation than the corresponding unmodified PUFAs. The oxidation of linoleic acid was effectively suppressed by the addition of the unmodified ascorbic acid or linoleoyl ascorbate. The oxidation processes of enzymatically synthesized 6-*O*-monolinoleoyl trehalose in water at various concentrations were measured based on both the decrease in the linoleoyl residue and oxygen consumption. It was suggested that the migration of oxygen into the hydrophobic core through the hydrophilic layer of the linoleoyl trehalose micelles affected the overall oxidation rate of linoleoyl residue. Oxidation of methyl linoleate in oil-in-water emulsions having droplets of median diameters ranging from 17 nm to 8.0 mm was carried out. The stoichiometry between methyl linoleate and oxygen was observed to be independent of both the size of oil droplet and the type of the surfactant, and was found to be unity during the early stage of the oxidation. Linoleic acid was encapsulated with various wall materials, such as gum arabic and maltodextrin, by drying the emulsion and its oxidation process was evaluated. Encapsulated linoleic acid of small droplet size oxidized more slowly than that of large droplet size.

1. Oxidation Kinetics of Fatty Acids

Lipid oxidation causes deterioration in food quality. The oxidation is a complicated process involving three steps: initiation, propagation and termination; its kinetics for each step has been studied [1-3]. If a simple equation that is a function of the amount of unoxidized substrate is available to describe the entire oxidation process of lipids, it would be possible to predict this process and the resultant deterioration of the lipid. Özilgen and Özilgen [4] reported that a kinetic expression of autocatalytic type in terms of the fraction of unoxidized substrate can describe the entire oxidation process of some lipids. The authors showed that the expression was successfully applicable to the entire oxidation process of n-6 fatty acids and their esters, and estimated the kinetic parameters. The expression was also usable for the first half of the oxidation process of n-3 fatty acids and their esters, but the latter half could not be described by the expression, though first-order kinetics could empirically be used to describe the oxidation [5]. Most fatty acids exist in the form of acylglycerol in food; therefore, the oxidation kinetics for acylglycerols is important in determining the deterioration of food quality. In order to examine whether or not the kinetic equations adopted for the oxidation of n-6 and n-3 fatty acids and their ethyl (or methyl) esters could be applicable to oxidation of acylglycerols, the oxidation processes of mono- and triacylglycerols of linoleic acid (n-6) and α-linolenic acid (n-3) at various temperatures were measured [6]. An acylglycerol was dissolved in hexane. That solution was placed in a flat-bottomed glass cup, and hexane was evaporated by allowing the cup to stand in the ambient temperature. The cups were placed in a desiccator in which a beaker filled with a saturated sodium chloride was placed to regulate relative humidity at about 75%. The desiccator was stored in the dark in a temperature-controlled chamber. At appropriate intervals, a cup was taken out, and the amount of unoxidized substrate was analyzed by gas chromatography. The amount of unoxidized substrate was analyzed according to the method of Craig and Murty [7].

Figures 1(a) and 2(a) show the oxidation processes of mono- and trilinolein and mono- and trilinolenin, respectively, at different temperatures. The weight loss of ethyl docosahexaenoate at 80°C under a nitrogen atmosphere by thermogravimetry was measured, and it showed that the loss was 1 to 2% for 180 h [8]. Therefore, disappearance of any substrate during measurements at high temperature such as 80°C would be insignificant. Each substrate oxidized faster at the higher storage temperature. Monolinolenin with three unsaturated bonds was much more rapidly oxidized than monolinolein with two unsaturated bonds at the same temperature. The similar tendency was observed between trilinolenin and trilinolein. Trilinolein was more slowly oxidized than monolinolein at the same temperature. Authors proposed the following kinetic equation to describe the entire autoxidation process of n-6 polyunsaturated fatty acids and their esters [5]:

$$\frac{dY}{dt} = -kY(1-Y) \tag{1}$$

where Y is the fraction of the unoxidized substrate, t is the time, and k is the rate constant. The equation was also applicable to the first-half of the oxidation process for n-3 polyunsaturated fatty acids and their esters. Under the conditions of $Y = Y_0$ at $t = 0$ integration of Eq. (1) gives:

$$\ln\frac{1-Y}{Y} = kt + \ln\frac{1-Y_0}{Y_0} \tag{2}$$

where Y_0 is a parameter, which was introduced for convenience to solve Eq. (1) and reflected the initial state of the substrate. The applicability of the kinetic expression of autocatalytic type (Eq. (1)) to the oxidation processes of each substrate at different temperatures was examined by plotting $\ln[(1-Y)/Y]$ versus t. As shown in Fig. 1(b), all the entire oxidation processes of monolinolein at various temperatures could be satisfactorily described by the expression. This was also true for the oxidation processes of trilinolein. The rate constant k and the parameter Y_0 were estimated from the slope and the intercept, respectively, of each line. The solid curves in Fig. 1(a) were drawn using the parameters estimated. Figure 2(b) shows the plots for monolinolenin. As shown by the solid lines, the first half of oxidation obeyed the expression of the autocatalytic type at any temperature; however, the latter half of oxidation deviated from the expression as shown by the broken line. The latter half ($Y < 0.5$) of the oxidation process of n-3 fatty acids and their esters was empirically expressed by the first-order kinetics [5]. The point at which the experimental points began to deviate from the line of Eq. (2) was not exactly 0.5 and was dependent on the temperature for autoxidation of monolinolenin and trilinolenin. Therefore, authors regarded the point, Y_c, as a parameter, and the first-order kinetics was adopted in the region of $Y < Y_c$.

$$\frac{dY}{dt} = -k_2 Y \tag{3}$$

Integration of Eq. (3) under the condition of $Y = Y_c$ at $t = t_c$ gives

$$\ln\frac{Y}{Y_C} = -k_2(t - t_C) \tag{4}$$

where t_c was calculated from Eq. (2) as follows:

$$t_C = \frac{1}{k}\ln\left[\frac{1-Y_C}{Y_C}\cdot\frac{Y_0}{1-Y}\right] \tag{5}$$

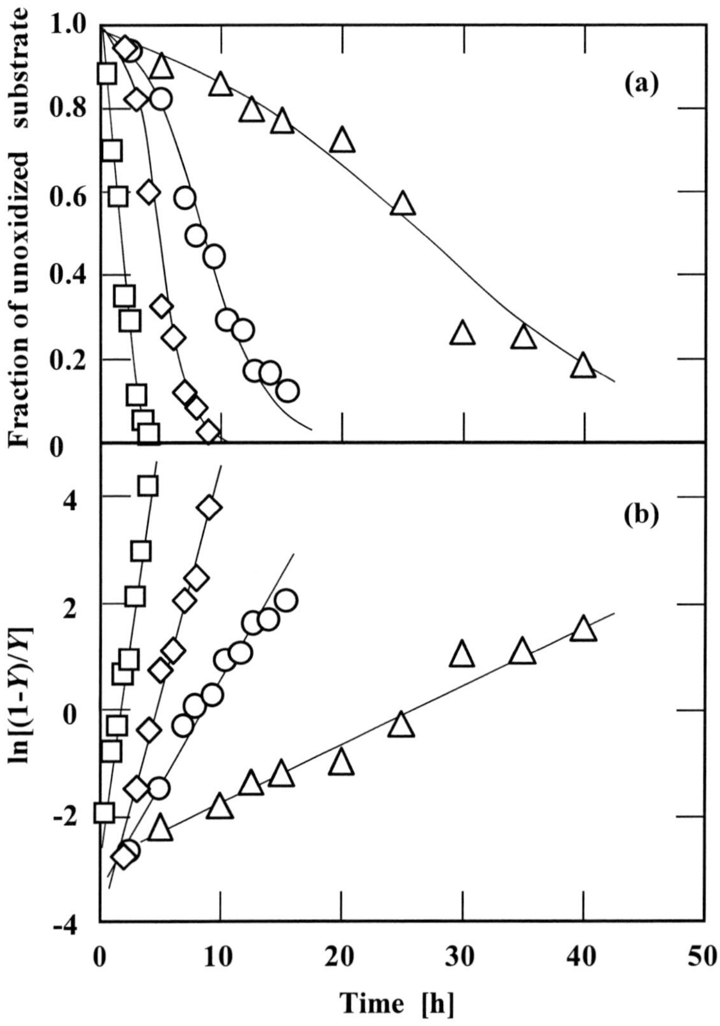

Figure 1. (a) Oxidation processes of monolinolein at 37°C (△), 50°C (○), 65°C (◇) and 80°C (□) and (b) applicability of Eq. (2) to the processes. The relative humidity was controlled at about 75%. The solid curves were calculated using the estimated values of k and Y_0 for the entire oxidation process.

The parameters were evaluated as follows: first the plots of ln[(1-Y)/Y] versus t were made, and an approximate Y_c value was empirically estimated. Near the Y_c value, some different Y_c values were assumed. For the experimental points of $Y > Y_c$, Eq. (2) was applied to estimate the k and Y_0 values. The t_c corresponding to Y_c was calculated from Eq. (5). Then, Eq. (4) was adopted for the experimental points of $Y < Y_c$ to estimate the k_2 value. The residual sum of squares for the entire autoxidation process was then calculated between the experimental points and the curves calculated using the parameters estimated above. The optimal Y_c value was determined to minimize the residual sum of squares, and the k, Y_0 and k_2 values were obtained for the Y_c value. The Y_c value below which Eq. (1) was not applicable was empirically fixed at 0.5 [5]. It seemed, however, that the Y_c value was not a constant and depended on the storage temperature; therefore, this value was regarded as a parameter. The most adequate Y_c value for each autoxidation was calculated, then the k and Y_0 values were determined for the points of $Y > Y_c$. For the points of $Y < Y_c$, the first-order kinetics was adopted to estimate the rate constant k_2. The oxidation processes of trilinolenin were also divided into the two regions, and the Y_c value depended on the temperature. The solid curves in Fig. 2 were calculated by substituting the k, Y_0, Y_c and k_2 values estimated to Eqs. (2) and (4). The broken curves in Fig. 2(a) indicate oxidation processes calculated by applying Eq. (2) to the latter half of each autoxidation. For both mono- and trilinolenin, the Y_c values were smaller at the higher storage temperatures.

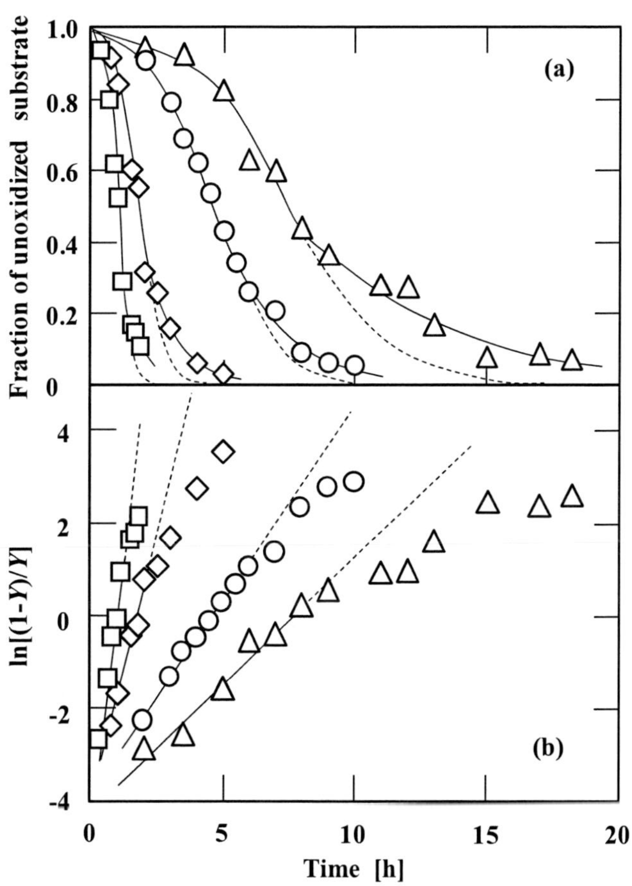

Figure 2. (a) Oxidation processes of monolinolenin at 37°C (△), 50°C (○), 65°C (◇) and 80°C (□) and (b) applicability of Eq. (2) to the processes. The relative humidity was controlled at about 75%. The solid curves were calculated using the estimated values of k and Y_0 for the entire oxidation process.

Figure 3 shows the Arrhenius plots for the k values of mono- and trilinolein and for the k and k_2 values of mono- and trilinolenin. The plots gave a straight line for each parameter of a substrate according to the Arrhenius equation:

$$k = k_0 \exp\left(-\frac{E}{RT}\right) \tag{6}$$

where k_0 is the frequency or pre-exponential factor, E is the activation energy, R is the gas constant, and T is the absolute temperature. The E and k_0 values were estimated from the slope and the intercept, respectively, of the line. The E values for the substrates tested here were almost equivalent to or a little less than those for fatty acids and their ethyl (or methyl) esters [5]. Although the oxidation of fatty acid or its ester is a complicated process, oxidation of a substrate proceeds through addition of oxygen to unsaturated bond to produce hydroperoxide. This step is common to autoxidation of all lipids [3]. Therefore, it would be expected that the enthalpy-entropy compensation holds in oxidation of fatty acids and their esters. The following equation is one of the expressions describing the compensation [9, 10]:

$$E = RT_\beta \ln k_0 + \gamma \tag{7}$$

where T_β is a parameter called isokinetic temperature and γ is a constant. The plots of the E values against the natural logarithms of the frequency factors $\ln k_0$ for the k and k_2 of the tested substrates and of fatty acids and their esters [5] lay almost on a straight line, and the isokinetic temperature T_β was evaluated to be 357K. This indicated that the oxidation process of each substrate, at least for the substrate disappearance experimentally observed here, proceeded essentially by the same mechanism without distinction of the type of fatty acid (n-3 or n-6).

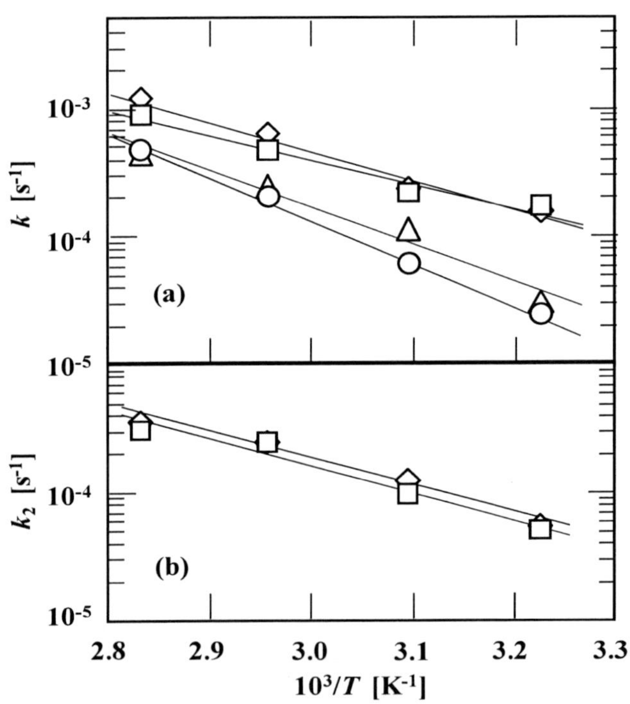

Figure 3. Estimation of the apparent activation energies and the frequency factors for the rate constants (a) k and (b) k_2 of mono- (△) and trilinolein (○) and mono- (◇) and trilinolenin (□).

2. Oxidation of Linoleoyl or Oleoyl Residue of its Esters with Hydrophobic Substance

Polyunsaturated fatty acids (PUFA), for example linoleic acid, have physiologic functions, and are essential to the human body [11]. But, they are easily oxidized in the air. The oxidants produced during its oxidation not only impair the flavor of foods, but can also cause diseases. Therefore, understanding the oxidation behavior of PUFA is important. Although many studies have reported the oxidation for PUFA, they examined fatty acid, methyl ester, or acylglecerols as PUFA sample in their research [5, 6, 12]. However, naturally-occurring fatty acids are combined with other material, such as saccharide, protein, etc. In human body, fatty acids form lipoproteins with protein, phospholipids with phosphoric acid and glycolipids with polysaccharide. The relationship between the oxidation rate of fatty acids and the binding materials has not been clearly researched enough.

We examined the effect of the molecular weight of hydrophobic substances esterified with linoleoyl residue on the oxidation of linoleoyl residue. Phenol, 2-naphtol, 1-undecanol, stearyl alcohol, and cholestanol were respectively used as hydrophobic substance to synthesize linoleoyl compounds with linoleic acid. Linoleic acid, methyl linoleate, ethyl linoleate and isopropyl linoleate, which are available in the market, were also used as the experimental samples. The relationships between the oxidation rate of linoleoyl residue and the binding hydrophobic substance were investigated experimentally by measuring the oxidation process of the linoleoyl residue of the sample.

Linoleid acid (Li), methyl linoleate (Li-Me), ethyl linoleate (Li-Et) and isopropyl linoleate (Li-Isop) were purchased. Phenol, 2-naphtol, 1-undecanol and stearyl alcohol were used in the synthesis of phenyl linoleate (Li-Ph), undecyl linoleate (Li-Un) and stearyl linoleate (Li-St), respectively. Cholestanol was purchased for the synthesis of cholestanol linoleate (Li-Cholesta). Oxalyl chloride and linoleic acid were mixed in a flask, and the reaction was carried out at 80°C using oil bath. After 1 hour, residual oxalyl chloride was removed under reduced pressure, while synthesized linoleoyl chloride remained in the flask. The binding substance (Phenol, 2-naphtol, 1-undecanol, stearyl alcohol, or cholestanol), pyridine and toluene were added to the flask constituents. They were reacted for 24 hours. After the reaction, they were dissolved in 100 mL of ethyl acetate. The mixture was washed with distilled water, 5% HCl and saturated saline solutions using a separating funnel. They were dried by magnesium sulfate, and were concentrated by the evaporator. After concentration, the target material was purified by column chromatography. A linoleoyl compound (about 30 mg) was dissolved in 1 mL of hexane. Ten microliters of that solution were placed in a flat-bottomed vial (20 mm i.d. and 50 mm height) using a microsyringe. Hexane was removed by dry air. After removal of hexane, the vial was covered with a screw-cap as soon as possible. About 20 vials were prepared for the oxidation of each compound at 80°C. The vials were placed in a desiccator, and the desiccator was stored in the dark in a temperature-controlled chamber (80°C). At regular intervals, a vial was removed to analyze the amount of unoxidized linoleoyl residue by gas chromatography. Adequate volumes of methyl palmitate, dissolved in hexane at a concentration of 30 mg/mL, were added to the flask/vial as the internal standard for GC analysis. Any unoxidized linoleoyl residue was trans-esterified to the corresponding methyl esters according to the previous method [7]. One milliliter of methanol and 0.1 mL of sodium methoixide, dissolved in methanol at a concentration of 0.5 g/L, were added to the flask/vial. The trans-esterification was continued at 80°C over 30 min and stopped by adding 0.05 mL of acetic acid to the flask/vial. Methanol was removed under reduced pressure. The remaining residue was dissolved in 1 mL of hexane and used for the GC analysis. In the case of Li-Me, Li-Et and Li-Isop, they were used for the analysis without the trans-esterification. Methyl linoleate derived from the unoxidized linoleoyl residue in Li, Li-Ph, Li-Naph, Li-Un, Li-St and Li-Cholesta, ethyl linoleate (Li-Et) and isopropyl linoleate (Li-Isop) were analyzed using a gas chromatograph equipped with a FID and a column (3.2 mm i.d. and 4.2 m length) packed with Thermon-3000 on Shincarbon A. The analytical conditions were as follows: the volume of sample injected was 5 μL, the temperatures of the injector and column were 230°C and 200°C, respectively, and the flow rate of N_2 as the carrier gas was 50 mL/min. The amount of unoxidized esters of linoleic acid and methyl palmitate were determined from the peak areas. The fraction of unoxidized linoleoyl residue of each compound was calculated from the ratio of the peak areas.

Figure 4 shows the changes with time in the fraction of the unoxidized linoleoyl residue of the samples investigated here at 80°C. Among all the samples, linoleic acid was oxidized at the fastest rate. There was a tendency that as the molecular weight of the hydrophobic substance increased, the linoleoyl residue underwent oxidation at a faster rate. As shown in Fig. 4, the oxidation of all the samples proceeded slowly during the early stage, was accelerated during the middle one, and was decelerated again during the later one. In other words, the oxidation processes of the all samples showed the reverse-sigmoidal pattern. These characteristics were similar to those for the oxidation of the polyunsaturated acyl residues [5, 6], which could be expressed by Eqs. (1) and (2). The applicability of this kinetic expression to the oxidation of the linoleoyl residue of the sample was examined by plotting $\ln((1-Y)/Y)$ versus t (Fig. 5). For any sample, the equation satisfactory expressed its oxidation, and the rate parameter, k and Y_0, were evaluated from the slope and intercept of the line. The solid curves in Fig. 4 were drawn using the evaluated k and Y_0 values. The oxidation rate constants, k values, were plotted versus the molecular weight of the hydrophobic substances esterified with linoleoyl residue in Fig. 6. As previously observed, the values tended to become smaller as the molecular weight of the hydrophobic substance became larger. However, for the molecular weights exceeding 150, the values of the rate constants were found to be similar. The oxidation process of the acyl residue can be considered to be divided into three periods: initiation, propagation and termination [13-15]. Initiation and termination showed radicalization of acyl residue and polymerization between oxidized substrate. Each period is only a part of the whole oxidation process. Propagation corresponded to the chain reaction between unoxidized and oxidized acyl residues, and is the main period of the oxidation process. Then, Eq. (1) mainly represents the propagation period. Y and $(1-Y)$ indicate the fraction of unoxidized and oxidized linoleoyl residue. The rate constant k represents the collision probability between the compound which has unoxidized linoleoyl residue and the other one which has oxidized residue since the samples in this study were all monolinoleoyl esters. As the molecular weight of the hydrophobic substance increased, the value of the rate constant decreased. This tendency indicated that the molecular movements are slowed down due to the increase in the whole molecular size. For the molecular weights exceeding 150, the values of rate constant were found to be similar. It was assumed that the movements among the linoleoyl residue esterified with substances with molecular weights over 150 were almost the same.

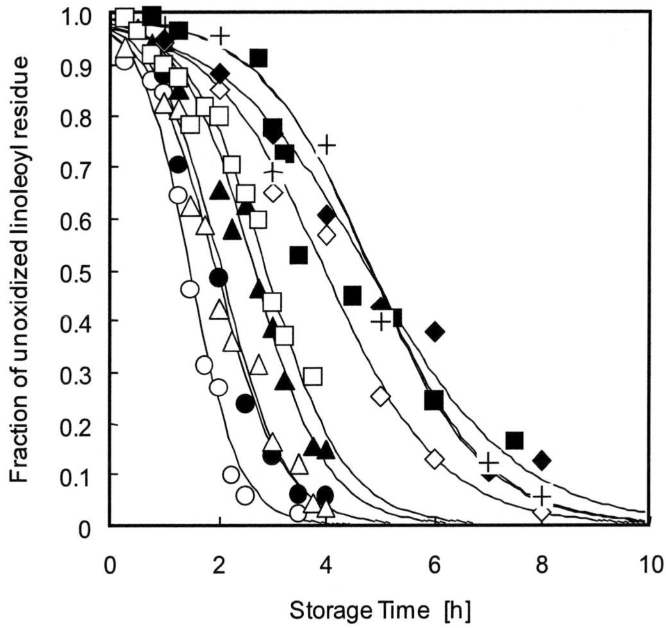

Figure 4. Oxidation processes of linoleoyl residue of different esters carried out at 80°C. The symbols and corresponding compounds are follows; (○) Li, (●) Li-Me, (△) Li-Et, (▲) Li-Isop, (□) Li-Ph, (■) Li-Naph, (◇) Li-Un, (◆) Li-St and (+) Li-Cholesta. The solid curves were calculated using the evaluated values of k and Y_0 for entire oxidation process.

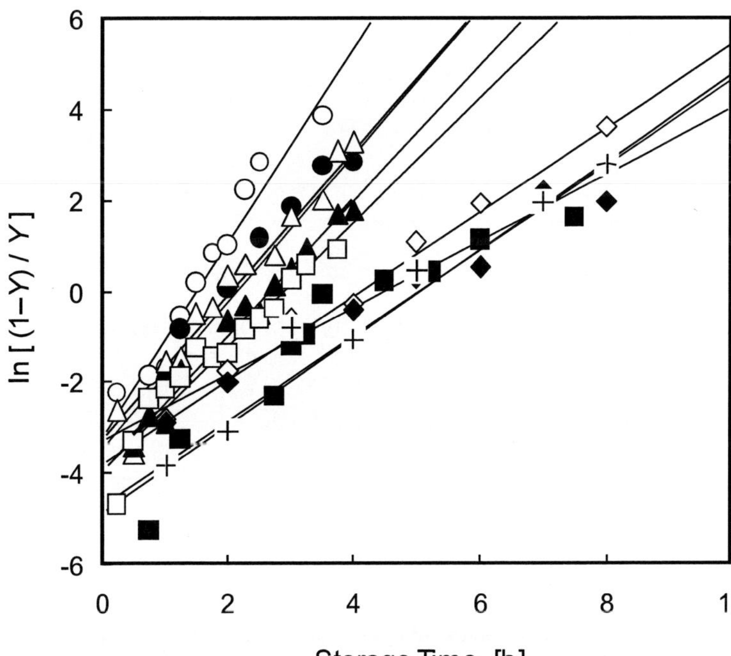

Figure 5. Applicably of the kinetic expression of the autocatalytic type to oxidation at 80°C. Symbols are the same as Fig. 4.

On the other hand, the oxidation processes of the other linoleoyl compounds, reported in a previous article, except for monolinoleoyl esters, did not follow this tendency. In the case of linoleoyl glycerols [6], the rate constant of monolinoleoyl glycerol approximately conformed with the result in this study. But the value of the constant of trilinoleoyl glycerol did not correspond with the result, and was remarkably large. This discrepancy indicated that the oxidation process of trilinoleoyl glycerol proceeded not only at intermolecular levels but also at intramolecular levels and the value of rate constant increased as a result. Moreover, the conformation of trilinoleoyl glycerol also affects the oxidation rate. The authors reported that the oxidation rate of acyl compound might be affected by intertwining among the molecules, which would depend on the molecular shapes or structures using oleoly residue [16]. The intertwining among the trilinoleoyl glycerol during the oxidation process could not affect this; hence the value of the rate constant becomes large. Therefore, the number of acyl residue and the conformation were necessary for the oxidation rate in the case of the compound having several acyl residues, and the results investigated here did not apply to the all acyl compounds.

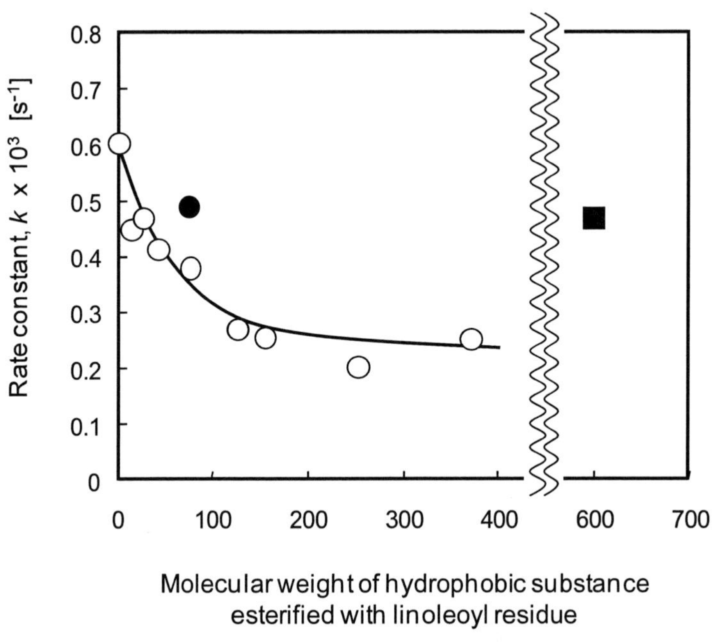

Figure 6. Relationship between the rate constant k and molecular weight of hydrophobic substance esterified with linoleoyl residue. White circle (○) represents the data acquired in this study, whereas the reference data for monolinolein and trilinolein is displayed by • and ■ respectively [12].

3. Oxidation of Linoleic Acid Coexistent with Lipids and Antioxidants

Studies on the oxidation of PUFA have usually been done using PUFA alone. However, actual food lipid is a mixture of acylglycerols consisting of a variety of saturated and unsaturated fatty acids. Therefore, authors measured the oxidation processes of linoleic acid and methyl linoleate in the presence of a saturated fatty acid or its methyl ester as a very simple model system of a lipid, and investigated the applicability of the kinetic equation to linoleic acid and methyl linoleate mixed with a saturated fatty acid or its methyl ester [17]. The dependency of the rate constant on the molar fraction of linoleic acid or methyl linoleate in the mixture was examined, and the temperature dependence of the rate constant was also investigated. The oxidation processes of linoleic acid mixed with lauric acid or methyl laurate at the weight ratios of 1:3, 1:1 and 3:1 were measured. In both cases, linoleic acid was oxidized more slowly at the lower ratios, and the oxidation process in the presence of lauric acid was similar to that in the presence of methyl laurate at any given ratio. Methyl linoleate was also oxidized more slowly at the lower ratios. However, there was a difference in the oxidation process based on the type of coexisting saturated fatty acid. That is, methyl linoleate mixed with lauric acid was oxidized faster than one mixed with methyl laurate at any ratio. The oxidation processes of linoleic acid and methyl linoleate were observed in the presence of myristic acid, methyl myristate, palmitic acid and methyl palmitate. Linoleic acid mixed with any fatty acid or its methyl ester was oxidized more slowly at the lower ratios. Methyl linoleate mixed with myristic acid or palmitic acid was oxidized faster than one mixed with methyl myristate or methyl palmitate. The applicability of Eq. (2) to these oxidation processes of linoleic acid and methyl linoleate mixed with lauric acid or methyl laurate was examined. In every case, the plots gave a straight line, and the rate constant k was evaluated. Figures 7(a) and (b) show the relationships between the molar fractions of linoleic acid and methyl linoleate, respectively, in the mixture and their rate constants. As shown in Fig. 7(a), the rate constant was proportional to the molar fraction of linoleic acid in both cases when the fatty acids and their methyl esters coexisted. This was true for the oxidation of methyl linoleate in the presence of the fatty acid methyl esters, as shown in Fig. 7(b). The rate expression (1) was derived under the assumption that the oxidation rate of a PUFA was proportional to both the concentrations of the unoxidized and oxidized substrates:

$$\frac{dC_{\mathrm{LH}}}{dt} = -k'C_{\mathrm{LH}}(C_{\mathrm{LH,t}} - C_{\mathrm{LH}}) \tag{8}$$

where C_{LH} is the concentration of the unoxidized substrate, k' is the rate constant, and the subscript t indicates the total of unoxidized and oxidized substrates. Eq. (1) can be obtained by dividing both sides of Eq. (8) by $C_{\mathrm{LH,t}}$, and there is the following relation between the rate constants k and k':

$$k = k'C_{\mathrm{LH,t}} \tag{9}$$

Equation (9) indicates that the rate constant, k, is proportional to the concentration of the substrate to be oxidized. When linoleic acid or methyl linoleate is mixed with a saturated fatty acid or its methyl ester, $C_{\mathrm{LH,t}}$ is proportional to the molar fraction of the substrate because the densities of the unsaturated and saturated fatty acids (or their methyl esters) are almost the same. Therefore, the linear relationships shown above indicated that the saturated fatty acid or its methyl ester would function merely as a diluent for the substrate to be oxidized. As shown in Fig. 7(b), the relationship between the k value and the molar fraction of methyl linoleate mixed with the saturated fatty acid was convex. This indicated that the saturated fatty acid promoted the oxidation of methyl linoleate. Prooxidant activity of free fatty acid has been reported [12, 18-19]. It was suggested that the carboxyl group of the saturated fatty acid catalyzed the decomposition of the hydroperoxide and that free radicals formed by the decomposition promoted the oxidation of methyl linoleate [12]. The results in Fig. 7 are consistent with the suggestions. The oxidation processes of linoleic acid and methyl linoleate mixed with lauric acid at the weight ratio of 1:1 were observed at several different temperatures. The dependency of the rate constant k on temperature was analyzed based on Eq. (6). The E values for linoleic acid and methyl linoleate were 54.4 kJ/mol and 49.5 kJ/mol, respectively, which were almost equivalent to those for the PUFAs and their methyl or ethyl esters [5].

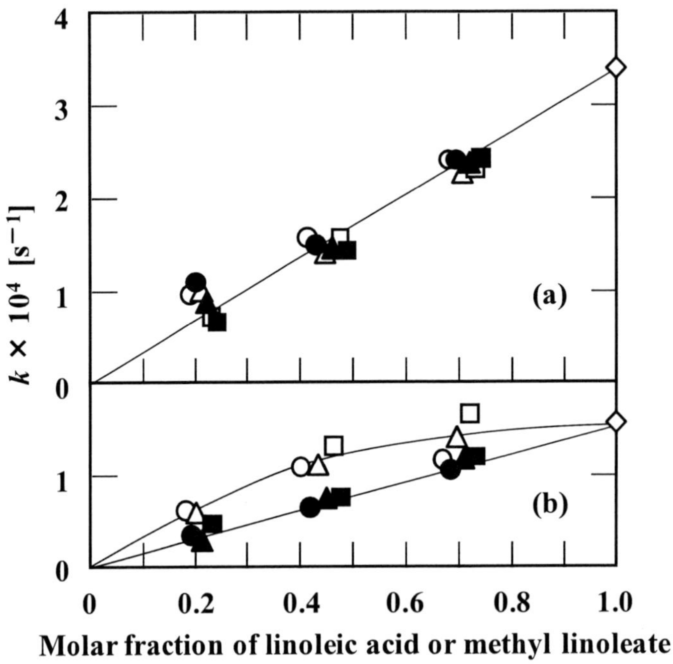

Figure 7. Effect of the molar fractions of (a) linoleic acid or (b) methyl linoleate on the rate constant. Linoleic acid or methyl linoleate was mixed with (○) lauric acid, (△) myrstic acid, (□) palmitic acid, (●) methyl laurate, (▲) methyl myristate, and (■) methyl palmitate. The symbol ◇ represents the rate constant of linoleic acid and methyl linoleate themselves.

Two PUFAs or their esters, such as linoleic and arachidonic acids, methyl linoleate, and ethyl arachidonate, were mixed, and their oxidation processes were measured at 65°C and *ca.* 0% relative humidity [20]. Except when a PUFA ester was mixed with a free PUFA, the oxidation of the less-oxidative PUFA was promoted as its content in the mixture decreased, while the oxidation of the more-oxidative PUFA was delayed with a decrease in its content. A kinetic model is proposed whereby a PUFA acts as the diluent for another PUFA, and the oxidation rate of the PUFA is proportional to the product of the unoxidized PUFA concentration and the sum of the concentrations of the oxidized PUFA and the other oxidized PUFA. This model clearly expressed the oxidation processes of the PUFAs in their mixed system. The oxidation process of a polyunsaturated acylglycerol mixed with a saturated or unsaturated acylglycerol was measured at the above-mentioned temperature and humidity

[21]. When two polyunsaturated acylglycerols were mixed, their oxidation processes were expressed by the kinetic model in which one acylglycerol acts as a diluent for another acylglycerol, and the oxidation product of the acylglycerol participates in the oxidation of another acylglycerol. However, the oxidation process of 1-monolinolein mixed with a saturated or monounsaturated acylglycerol was not expressed by the model but obeyed the kinetics of an autocatalytic type. The rate constant in the mixed system was greater than the constant which was predicted under the assumption that the saturated or monounsaturated acylglycerol merely acted as a diluent.

L-Ascorbic acid (AsA), which is known as vitamin C, is a water-soluble vitamin and widely used as an additive in foods and cosmetics due to its strong reducing ability. Acyl ascorbate is an amphiphilic antioxidant, because it consists of ascorbic and fatty acid as a hydrophilic antioxidant and lipophilic group, respectively [22]. When compared to a chemical method, the enzymatic synthesis of acyl ascorbate through the condensation of ascorbic and fatty acids using a lipase in an organic solvent has some advantages, such as the simplicities of the reaction and purification processes and its high regioselectivity [23-25]. Acyl ascorbate has not only an equivalent antioxidative activity [26, 27] but a good emulsifying ability [28-30]. The oxidation processes of linoleic acid in the presence of ascorbic acid or saturated acyl ascorbate were analyzed by applying a kinetic equation of the autocatalytic type to the processes [31]. A specific AsA and octanoic, lauric or palmitic acid were added into an amber glass bottle with a screw-cap, and the immobilized lipase from *Candida antarctica* and acetone as a catalyst and solvent, respectively, were further added to the bottle. The headspace of the bottle was filled with N_2, and the bottle was tightly sealed. The bottle was then immersed in a water-bath at 55°C with vigorous shaking. After *ca.* 24 h, each 6-*O*-acyl L-ascorbate was isolated from the reaction mixture according to the previous procedures [25] with a slight modification. Linoleic acid and AsA or octanoyl, lauroyl or palmitoyl ascorbate were mixed at the molar ratio from 0.025 to 0.2 (AsA/ linoleic acid), and preserved at relative humidity of 12%. The container was stored in the dark at a given temperature (37, 50, 65 or 80°C). Samples were periodically taken, and the amount of unoxidized linoleic acid was measured by the GC analysis with an FID [32, 33]. The oxidative stabilities at 37°C and 12% relative humidity of linoleic acid coexistent with AsA and octanoyl ascorbate at various molar ratios were measured. The higher the molar ratio was, the more strongly the oxidation of linoleic acid was suppressed in both cases. Octanoyl ascorbate had stronger antioxidative ability than AsA. The oxidation of linoleic acid mixed with octanoyl ascorbate at the molar ratio of 0.1 was suppressed for at least 130 h. The oxidation processes of linoleic acid mixed with lauroyl and palmitoyl ascorbates showed similar results. The induction period for the oxidation of linoleic acid was prolonged by the addition of the ascorbates. Figure 8 shows the oxidation processes at 80°C and 12% relative humidity of linoleic acid with no additive and that with AsA or octanoyl, lauroyl, or palmitoyl ascorbate at the molar ratio of 0.05. Linoleic acid without additive was quickly oxidized, whereas the oxidative stability of linoleic acid was slightly improved by its coexistence with AsA. Octanoyl, lauroyl, and palmitoyl ascorbates retarded the oxidation of linoleic acid more than AsA. The entire oxidation process of linoleic acid could be expressed by Eq. (1). The k and Y_0 values for the oxidation processes of linoleic acid at 37, 50 and 65°C were also estimated. Figure 9 shows the relationship between the acyl chain length of the ascorbates and the k value at various temperatures. At any temperature, the k value for linoleic acid with no additive was greater than that for linoleic acid with AsA or acyl ascorbate. There was a tendency for the k value in the presence of ascorbate with a larger acyl chain length to be slightly smaller. The k value for linoleic acid with AsA (the acyl chain length equal to zero) seemed to be greater than that for linoleic acid with the acyl ascorbates at any temperature. The Y_0 values for the additives were greater than that for linoleic acid with no additive although there were some exceptions. This indicated that the addition of an additive delayed the induction period in the oxidation process of linoleic acid. The temperature dependence of the rate constant k was analyzed based on the Arrhenius equation as Eq. (6). The E values for linoleic acid mixed with every ascorbate were at the range of 50 to 70 kJ/mol and there was a tendency for E value to decrease with increasing acyl chain length. The k_0 values for linoleic acid in the presence of the ascorbates were smaller than that for linoleic acid with no additive or AsA. The k_0 value also decreased with increasing acyl chain length. This indicates that the presence of acyl ascorbate lowers both the height of the energy barrier for the oxidation of linoleic acid and the probability of the reaction resulting in the oxidation of linoleic acid.

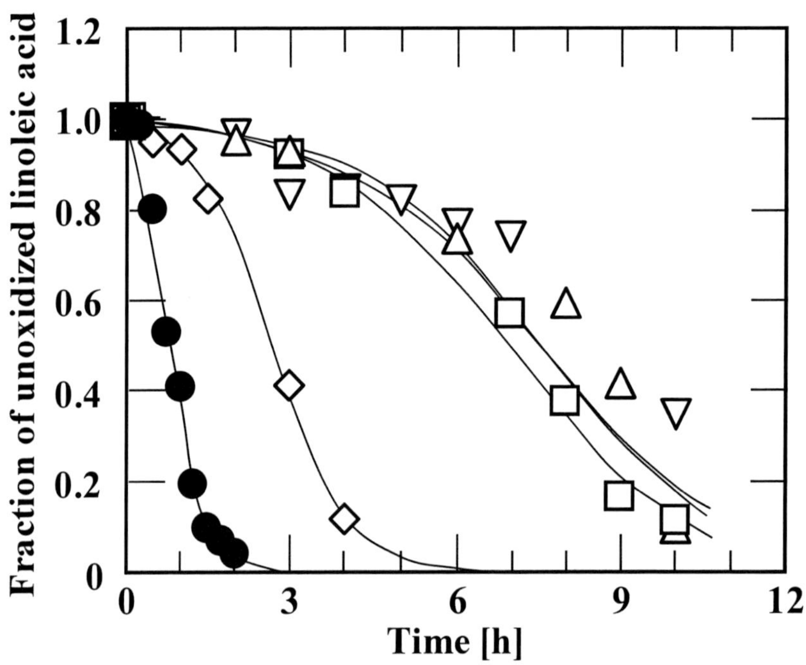

Figure 8. Oxidation processes of linoleic acid with (●) no additive and that mixed with (◇) ascorbic acid, (□) octanoyl ascorbate, (△) lauroyl ascorbate or (▽) palmitoyl ascorbate at the molar ratio = 0.05 and at 80°C. The solid curves were drawn using the k and Y_0 values calculated.

Ferulic acid, 3-(4-hydroxy-3-methoxyphenyl)-2-propenoic acid, occurs as esters in rice, wheat, barley, citrus fruits, and many other plants, and is an efficacious radical scavenger which readily forms a resonance stabilized phenoxy radical because of its phenolic nucleus and its extended side chain conjugation [34]. Due to its radical scavenging ability, it is used as an additive in foods to prevent lipid oxidation. However, the low solubility of ferulic acid in lipids restricts its application in the food industry. Lipophilic antioxidants are supposed to be more effective for the suppression of lipid oxidation than hydrophilic ones [35, 36]. Alkyl ferulates, which should be more lipophilic than unmodified ferulic acid, have recently been utilized in the food and cosmetic industries as antioxidants and radical scavenging agents [37, 38]. The oxidation processes of linoleic acid in the presence of ferulic acid, and 1-pentyl, 1-hexyl and 1-heptyl ferulates were observed at various temperatures and different molar ratios of each additive to linoleic acid [39]. The processes were analyzed based on the kinetic equation of the autocatalytic type (Eq. (1)) to evaluate the k and Y_0 values by the latter of which the initiation period for the oxidation of linoleic acid was mainly governed. The k values for linoleic acid mixed with the alkyl ferulates were smaller than that for linoleic acid mixed with ferulic acid. The greater suppressive effect of the alkyl ferulates would be ascribed to their higher solubility in linoleic acid. Both the E and k_0 values in Eq. (6) for the oxidation of linoleic acid mixed with ferulic acid or pentyl ferulate decreased with the increasing molar ratio of the additive to linoleic acid.

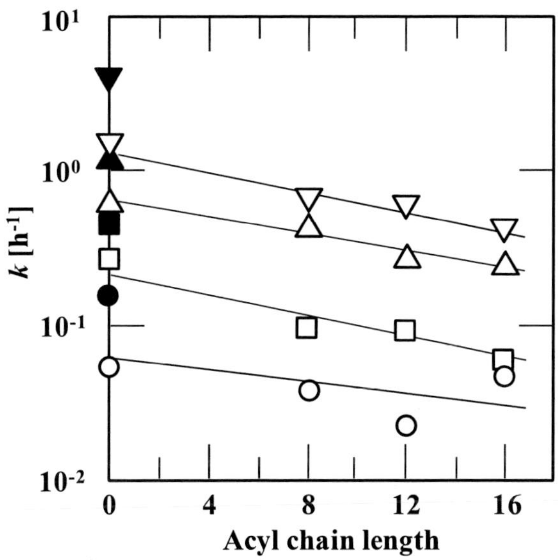

Figure 9. Relationship between acyl chain length of ascorbates and the rate constant, k, at (○) 37, (□) 50, (△) 65 and (▽) 80°C. Open symbols represent the rate constants for the oxidation of linoleic acid mixed with various ascorbates, and the closed symbols that for no additive.

4. Stability of Linoleoyl Ascorbate in a Bulk System

Conjugated linoleic acid (CLA) is a group of positional and geometric isomers of linoleic acid and has attracted considerable attention due to its physiological characteristics such as its antioxidant properties [40, 41]. CLA is potentially valuable as a raw material for functional food but is quite susceptible to oxidation. The oxidation causes deterioration of food. An effective method has been developed for fractionating CLA isomers through selective esterification using *Candida rugosa* lipase to produce *cis*-9,*trans*-11- (*c*9,*t*11) and *trans*-10,*cis*-12-conjugated linoleic acid (*t*10,*c*12CLA) isomers in purities of about 80% [42]. Using these isomers, we also reported the oxidation kinetics for *c*9,*t*11 and *t*10,*c*12CLA isomers [43]. Furthermore, conjugated linoleoyl ascorbates (CLA-AsA) were synthesized through the condensation of *c*9,*t*11CLA or *t*10,*c*12CLA with AsA using immobilized lipase from *C. antarctica* in an organic solvent, and the oxidation processes for CLA moiety in synthesized CLA-AsAs and unmodified CLAs were also measured at 65°C and 75% relative humidity (Fig. 10) [44]. The unmodified CLA isomers were almost completely oxidized within 4 h, whereas all the CLA-AsAs were significantly resistant to oxidation. The oxidation kinetics was empirically expressed by the Weibull equation [45]:

$$Y = \exp[-(kt)^n] \tag{10}$$

where n is the shape constant. The k values for CLA-AsAs and linoleoyl ascorbate were about 1/30 and 1/60, respectively, of that for the corresponding unmodified CLA isomers. Although it is reported that *t*10,*c*12CLA is more easily oxidized than *c*9,*t*11CLA [43], there was no significant difference in the susceptibility to oxidation between the CLA isomers esterified with AsA. The n values were greater than one for all the unmodified CLA isomers, whereas the values for CLA-AsAs were less than one. This indicated that there were induction periods, which reflected the slow progress of the oxidation during the early stage of storage, for unmodified CLA isomers, whereas the oxidation for CLA-AsAs progressed very slowly without an induction period. Therefore, it was quantitatively demonstrated that the oxidation process for conjugated linoleoyl moiety of CLA-AsA was different from that for unmodified CLA.

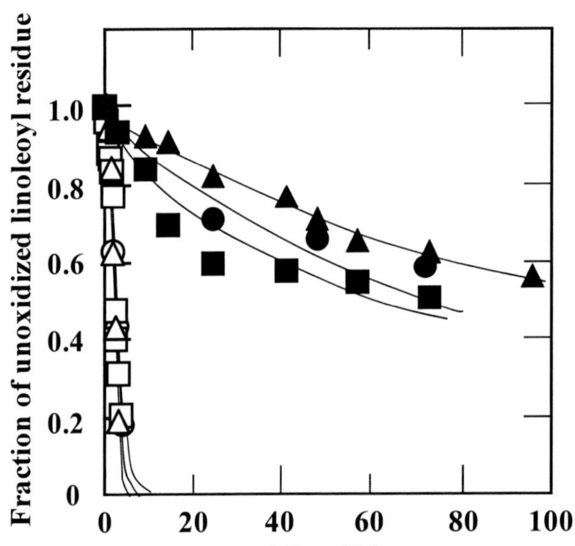

Figure 10. Oxidation processes of (○) *c*9,*t*11CLA, (□) *t*10,*c*12CLA, (△) LA, (●) *c*9,*t*11CLA-AsA, (■) *t*10,*c*12CLA-AsA, and (▲) LA-AsA at 65°C and 75% relative humidity. The solid curves were calculated using the estimated kinetic parameters of the Weibull model.

The condensation between AsA and various PUFAs, such as α- and γ-linolenic, dihomo-γ-linolenic, arachidonic, eicosapentaenoic, and docosahexaenoic acids, were catalyzed by the immobilized lipase to produce polyunsaturated acyl ascorbates (PUFA-AsAs) [27, 46]. The oxidation processes of the unmodified PUFA and the polyunsaturated acyl moiety of the PUFA-AsAs at 65°C and nearly 0% relative humidity were measured. The unmodified PUFAs were almost completely autoxidized within 5 h, whereas all the PUFA-AsAs were significantly resistant to the oxidation. The polyunsaturated acyl moiety of 90% or more remained in the unoxidized state during the test period for every ascorbate. Introduction of PUFA to AsA significantly improved its oxidative stability. The oxidation process of eicosapentaenoyl ascorbate was almost the same as that of eicosapentaenoic acid mixed with an equimolar amount of ascorbic acid.

5. Oxidation of Linoleoyl Residue of its Disaccharide Ester in a Micelle System

In food, lipids also exist in disperse systems such as the oil-in-water (O/W) emulsion, water-in-oil (W/O) emulsion and micelle, and the state in which the lipid exists could affect its oxidative stability. The effects of the type of emulsifier and other factors on the lipid oxidation in the O/W emulsion systems have been extensively investigated [47-49]. For the lipid oxidation in a micelle system, an interesting phenomenon that a fatty acid with a higher unsaturation is oxidized more slowly was found [50, 51]. In these experiments, the oxidation of an unsaturated fatty acid was initiated by adding a radical, and an excess amount of an emulsifier to form the micelle of the unsaturated fatty acid. Furthermore, the initial mole of oxygen was less than that of the unsaturated fatty acid. This fact suggested the possibility that oxygen was the rate-limiting component. Linoleic acid was regiospecifically condensed with trehalose using a lipase in an organic solvent to produce the 6-*O*-monoacyl trehalose [52]. The ester could form a micelle in aqueous solution with no addition of other emulsifiers. The oxidation of the linoleoyl residue was measured under the assumptions that the initial mole of oxygen was more than that of the linoleoyl residue and that no radical was added at the various initial concentrations of the linoleoyl trehalose. Monolinoleoyl trehalose was dissolved in distilled water at various concentrations. A portion of each solution was put into an amber glass vessel, in which an oxygen electrode was installed. The initial amount of oxygen was estimated assuming that the ideal gas law held in the air phase and that the aqueous phase was equilibrated with air. The initial molar ratio of oxygen to linoleoyl trehalose was greater than 3, indicating that the oxygen was not a rate-limiting component. The vessel was immersed in a water bath at 35°C. The linoleoyl trehalose was allowed to oxidize with magnetic stirring, and the oxygen concentration in the air phase was then determined using the oxygen electrode and recorded. The solution of a given concentration was put into amber vials to provide the same volume ratio of the air phase to the aqueous one as in the previous experiment. The vials were placed in a water bath at 35°C then shaken. At appropriate intervals, a vial was removed to determine the concentration of the unoxidized linoleoyl trehalose using an HPLC and a UV detector (220 nm). For the linoleoyl trehalose concentrations higher than its critical micelle concentration (CMC), which was *ca.* 0.35 mmol/L [53], the size distribution of the micelles was measured using dynamic light scattering spectrophotometer to estimate the median diameter based on the weight fraction.

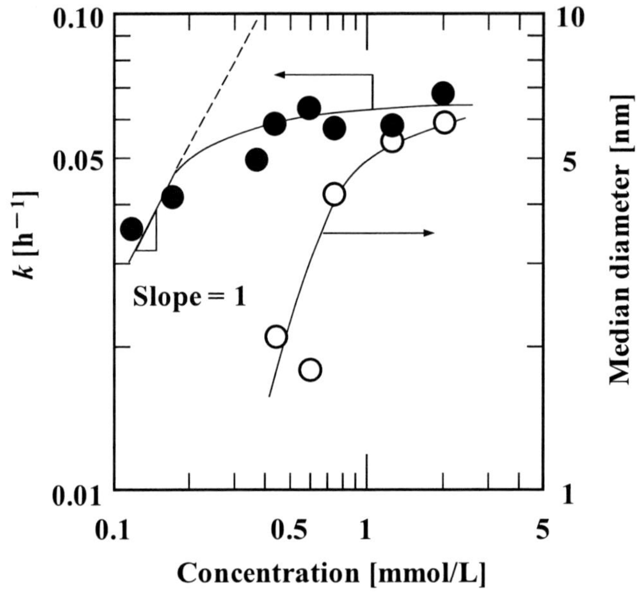

Figure 11. Concentration dependences of the rate constant *k* for the oxidation of linoleoyl trehalose and of the median diameter of micelles in an aqueous solution. The solid curves were drawn by connecting the data points. The broken line was drawn under the assumption that the rate constant *k* is in proportion to the substrate concentration.

First, the oxygen consumption during the oxidation at 35°C of the linoleoyl residue of its trehalose ester at various concentrations was measured. Because the molar ratio of oxygen to the linoleoyl residue was greater than one in every case, a significant amount of oxygen remained when the linoleoyl residue was fully oxidized. The oxidation at the same temperature of the linoleoyl trehalose ester proceeded slower at the lower concentrations. More specifically, the oxidation was significantly retarded at the concentrations lower than the CMC of the linoleoyl trehalose. In order to assess the oxidation of an unsaturated fatty acid based on the oxygen consumption, the stoichiometric relationship between oxygen and the linoleoyl residue is important. The plots of the moles of consumed oxygen versus those of the oxidized linoleoyl residue, except for the late stage of oxidation, were scattered on a line with a uniformed slope, indicating that the stiochiometric coefficient of oxygen to the linoleoyl residue is same during the early and middle stages of the oxidation. The same value was obtained for the oxidation of linoleic acid in a bulk system [8]. The oxidation of the linoleoyl residue slowly proceeded during the early stage, rapidly during the middle stage, and again slowly during the late stage. The applicability of Eq. (1) or (2) to the oxidation process was examined. The plots of $\ln[(1-Y)/Y]$ versus t gave a straight line at every concentration of the linoleoyl trehalose. The rate constant, k, was evaluated from the slope of the line. The k values are plotted versus the concentration of the linoleoyl trehalose in Fig. 11. The diameter of the micelles was estimated assuming that the linoleoyl trehalose forms a spherical micelle, as no information is available on the shape. In a homogeneous system, the k value should be proportional to the substrate concentration [17, 21]. It seemed that the k value was in proportion to the concentration at the substrate concentrations lower than the CMC, though there were only two points. At these concentrations, the substrate molecules should exist as a monomer in the solution. However, the k value was not in proportion to the substrate concentration at the concentrations higher than the CMC, and the plots for the *k* values lay under the dotted line for the monomer system. At the concentrations higher than the CMC, the substrate molecules existed in both forms of the monomer and micelle. If linoleoyl trehalose molecules form a spherical micelle, the hydrophilic trehalose moieties would form a shell. Because the oxygen molecule has a hydrophobic property, the shell would act as the barrier for the oxygen molecule to penetrate into the core consisting of the linoleoyl residues. It is not conclusive, but there is a possibility that the mass transfer resistance plays an important role in the oxidation of the linoleoyl residue in a micelle system though the particle size is on the order of nanometer.

6. Oxidation of Methyl Linoleate in O/W Micro- and Nanoemulsion Systems

An emulsion is a common structure in lipid-containing foods from home cooking to industry. Many factors, such as the addition of an antioxidant [54-57], protein [58-60], metal ion [61] and chelator [47, 57], emulsifier type [47, 62], and homogenization conditions [63, 64], affect the lipid oxidation in the emulsion system. Oil-droplet size of the emulsion is also an important factor affecting the oxidation [62, 64-66]. Although the oil-droplet sizes were in almost the same range (from 0.2 μm to 30 μm) in these studies, their conclusions were quite conflicting. Lethuaunt *et al.* [65] reported that the rates of oxygen consumption and conjugated diene formation were higher for the small oil-droplets. On the other hand, Nakaya *et al.* [66] reported that the hydroperoxide content in the emulsion with a smaller droplet size was significantly lower than that in the emulsion containing large droplets. However, Osborn and Akoh [62] concluded that the oil-droplet size had no effect on the lipid oxidation in structured lipid-based oil-in-water emulsions. Rapid developments in nanotechnology have allowed us to focus on its application to foods. A nanoemulsion has several interesting properties. The emulsion looks bluish transparent because the droplets are too small to scatter visible light. Droplets in the emulsion have much higher specific surface areas than the common emulsion that has a larger droplet size. The high surface area would elicit an effect at the interface between the oil and aqueous phases on phenomena occurring in the emulsions, including the lipid oxidation. Authors prepared O/W emulsions having the oil-droplet sizes of 17 nm to 8.0 μm in the same compositions of oil and surfactant in order to exclude the effects of the composition on the oxidation [67]. The oxidation processes of methyl linoleate in the emulsions were measured in order to examine the effect of the oil-droplet size on the oxidation kinetics over a wider range of oil-droplet size compared to the previous studies [62, 64-66]. The O/W emulsions with various oil-droplet diameters using the Q-12Y or ML-750 surfactant, which were both categorized as decaglycerol monolaurate, were prepared. Phosphate buffer (50 mmol/L, pH 7.4) was used as the water phase. A surfactant was dissolved in purified water at 20 or 30% (w/v). Methyl linoleate as an oil phase was added to the surfactant solution. The mixture was then homogenized using a rotor/stator homogenizer. In order to produce emulsions having small oil droplets, a coarse emulsion was further homogenized twice using a high-pressure homogenizer. The O/W emulsions were diluted with a phosphate buffer. The concentrations of the surfactant and methyl linoleate were 3% (w/v) and 0.75% (v/v), respectively, for all the emulsions. The emulsion was placed in amber vials and each vial was tightly sealed with a silicone cap. The vials were maintained at 40°C in a thermo-controlled oven. The emulsions in the vials were mixed with a magnetic stirrer in order to promote the supply of oxygen from gas phase to the emulsion phase and to prevent creaming of the emulsions. At appropriate intervals, one of the vials was removed from the oven to measure the amount of unoxidized methyl linoleate using a gas chromatograph. The partial oxygen pressure in the emulsion was measured in an amber vial tightly sealed with a lid equipped with an oxygen sensor.

The oil-droplet size significantly affected the oxidation process of methyl linoleate in the emulsions prepared using the Q-12Y surfactant. There was a tendency that the period of the induction step was longer and the oxidation rate during the propagation step was higher for the emulsion containing the larger droplet. On the other hand, the effect of the initial oil-droplet size on the oxidation process was not remarkable for the emulsions prepared using the ML-750 surfactant. The oxidation process for the emulsion having any oil-droplet size was analyzed on the basis of the rate equation of the autocatalytic type (Eqs. (1) and (2)), and the k and Y_0 values were estimated. The induction period, t_{ind}, for the methyl linoleate was defined as the time at which the tangent at $Y = 0.5$ crossed the line of $Y = 1$, that can be calculated from the k and Y_0 values using the following equation:

$$t_{ind} = \frac{1}{k}\left(\ln\frac{Y_0}{1-Y_0} - 2\right) \tag{11}$$

Figure 12 shows the dependencies of the k and t_{ind} values on the initial diameter of the oil droplets in the emulsions. For the emulsions prepared using the Q-12Y surfactant, both the k and t_{ind} values were smaller for the emulsions having smaller oil droplets. On the other hand, there were no significant dependencies of the k and t_{ind} values on the initial oil-droplet size of the emulsions prepared using the ML-750 surfactant. The oil-droplet size hardly changed for the emulsions with the Q-12Y surfactant, but it significantly changed for those prepared using the ML-750 surfactant. The difference in the stability between the emulsions prepared using the Q-12Y and ML-750 surfactants seemed to result in the different dependencies of the k and t_{ind} values on the initial oil-droplet size. The specific surface area of the oil-droplet is higher for the smaller oil-droplets. The increase in the specific surface area seems to promote the oxidation of methyl linoleate when the diffusion of oxygen through the interface is rate-limiting or to maintain the k value constant when the rate-limiting step is the oxidation reaction itself. The k value was, however, smaller for the emulsion containing smaller oil-droplets. Authors proposed the model which describes the dependence of the k value on the oil-droplet size of the emulsion. This model is based on the property of the autocatalytic-type rate expression and dilution of methyl linoleate by a hydrophobic moiety of the surfactant and is expressed by Eqs. (8) and (9) [17]. Surfactant molecules cover the surface of the oil droplets, and the surfactant molecule penetrates its hydrophobic moiety into the oil phase. The hydrophobic moiety of the Q-12Y surfactant is the lauroyl residue, which is a saturated acyl chain. The penetration of the saturated lauroyl residue into the methyl linoleate phase should dilute the substrate, which would result in the lowering of the k value based on Eq. (9). Assuming that an oil-droplet having a diameter, D_O, is fully covered with surfactant molecules to form the hydrophilic layer, the thickness of which is D_H, that the volume of a hydrophobic moiety is V_L, and that the residual area per surfactant molecule is a. Based on these assumptions, the k value for an oil-droplet covered with surfactant is given by Eq. (12):

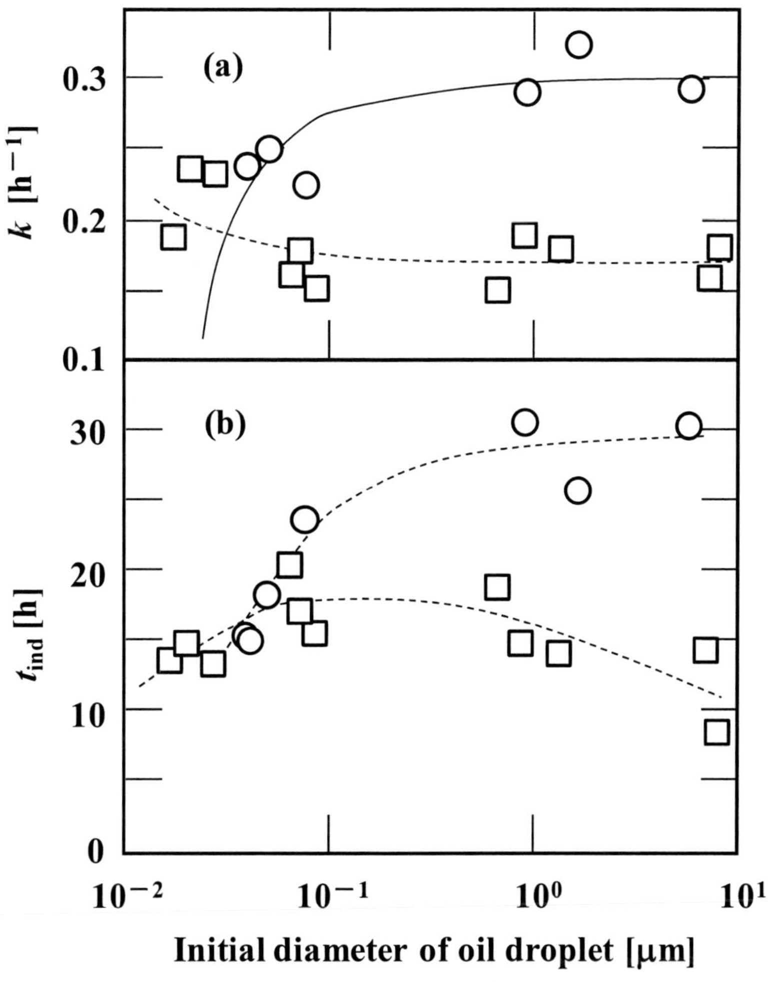

Figure 12. Dependencies of the kinetic parameters, k (●, ○) and t_{ind} (▲, △), for the oxidation of methyl linoleate on the initial oil-droplet size in O/W emulsions prepared using (closed symbols) Q-12Y and (open symbols) ML-750. The solid curve for Q-12Y was drawn based on the proposed model, while that for ML-750 was drawn by smoothly connecting the experimental points.

$$\frac{k}{k_n} = 1 - \frac{6V_L}{a(D_O - 2D_H)} \tag{12}$$

where k_n is the rate constant for methyl linoleate which is not covered by the surfactant. The hydrophilic and hydrophobic moieties of the Q-12Y surfactant are the decaglyceryl and lauroyl residues, respectively. Based on Kopp's rule [68], their volumes and the cross-sectional area of the HCOH group in the hydrophilic moiety were estimated. The D_H value was evaluated by dividing the volume of the hydrophilic moiety by its cross-sectional area. Furthermore, the k_n value was roughly estimated from the k values for the microemulsions. The k values for the emulsions having various oil-droplet sizes were calculated by substituting the estimated k_n, V_L, a, D_O, and D_H values into Eq. (12), and are shown in Fig. 12(a) by the solid curve. This curve expressed the experimental results well. This indicates that the dilution of the substrate oil by the saturated hydrophobic moiety of the surfactant plays an important role in the smaller k value for the emulsions having smaller oil droplets.

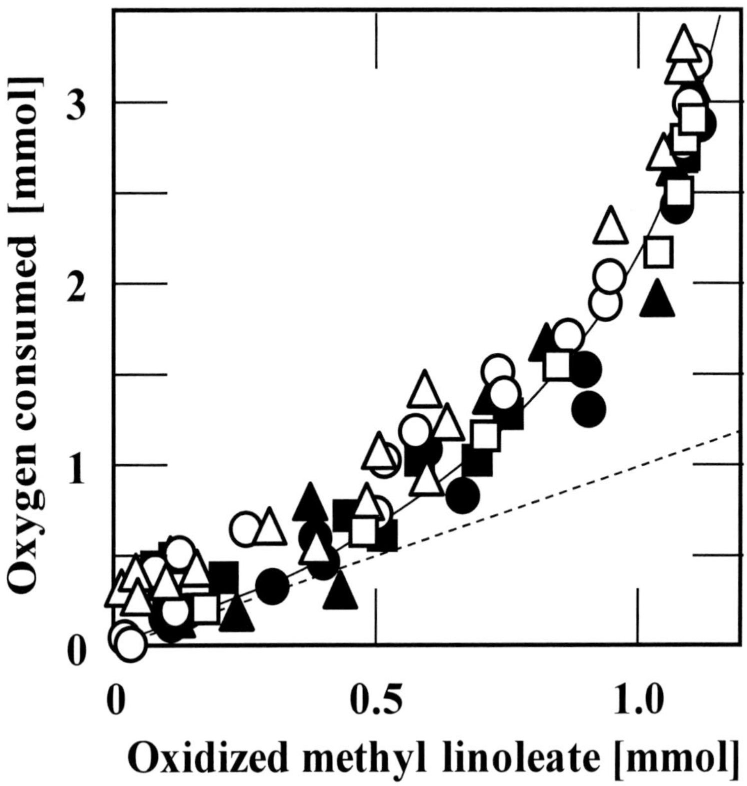

Figure 13. Relationship between the amount of consumed oxygen and that of oxidized methyl linoleate during the oxidation of methyl linoleate on the initial oil-droplet size in O/W emulsions prepared using (closed symbols) Q-12Y and (open symbols) ML-750. The initial median diameters of the oil droplets in the emulsions were 52 nm (●), 79 nm (▲), 0.92 μm (■), 17 nm (○), 88 nm (△) and 1.3 μm (□).

Each oxygen consumption behavior during the oxidation of methyl linoleate in the emulsions prepared using the Q-12Y or ML-750 surfactant was similar to the decrease in the fraction of the remaining methyl linoleate. The molar amount of the consumed oxygen was estimated on the basis of the ideal gas law, and the molar amount of the consumed methyl linoleate was calculated from the fraction of the remaining substrate. Figure 13 shows the stoichiometric relationship between the oxidized substrate and the consumed oxygen for the emulsions with various initial oil-droplet diameters. All the plots lie on a curve. The plots during the early stage of the oxidation lie on a straight line with uniformed slope, indicating that the stoichiometric coefficient between methyl linoleate and oxygen was same. This result was similar to our previous one for the oxidation of methyl linoleate in a bulk system [8]. During the later stage of oxidation, more oxygen was consumed in order to oxidize the methyl linoleate. Both the oil-droplet size and the surfactant type did not affect the stoichiometric relationship.

The changes in the oil-droplet size of the emulsions with various initial oil-droplet sizes prepared using the Q-12Y and ML-750 surfactants were measured. Irrespective of the initial oil-droplet size, the oil-droplet sizes of the emulsions prepared using the Q-12Y surfactant hardly changed except during the later stage of the storage in which the methyl linoleate was almost completely oxidized. On the other hand, the oil-droplet size of the emulsions prepared using the ML-750 surfactant significantly changed during the storage. The size of the small oil-droplets gradually increased and leveled off at about ten times the initial size. The large oil-droplets quickly became small droplets, then they became larger, similar to the oil-droplets having the small initial size. Both the Q-12Y and ML-750 surfactants are chemically decaglyceryl laurate. The hydrophilic moiety is not strictly the decaglyceryl residue, but there is a distribution in the degree of polymerization of the glyceryl residues. The precise distributions for the surfactants have not been provided by the manufacturers and depend on the lot number of a surfactant. The distribution of the Q-12Y surfactant would be different from that of the ML-750 surfactant, and this difference seemed to be a reason for the difference in the stability between the emulsions prepared using the surfactants.

7. Microencapsulation of Linoleic Acid and its Oxidative Stability

Microencapsulation of a lipid as a core material with a wall material can provide the core material with some new functions [69] and is a promising technology in food and other industries [70]. One of the functions is suppression or retardation of oxidation of an encapsulated PUFA [71, 72]. Microencapsulation consists of two steps: one is emulsification of a core material with a dense solution of a wall material, and the second is the drying of the emulsions.

Spray-drying is the most popular technique to prepare microcapsules [73]. Therefore, properties of emulsions such as stability and droplet size would affect the characteristics of the microcapsules prepared by spray-drying. Linoleic acid was emulsified with a dense solution of gum arabic or maltodextrin with a dextrose equivalent of 2-5 in the presence or absence of a small-molecule emulsifier (Tween 20 (polycxyethylene sorbitan monolaurate, HLB = 16.7), Tween 85 (polyethylene sorbitan trioleate, HLB = 11.0) or Span 20 (sorbitan monolaurate, HLB = 8.6)), and the median diameter of the oil droplets and the stability of the emulsions were measured [33].

The emusions were spray-dried toproduce microcapsules. The encapsulation efficiency was estimated, and the oxidation of the encapsulated linoleic acid was also measured.

Gum arabic or maltodextrin was dissolved in distilled water at a concentration of 15% (w/v) with slight heating. Linoleic acid was mixed with the polysaccharide solution to produce a weight ratio of the acid to the polysaccharide of 0.1, 0.2, 0.5, 1.0 or 2.0. When an emulsifier was further added in the aqueous phase at a ratio of the acid to maltodextrin = 0.2, its amount was fixed at 10% by weight of the acid. The amount corresponded to overall concentrations of 2.5, 1.6 and 8.5 mmol/L for Tween 20, Tween 85 and Span 20, respectively, at a weight ratio of 0.2. Because the surface excess of Tween 20 was 2.8×10^{-3} g/m^2 [74], the amount of added Tween 20 would be sufficient to achieve saturation coverage of oil droplets with a diameter of 1 μm or smaller.

Although the surface excess of other emulsifiers are unknown, their amounts added seem to be sufficient for covering the surface of the oil droplets. The mixture was emulsified with a rotor/stator homogenizer for 2 min.

This single-step emulsification was denoted as method A. To prepare an emulsion with a smaller diameter, the emulsion was further homogenized three times with a high-pressure homogenizer at 500 kgf/cm^2 (method B). Except for examination of the effect of droplet size on the oxidative stability, method A was adopted for preparation of the emulsions. The particle size distribution of the emulsions was measured using a centrifugal particle analyzer after appropriate dilution with 1.0% (w/v) sodium dodecyl sulphate (SDS).

The stability of the emulsions was estimated by a turbidimetric method [75]. The emulsion was stored at 25°C with gentle stirring. At appropriate intervals, an aliquot (10μL) of the emulsion was pipetted out and diluted with 2.0 mL of 1.0% (w/v) SDS. The absorbance at 500 nm of the diluted emulsion was measured. The emulsion was fed into a spray-dryer at a flow rate 3.0 kg/h and was atomized by a centrifugal atomizer operated at 3×10^4 rpm. The emulsion in the reservoir was gently magnetically-stirred to prevent flotation of the emulsion droplets. The temperatures of air at the inlet and outlet were 200°C and 100-110°C, respectively. The flow rate of air was ~7.5 m^3/min. The microcapsules were prepared and collected in a cyclone.

Ten milligrams of spray-dried microcapsules were weighed into a flat-bottom glass cup. About 20 cups were prepared for each sample. The cups were place in a desiccator, in which a Petri dish filled with a saturated lithium chloride solution was placed to regulate the relative humidity at 12%.

The desiccator was stored in the dark at 37°C. At appropriate intervals, a cup was taken out of the desiccator, and the sample was dissolved with 0.1 mol/L NaOH in a vial. Methanol and chloroform, in which methyl palmitate was dissolved at a concentration of 0.01% (w/v) as an internal standard in gas chromatographic analysis, were then added to extract lipophilic substances. After vigorous agitation, 0.1 mol/L HCl and distilled water were added, and the vial was then agitated.

After centrifugation to separate the organic and aqueous phases, the lower organic phase was pipetted out [76]. After evaporation, the residue was mixed with methanol, benzene, and 2.0 mol/L (trimethylsilyl)diazomethane. The mixture was kept at room temperature for 30 min to convert linoleic acid to methyl linoleate [32]. After evaporation of the solvents, the remainder was dissolved in hexane. The unoxidized lnioleic acid in the solution was determined by a gas chromatography with a hydrogen ionization detector. If linoleic acid is fully encapsulated with a polysaccharide, its amount in a given weight of microcapsules can be calculated from the composition of emulsion used for preparing the microcapsules. However, the acid subjected to microencapsulation would not be fully encapsulated in practice.

The actual amount of linoleic acid in 10 mg of fresh microcapsules was determined according to the above-mentioned GC analysis. Then, the encapsulation efficiency was defined as a ratio of the actual amount of the acid in the microcapsules to the calculated one.

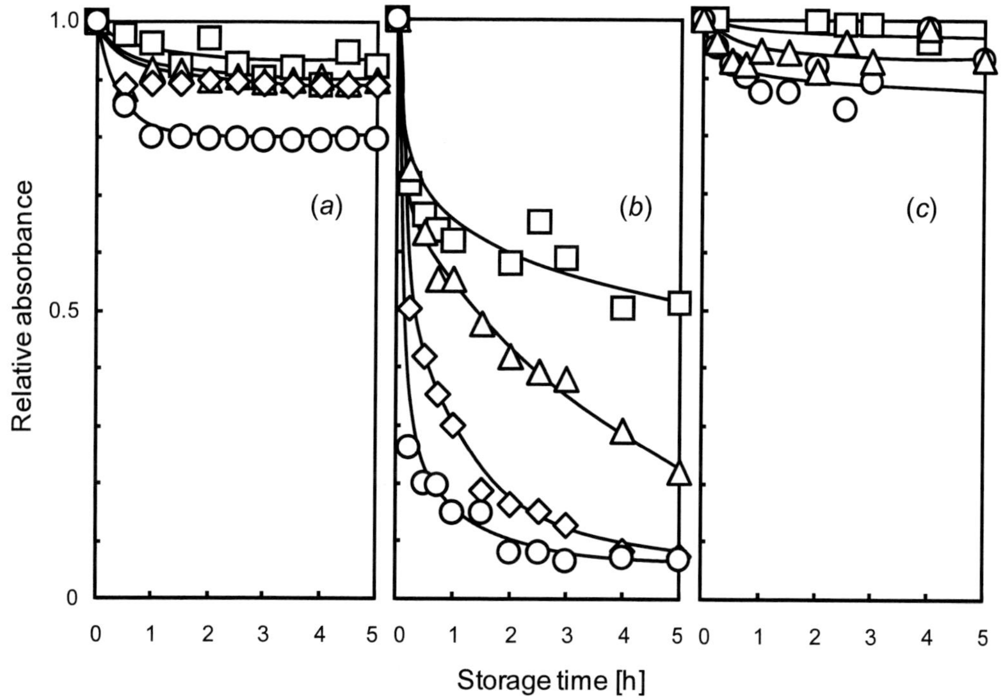

Figure 14. Stability of emulsions prepared with (*a*) gum arabic and (*b*) maltodextrin at different weight ratios of linoleic acid to the polysaccharide, and (*c*) of emulsions prepared with maltodextroin at the ratio of 0.2 in the presence of a small-molecule emulsifier. Symbols □, △, ◇ and ○ in (*a*)and (*b*) represent the weight ratios of 0.2, 0.5, 1.0 and 2.0, respectively. Symbols □, ○ and △ in (*c*) indicate Tween 20, Tween 85 and Span 20.

Table 1. Change in median diameter of oil droplet with time for linoleic acid emulsions prepared with gum Arabic and mattodextrin, and encapsulation efficiency after encapsulation by spray drying

			Emulsifier[b]		
Wall material[a]	**Gum arabic**	**Maltodextrin**	**Tween 20**	**Tween 85**	**Span 20**
Storage time (h)			**Median diameter (μm)**		
0	0.68	1.68	1.30	1.46	1.30
2	0.81	ND[c]	1.32	1.40	1.29
5	0.83	ND[c]	1.28	1.70	1.29
Encapsulation efficiency	0.97	0.49	0.67	0.58	0.82

[a] The weigt ratio of linoleic acid and wall material was fixed at 0.2.

[b] The amount of added emulsifier was 10% by weight of linoleic acid.

[c]. ND: not determined.

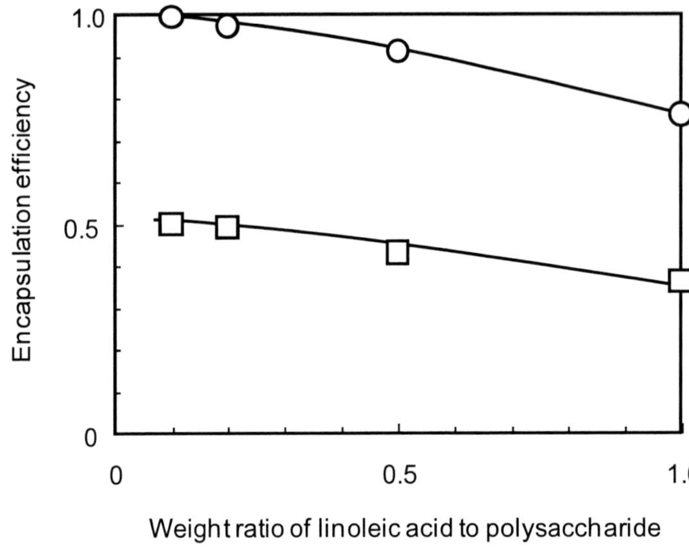

Figure 15. Dependence of encapsulation efficiency of linoleic acid encapsulated with (○) gum arabic or (□) maltodextorin on the weight ratio of the acid to the polysaccharide.

Figure 14(a) and (b) show the stability of O/W emulsions, which contained gum arabic and maltodextrin, respectively, in the outer aqueous phase at a concentration of 15%(w/v). The emulsions were prepared at various weight ratios of linoleic acid to polysaccharide. The vertical axis represents the absorbance normalized by the initial value. When the outer phase contained gum arabic, the emulsions were stable at any ratio except at the ratio of 2.0. However, when maltodextrin was added to the outer aqueous phase, the emulsions were unstable. The stability decreased with an increase of the weight ratio of linoleic acid to maltodextrin. Gum arabic is a small content of proteineous residue in the carbohydrate chain [77, 78]. The residue attached on the oil surface acts as an emulsion stabilizer. On the other hand, maltodextorin is a relatively linear homopolymer of glucose and has little ability as an emulsifier. Matsumura *et al.* measured the interfacial tension and viscosity at the oil surface in an emulsion system containing gum arabic, maltodextrin or pullulan, and showed that only gum arabic was adsorbed on the surface to form a viscoelastic layer [79]. This would be the reason why the emulsions containing gum arabic were more stable than those containing maltodextrin. Figure 14(c) shows the stability of emulsions prepared by adding Tween 20, Tween 85 or Span 20 together with maltodextrin. The weight ratio of linoleic acid to maltodextrin was fixed at 0.2. The addition of emulsifier improved the stability of the emulsion. Among the emulsifiers tested, Tween 20, which has the highest HLB value, that is, the most hydrophilic, was the most effective for the stabilization of emulsion, and Tween 85 and Span 20 followed. The order corresponded well to the HLB values of the emulsifiers. Table 1 shows the change in median diameter of the oil droplets with time. The emulsions were prepared at the weight ratio of 0.2. The emulsion prepared with gum arabic had the smallest diameter, although the diameter became larger with storage time. The diameter of emulsion prepared with maltodextrin was 2.5 times that of the emulsion prepared with gum arabic. Since the emulsion prepared with maltodextrin phase-separated during the storage, one could not measure the change in the diameter with time. Addition of an emulsifier in the aqueous phase during the preparation of the emulsion with maltodextrin slightly reduced the diameter, and the diameter scarcely changed during the test period. Thus, the addition of a small-molecule emulsifier could improve the stability of an emulsion with maltodextrin. Encapsulation efficiency is one of the important parameters in microencapsulation, as well as surface oil present. Only the encapsulation efficiency was measured in this study. Figure 15 shows the dependence of encapsulation efficiency on the weight ratio of linoleic acid to gum arabic or maltodextrin for microcapsules prepared by spray-drying. The efficiency of microcapsules prepared with gum arabic was high, while that of microcapsule prepared with maltodextrin was low. The high efficiency of gum arabic could be ascribed to the properties of gum arabic that were mentioned above. The efficiency of gum arabic decreased as the weight ratio increased. McNamee *et al.* reported a similar dependency for microcapsules prepared with soy oil and gum arabic by spray-drying [80]. At higher ratios, a quantity of gum arabic as a wall material would be insufficient to fully cover the oil droplets. The insufficiency might result in a decrease in the efficiency. When the emulsion prepared with maltodextrin was spray-dried, only half of the linoleic acid was encapsulated, even at the weight ratio of 0.1. Maltodextrin has little or no surface activity [79, 81]. Therefore, coalescence of the emulsion droplets was likely to occur in the reservoir to the atomizer, although the emulsion in the reservoir was magnetically stirred and phase-separation did not occur, and would result in the low encapsulation efficiency. Since the wall of the dryer was oily after operation, linoleic acid that was not encapsulated would scatter during spray-drying. The encapsulation efficiencies of the microcapsules prepared in the presence of an emulsifier are listed in Table 1. The weight ratio of linoleic acid and maltodextrin was 0.2, and the emulsifier content was 10% by weight of the acid. The addition of an emulsifier improved the efficiency. However, one cannot discuss the effect of the type of emulsifier on the efficiency, because only three kinds of emulsifier were examined. Figure 16 shows the oxidative processes of linoleic aicd encapsulated with gum arabic and maltodextrin at various ratios. The oxidative process of linoleic acid en capsulated with gum arabic largely depended on the ratio, and the acid oxidized faster at a higher ratio. In the case where linoleic acid was encapsulated with maltodextrin, the ratio scarcely affected the oxidative process, and the acid was easily oxidized at any ratio. Similar tendencies were observed for the microcapsules prepared with gum arabic and maltodextrin by hot-air-drying of a single droplet of the emulsion, where the diameter of the prepared microcapsules was 1-2 mm [72]. As shown in Fig. 16, linoleic acid encapsulated with gum arabic, which was surface-active, was more stable toward oxidation than that encapsulated with maltodextrin. Thus, it was examined whether addition of an emulsifier could improve the oxidative stability of linoleic acid encapsulated with maltodextrin (Fig. 17). The addition, however, exhibited no significant effect on improvement in oxidative stability, regardless of the type of emulsifier. Pongincbbi *et al.* reported that addition of an emulsifier retarded the oxidation of linoleic acid in an emulsion. The effect of an emulsifier on the oxidative stability of linoleic acid might differ between in the dehydrated state (microcapsule) and in an emulsion containing much water [82]. The size of the oil droplet would be a factor affecting the stability of the encapsulated liquid. Emulsions with different median diameters prepared by methods A and B were spray-dried to produce microcapsules. The aqueous solution was 15% (w/v) maltodextrin, and Tween 85 was added to the aqueous phase at a ratio of 10% by weight of linoleic acid. The median diameters of the droplets prepared by method A and B were 1.59 ± 0.5 μm (mean ± SD) and 0.98 ± 0.2 μm, respectively. The oxidative processes of linoleic acid in the microcapsules are shown in Fig. 18. Linoleic acid in the microcapsules prepared by method B (smaller droplets) oxidized more slowly than that in the microcapsules prepared by method A. Reineccius showed a higher retention of orange oil in carbohydrate microcapsules for a smaller core material [83]. The observation was consistent with this result. It has been shown that lnioleic acid led to the surface of the microcapsules being easily oxidized [72]. When the droplet of linoleic acid is large, the acid would likely be exposed on the surface of the microcapsule during drying.

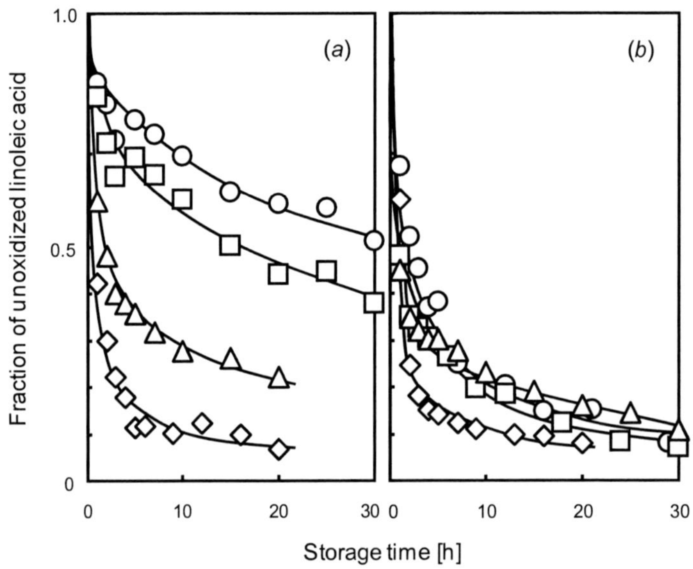

Figure 16. Oxidative process of linoleic acid encapsulated with (*a*) gum arabic and (*b*) maltodextrin at 37ºC and a relative humidity of 12%. The weight ratios of the acid to the polysaccharide were (○) 0.1, (□) 0.2, (△) 0.5 and (◇) 1.0.

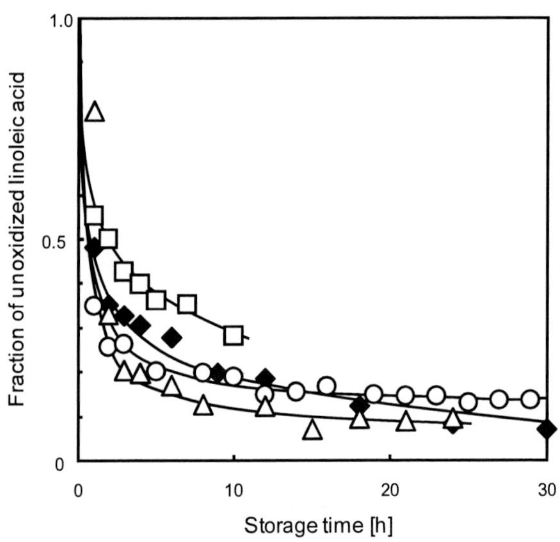

Figure 17. Oxidative process at 37°C and 12% relative humidity for linoleic acid encapsulated with maltodextroin in the presence of (□) Tween 20, (○) Tween 85, (△) Span 20 and (◆) in the absence of any emulsifier.

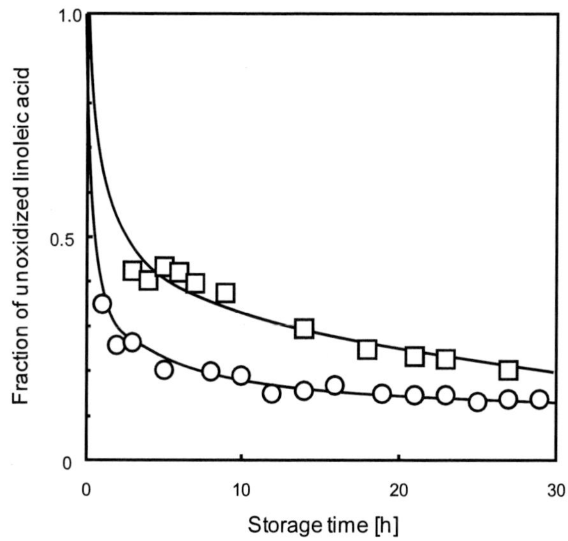

Figure 18. Effect of oil-droplet size in emulsion on oxidative stability of linoleic acid encapsulated with maltodextrin in the presence of Tween 85. The symbols ○ and □ indicate that the emulsions were prepared by method A and B, repectively. The median diameters of the emulsions by method A and B were 1.59 and 0.98 μm, respectively.

Acknowledgments

Most of this study was supported by the Program for the Promotion of Basic Research Activities for Innovative Biosciences (PROBRAIN), Japan.

The authors are very grateful to Dr. Ryuichi Matsuno, Professor Emeritus of Kyoto University and the President of Ishikawa Prefectural University, for his valuable discussions and advise throughout this study, and sincerely appreciate and take pride in the late Dr. Eiichiro Ishido for his patient efforts in this study. The authors would like to thank all the staff of the Laboratories of Department of Biotechnology and Chemistry, Faculty of Engineering, Kinki University, Department of Applied Chemistry and Chemical Engineering, Toyama National College of Technology, and Division of Food Science and Biotechnology, Graduate School of Agriculture, Kyoto University.

References

[1] Labuza, T. P. Kinetics of lipid oxidation in foods. *Crit. Rev. Food Technol.* 1971, 2, 355-404.

[2] Brimberg, U. I. On the kinetics of the autoxidation of fats. *J. Am. Oil Chem. Soc.* 1993, 70, 249-254.

[3] Simic, M. G.; Jovanovic, S. V.; Niki, E. *In Lipid Oxidation in Food (ACS Symposium Series 500)*; Angelo, A. J.; Ed.; Mechanisms of lipid oxidative processes and their inhibition; Washington, D.C., 1992; pp 14-32.

[4] Özilgen, S.; Özilgen, M. Kinetic model of lipid oxidation in foods. *J. Food Sci.* 1990, 55, 498-501, 536.

[5] Adachi, S.; Ishiguro, T.; Matsuno, R. Autoxidation kinetics of fatty acids and their esters. *J. Am. Oil Chem. Soc.* 1995, 72, 547-551.

[6] Minemoto, Y.; Ishido, E.; Adachi, S.; Matsuno, R. Autoxidation kinetics for polyunsaturated acylglycerols. *Food Sci. Technol. Res.* 1999, 5, 104-107.

[7] Craig, B. M.; Murty, N. L. Quantitative fatty acid analysis of vegetable oils by gas-liquid chromatography. *J. Am. Oil Chem. Soc.* 1959, 36, 549-552.

[8] Adachi, S.; Ishiguro, T.; Matsuno, R. Thermal analysis of autoxidation of ethyl esters of n-3 and n-6 fatty acid. *Food Sci. Technol., Int.*1995, 1, 1-4.

[9] Leffler, J. E. The enthalpy-entropy relationship and its implications for organic chemistry. *J. Org. Chem.* 1955, 20, 1202-1231.

[10] Exner, O. Concerning the isokinetic relationship. *Nature*, 1964, 201, 488-490.

[11] Yamamoto, S. Physicolosical eicosanoids – one side of the function of essential fatty acids (in Japanese). *Vitamines* 1998, 72, 699-708.

[12] Miyashita, K.; Takagi, T. Study on the oxidative rate and prooxidant activity of free fatty acids. *J. Am. Oil Chem. Soc.* 1986, 63, 1380-1384.

[13] Portar, N. A. Mechanisms for autoxdation of polyunsaturated lipids. *Acc. Chem. Res.* 1986, 19, 262-268.

[14] Cosgrove, J. P.; Church, D. F.; Proyor, W. A. The kinetics of the autoxidation of polyunsaturated fatty acids. *Lipids* 1987, 22, 299-304.

[15] Frankel, E. N. Recent advances in lipid oxidation. *J. Sci. Food Agric.* 1991, 54, 495-511.

[16] Minemoto, Y.; Kometani, T.; Piao, J.; Adachi, S. Oxidation of oleolyl residue of its esters with ethylene glycol, glycerol and erithritol. *Lebensm. Wiss. Technol.* 2006, 39, 1-5.

[17] Ishido, E.; Minemoto, Y.; Adachi, S.; Matsuno, R. Autoxidation process of linoleic acid and methyl linoleate mixed with saturated fatty acid or its methyl ester. *Lebensm. Wiss. Technol.* 2001, 34, 234-238.

[18] Kiritsakis, A.; Tsipeli, A. Relationship of the acidity of olive oil to its resistance to oxidation. *La Rivista Italiana delle Sostanze Grasse*, 1992, 69, 513-515.

[19] Frega, N.; Mozzon, M.; Lercker, G. Effects of free fatty acids on oxidative stability of vegetable oil. *J. Am. Oil Chem. Soc.* 1999, 76, 325-329.

[20] Ishido, E.; Adachi, S.; Minemoto, Y.; Matsuno, R. Kinetic expression for the oxidation of linoleic and arachidonic acid esters in their mixed system. *Biosci. Biotechnol. Biochem.* 2002, 66, 73-77.

[21] Ishido, E.; Minemoto, Y.; Adachi, S.; Matsuno, R. Oxidation of polyunsaturated acylglycerol mixed with saturated or unsaturated acylglycerol. *Food Sci. Technol. Res.* 2002, 8, 353-356.

[22] Watanabe, Y.; Adachi, S. *In Biochemical Engineering;* Dumont, F. E.; Sacco, J. A.; Ed.; Chapter 2 Enzymatic synthesis of acyl ascorbate and its function as a food additive; Nova Science Publishers, Inc.: New York, NY, 2009; pp 41-77.

[23] Humeau, C.; Girardin, M.; Coulon, D.; Miclo, A. Synthesis of 6-*O*-palmitoyl L-ascorbic acid catalyzed by *Candida antarctica* lipase. *Biotechnol. Lett.* 1995, 17, 1091-1094.

[24] Watanabe, Y.; Adachi, S.; Nakanishi, K.; Matsuno, R. Condensation of L-ascorbic acid and medium-chain fatty acids by immobilized lipase in acetonitrile with low water content. *Food Sci. Technol. Res.* 1999, 5, 188-192.

[25] Yan, Y.; Bornscheuer, U. T.; Schmid, R. D. Lipase-catalyzed synthesis of vitamin C fatty acid esters. *Biotechnol. Lett.* 1999, 21, 1051-1054.

[26] Watanabe, Y.; Adachi, S.; Nakanishi, K.; Matsuno, R. Lipase-catalyzed synthesis of unsaturated acyl L-ascorbates and their ability to suppress autoxidation of polyunsaturated fatty acid. *J. Am. Oil Chem. Soc.* 2001, 78, 823-826.

[27] Watanabe, Y.; Kuwabara, K.; Adachi, S.; Nakanishi, K.; Matsuno, R. Production of saturated acyl L-ascorbate by immobilized lipase using a continuous stirred tank reactor. *J. Agric. Food Chem.* 2003, 51, 4628-4632.

[28] Watanabe, Y.; Adachi, S.; Fujii, T.; Nakanishi, K.; Matsuno, R. Surface activity of 6-*O*-hexanoyl, octanoyl, decanoyl and dodecanoyl ascorbates. *Jpn J. Food Eng.* 2001, 2, 73-75.

[29] Kuwabara, K.; Watanabe, Y.; Adachi, S.; Nakanishi, K.; Matsuno, R. Emulsifier property of saturated acyl L-ascorbate in O/W emulsion. *Food Chem.* 2003, 82, 191-194.

[30] Kuwabara, K.; Watanabe, Y.; Adachi, S.; Nakanishi, K.; Matsuno, R. Continuous production of acyl L-ascorbates using a packed-bed reactor with immobilized lipase. *J. Am. Oil Chem. Soc.* 2003, 80, 895-899.

[31] Watanabe, Y.; Ishido, E.; Fang, X.; Adachi, S.; Matsuno, R. Oxidation kinetics of linoleic acid in the presence of saturated acyl L-ascorbate. *J. Am. Oil Chem. Soc.* 2005, 82, 389-392.

[32] Hashimoto, N.; Aoyama, T.; Shioiri, T. A simple efficient preparation of methyl easters with trimethylsilyldiazomethane ($TMSCHN_2$) and its application to gas chromatographic analysis of fatty acids. *Chem. Pharm. Bull.* 1981, 29, 1475-1478.

[33] Minemoto, Y.; Hakamata, K.; Adachi, S.; Matsuno, R. Oxidation of linoleic acid encapsulated with gum arabic or maltodextrin by spray-drying. *J. Microencapsulation*, 2002, 19, 181-189.

[34] Graf, E. Antioxidant potential of ferulic acid. *Free Rad. Biol. Med.*, 1992, 13, 435-448.

[35] Watanabe, Y.; Fang, X.; Minemoto, Y.; Adachi, S.; Matsuno, R. Suppressive effect of saturated L-ascorbate on the oxidation of linoleic acid encapsulated with maltodextrin or gum arabic by spray-drying. *J. Agric. Food Chem.* 2002, 50, 3984-3987.

[36] Watanabe, Y.; Fang, X.; Adachi, S.; Fukami, H.; Matsuno, R., Oxidation of 6-*O*-arachidonoyl L-ascorbate microencapsulated with a polysaccharide by spray-drying. *Lebensm. Wiss. Technol.* 2004, 37, 395-400.

[37] Taniguchi, H.; Nomura, E.; Tsuno, T.; Minami, S. Ferulic acid ester antioxidant/UV absorbent. *Eur. Patent Appl.* 1998, 0681825A2.

[38] Suzuki, A.; Ochiai, R.; Tokimitsu, I. Compositions and methods for alleviating hypertension or preventing a rise in blood pressure. *U. S. Patent Appl.* 2002, 20020051810.

[39] Fang, X.; Shima, M.; Kadota, M.; Tsuno, T.; Adachi, S. Suppressive effect of alkyl ferulate on the oxidation of linoleic acid. *Biosci. Biotechnol. Biochem.* 2006, 70, 457-461.

[40] Berg, J. J. M.; Cook, N. E.; Tribble, D. L. Reinvestigation of the antioxidant properties of conjugated linoleic acid. *Lipids* 1995, 30, 599-605.

[41] Leung, Y. H.; Liu, R. H. *trans*-10,*cis*-12-Conjugated linoleic acid isomer exhibits stronger oxyradical scavenging capacity than *cis*-9,*trans*-11-conjugated linoleic acid isomer. *J. Agric. Food Chem.* 2000, 48, 5469-5475.

[42] Nagao, T.; Shimada, Y.; Yamauchi-Sato, Y.; Yamamoto, T.; Kasai, M.; Tsutsumi, K.; Sugihara, A.; Tominaga, Y. Fractionation and enrichment of CLA isomers by selective esterification with *Candida rugosa* lipase. *J. Am. Oil Chem. Soc.* 2002, 79, 303-308.

[43] Minemoto, Y.; Adachi, S.; Shimada, Y.; Iwata, T.; Yamaguchi, Y.; Yamamoto, T.; Kometani, T.; Matsuno, R. Oxidation kinetics for cis-9,trans-11 and trans-10,cis-12 isomers of conjugated linoleic acid. *J. Am. Oil Chem. Soc.* 2003, *80*, 675-678.

[44] Watanabe, Y.; Sawahara, Y.; Nosaka, H.; Yamanaka, K.; Adachi, S. Enzymatic synthesis of conjugated linoleoyl ascorbate in acetone. *Biochem. Eng. J.* 2008, 40, 368-372.

[45] Cunha, L. M.; Oliveira, F. A. R.; Oliveira, J. C. Optimal experimental design for estimating the kinetic parameters of processes described by Weibull probability distribution function. *J. Food Eng.* 1998, 37, 175-191.

[46] Watanabe, Y.; Minemoto, Y.; Adachi, S.; Nakanishi, K.; Shimada, Y.; Matsuno, R. Lipase-catalyzed synthesis of 6-*O*-eicosapentaenoyl L-ascorbate in acetone and its autoxidation. *Biotechnol. Lett.* 2000, 22, 637-640.

[47] Mancuso, J. R.; McClement, D. J.; Decker, E.A. The effects of surfactant type, pH, and chelators on the oxidation of salmon oil-in-water emulsions. *J. Agric. Food Chem.* 1999, 47, 4112-4116.

[48] Chaiyasit, W.; Silvestre, M. P. C.; McClements, D. J.; Decker, E. A. Ability of surfactant hydrophobic tail group size to alter lipid oxidation in oil-in-water emulsions. *J. Agric. Food Chem.* 2000, 48, 3077-3080.

[49] Kubouchi, H.; Kai, H.; Miyashita, M.; Matsuda, K. Effects of emulsifiers on the oxidative stability of soybean oil TAG in emulsions. *J. Am. Oil Chem. Soc.* 2002, 79, 567-570.

[50] Miyashita, K.; Nara, E.; Ota, T. Oxidative stability of polyunsaturated fatty acids in an aqueous solution. *Biosci. Biotechnol. Biochem.* 1993, 57, 1638-1640.

[51] Nagler, L. G.; Lankin, V. Z.; Kozachenko, A. I.; Gurevich, S. M. Rate of free radical oxidation of C18 diene and triene fatty acids in aqueous micellar solutions and effectiveness of β-carotene as an inhibitor of their oxidation. *Biochem. (Moscow)* 2003, 68, 203-208.

[52] Chen, J.; Kimura, Y.; Adachi, S. Oxidation of linoleoyl residue of its treharose ester in an aqueous solution. *Food Sci. Technol. Res.* 2006, 12, 163-166.

[53] Chen, J.; Kimura, Y.; Adachi, S. Synthesis of linoleoyl disaccharides through lipase-catalyzed condensation and their surface activities. *J. Biosci. Bioeng.* 2005, 100, 274-279.

[54] Frankel, E. N.; Huang, S. W.; Kanner, J.; German, J. B. Interfacial phenomena in the evaluation of antioxidants: bulk vs emultion. *J. Agric. Food Chem.* 1994, 42, 1054-1059.

[55] Hu, M.; McClements, D. J.; Decker, E. A. Antioxidant activity of a proanthocyanidin-rich extract from grape seed in whey protein isolate stabilized algae oil-in-water emulsions. *J. Agric. Food Chem.* 2004, 52, 5272-5276.

[56] Let, M. B.; Jacobsen, C.; Pharm, K. A.; Meter, A. S. Protection against oxidation of fish-oil-enriched milk emulsions through addition of rapeseed oil or antioxidants. *J. Agric. Food Chem.* 2005, 53, 5429-5437.
[57] Let, M. B.; Jacobsen, C.; Meter, A. S. Ascorbyl palmitate, gamma-tocopherol, EDTA affect lipid oxidation in fish oil enriched salad fressing differently. *J. Agric. Food Chem.* 2007, 55, 2369-2375.
[58] Huang, S. W.; Satué-Gracia, T.; Frankel, E. N.; German, J. B. Effect of lactoferrin on oxidative stability of corn oil emulsions and liposomes. *J. Agric. Food Chem.* 1999, 47, 1356-1361.
[59] Hu, M.; McClements, D. J.; Decker, E. A. Lipid oxidation in corn oil-in-water emulsions stabilized by casein, whey protein isolate, and soy protein isolate. *J. Agric. Food Chem.* 2003, 51, 1696-1700.
[60] Djordjevic, D.; Crecaci, L.; Alamed., J.; McClements, D. J.; Dicker, E. A. Chemical and physical stability of protein- and gum arabic-stabilized oil-in-water emulsions containing limonene. *J. Food Sci.* 2008, 73, C137-C172.
[61] Donnelly, J. L.; Decker, E. A.; McClements, D. J. Iron-catalyzed oxidation of Menhaden oil as affected by emulsifiers. *J. Food Sci.* 1998, 63, 997-1000.
[62] Osborn, H. T.; Akoh, C. C. Effect of emulsifier type, droplet size, and oil concentration on lipid oxidation in structured lipid-based oil-in-water emulsions. *Food Chem.* 2004, 84, 451-456.
[63] Let, M. B.; Jacobsen, C.; Sørensen, A. D.; Meter, A. S. Homogenization conditions affect the oxidative stability of fish oil enriched milk: lipid oxidation. *J. Agric. Food Chem.* 2007, 55, 1773-1778.
[64] Sørensen, A. D.; Baron, C. P.; Let, M. B.; Brüggenmann, D. A. Homogenization conditions affect the oxidative stability of fish oil enriched milk: oxidation linked to changes in protein composition at the oil-water interface. *J. Agric. Food Chem.* 2007, 55, 1781-1789.
[65] Lethuaut, L.; Métro, F.; Genot, C. Effect of droplet size on lipid oxidation rates of oil-in-water emulsions stabilized by protein. *J. Am. Oil Chem. Soc.* 2002, 79, 425-430.
[66] Nakaya, K.; Ushio, H.; Matsukawa, S.; Shimizu, M.; Ohshima, T. Effects of droplet size on the oxidative stability of oil-in-water emulsions. *Lipids* 2005, 40, 501-507.
[67] Imai, H.; Maeda, T.; Shima, M.; Adachi, S. Oxidation of methyl linoleate in oil-in-water micro- and nanoemulsion systems. *J. Am. Oil Chem. Soc.* 2008, 85, 809-815.
[68] Satoh, K. In: *Estimation methods of physical properties; Molecular volume at boiling point (in Japanese);* Maruzen, Tokyo, 1954; pp 150-152.
[69] Matsuno, R.; Adachi, S. Lipid encapsulation technology – techniques and applications to food. *Trends Food Sci. Technol.* 1993, 4, 256-261.
[70] Gibbs, B. F.; Kermasha, S.; Alli, I.; Mulligan, C. N. Encapsulation in food industry, a review. *Int. J. Food Sci. Nutr.* 1999, 50, 213-224.
[71] Imagi, J.; Muraya, K.; Yamashita, D.; Adachi, S.; Matsuno, R. Retarded oxidation of liquid lipids entrapped in matrixes of saccharides or proteins. *Biosci. Biotechnol. Biochem.* 1992, 56, 1236-1240.
[72] Minemoto, Y.; Adachi, S.; Matsuno, R. Autoxidation of linoleic acid encapsulated with polysaccharides of differing weight ratio. *Biosci. Biotechnol. Biochem.* 1999, 63, 866-869.

[73] Re, M. I. Microencapsulation by spray-drying. *Drying Technol.* 1998, 16, 1195-1236.

[74] McClements, D. J.; Dungan, S. R. Factors that affect the ration of oil exchange between oil-in-water emulsion droplets stabilized by a nonionic surfactant: droplet size, surfactant concentration, and ionic strength. *J. Phys. Chem.* 1993, 97, 7304-7308.

[75] Pearce, K. N.; Kinsella, J. E. Emulsifying properties of proteins: evalution of a turbidimetric technique. *J. Agric. Food Chem.* 1978, 26, 716-723.

[76] Bligh, E. G.; Dyer, W. J. A rapid method of total lipid extraction and purification. *Can. J. Biochem. Physiol.* 1959, 37, 911-917.

[77] Dickinson, E.; Murray, B. S.; Stainsby, G.; Anderson, D. M. Surface activity and emulsifier behaviour of some Acacia gums. *Food Hydrocolloids,* 1988, 2, 477-490.

[78] Randall, R. C.; Phillips, G. O.; Williams, P. A. The role of the proteinaceous component on the emulsifying properties of gum arabic. *Food Hydrocolloids,* 1988, 2, 131-140.

[79] Matsumura, Y.; Satake, C.; Egami, M.; Mori, T. Interaction of gum arabic, maltodextrin and pullulan with lipids in emulsions. *Biosci. Biotechnol. Biochem.* 2000, 64, 1827-1835.

[80] McNamee, B. F.; O'Riordan, E. D.; O'Sullivan, M. Emulsification and microencapsulation properties of gum arabic. *J. Agric. Food Chem.* 1998, 46, 4551-4555.

[81] Castle, J.; Dickinson, E.; Murray, B. S.; Stainsby, G. *In Physicochemical and Biochemical Studied ACS Symposium Series* 343; Brash, J. L.; Horbett, D. M.; ED.; Mixed-protein films adsorbed at oil-water interface, protein at interface; American Chemical Society: Washington, 1987; pp 118-134.

[82] Ponginebbi, L.; Nawar, W. W.; Chinachoti, P. Oxidation of linoleic acid in emulsion: effect of substrate, emulsifier and sugar concentration. *J. Am. Oil Chem. Soc.* 1999, 76, 131-137.

[83] Reineccius, G. A. Carbohydrates for flavour encapsulation. *Food Technology* 1991, 45, March, 144-149.

In: Linoleic Acids
Editor: Igho Onakpoya

ISBN: 978-1-62257-384-4
© 2012 Nova Science Publishers, Inc.

Chapter IV

Linoleic and Other Fatty Acids, Cryoresistance, and Fodder Value of Yakutian Plants

Klim A. Petrov, Aleksandr A. Perk and Valentin A. Chepalov
Institute for Biological Problems of the Cryolithozone,
Siberian Branch of Russian Academy of Sciences, Yakutsk, Russia

Abstract

The peculiarity of food preferences of people living in the circumpolar regions is the prevalence in their diet of the albumin-lipid components over hydrocarbon. This is of adaptive importance for the survival of humans in extreme climatic conditions (low temperature and short daylight in winter). Meat from domestic and wild animals is one of the main sources of essential fatty acids, including linoleic acid. Consumer properties of this product depend, first of all, on the quantity and quality of the used feed. We investigated fatty acid composition of the lipids in annual and perennial forage grassy plants (*Avena sativa* L., *Elytrigia repens* L. Nevski, *Equisetum variegatum* Schleich. ex Web., *Equisetum scirpoides* Michx.) during their vegetation and in transitional period in autumn into the frost resistant physiological state under the conditions of the extreme cold climate of the Central and North-Eastern (pole of cold of the Northern hemisphere) Yakutia. Formation of cryoresistance in *Equisetaceae* was accompanied by a significant increase in the level of polyunsaturated fatty acids, including essential fat acids (linoleic and linolenic). In this chapter, problems connected with the role of the linoleic and other polyunsaturated fatty acids in the formation and regulation of cryoresistance of living systems through the food chain are discussed.

Introduction

The peculiarity of food preferences of people living in the circumpolar regions is the prevalence in their diet of the albumin-lipid components over hydrocarbon. This is of adaptive importance for the survival of the humans in extreme climatic conditions (low temperature and short daylight in winter). Linoleic, linolenic and arachidonic fatty acids possess F-vitamin activity and are essential fatty acids in man. Meat of domestic and wild animals has previously, and still is one of the main sources of essential fatty acids for the native population. Consumer properties of this product depend on the quantity and quality of the used feed. More recently, imported vegetable oils (sunflower-seed, soy-bean oils and etc.) began to be used in this capacity, because these crops are not grown in the North conditions. The Yakutia region, which occupies more than 3.1 million square miles of the Russian Siberia is a traditional breeding ground for cattle, horses and reindeers.

Cryoresistance of Plants in the Yakutia Region

Plant growth is an integral process involving the formation of new elements, and the structure of plant organisms reflects the influence of complex environmental factors. Under natural conditions of growth, plants are subject to the influence of various factors, some of which are favorable for growth processes; while others are not, for example, low temperatures. Available evidence suggests that in conditions of the cryolithic zone, plants grow and develop under an extraordinary peculiar climatic situation, caused by the rarest combination of permafrost with high activity of the solar radiation, long daylight with sharp lowering of night temperatures and relatively warm, but short summer.

In this territory, situated exclusively in an area of permafrost (cryolithic zone), seasonal peak temperatures are severe, climatic conditions which are present nowhere else in the world. For example, in Central and North- East Yakutia (pole of cold of the Northern hemisphere) a frostless period lasts 90-110 days at the most, with average temperatures below -40 °C in January, and 18-19 °C in July. Minimal temperatures range from -64 to -68 °C, with maximum temperatures of 34-38 °C. Average annual temperature is -10 to -12 °C. The height of the snow cover is 20-40 centimeters, and the annual precipitation is 200-250 millimeters. Shortness of the vegetative period, evident by sharp rises in temperatures in spring and their fast drop in autumn makes for rapid passage of ontogenesis stages by aboriginal species of plants.

A general theory of plant hardening due to low temperatures under conditions of moderate latitudes was described by Tumanov [1]. According to this theory, herbaceous plants, in order to acquire properties of frost resistance should undergo three stages of preparation: slowing down and stopping of growth, then the first and second stages of hardening. The first stage of hardening occurs in temperatures above 0 °C and in the light (about 10 °C in the day and about 2 °C in the night); the second stage during the gradual decrease to sub-zero temperatures (from -1 to -10 °C) and moderate humidity. The role of photo-synthesis as the key triggering process during the development of cold and frost resistance mechanisms was also shown in the works by Tumanov [1] and was summarized by Levitt [2].

We have previously described the increased content (total and fractional) of lutein and zeaxanthin in the carotenoid composition of grassy and woody plants of Yakutia during hardening, which supports photosynthetic activity at low positive temperatures [3-5]. During cold hardening, because of excessive carbon use in growth processes, elevated amounts of

CO_2 promotes accumulation of certain groups of carbohydrates, proteins and lipids, tied to processes of hardening formation [6].

One of the important properties that confer frost resistance in dormant plants is the ability of cells to counteract the disturbance of membrane integrity. In cell membranes, the fatty acid moieties of lipid molecules regulate their adaptation to unfavourable factors. Large solute material accumulates during interaction of plant lipids with the environment [2, 7]. Adaptive changes of lipids involve the synthesis and dissociation of fatty acids [8], as well as spatial reorganization of its structure [9]; mechanisms that help in the regulation of the membrane fluidity.

Polyunsaturated fatty acids (PUFA) play a key role in the support of membranes' fluidity, their content and composition of which is regulated by the activity of the desaturases. Advances in molecular biology and genetic technology have made it possible to fix characteristics of the cyanobacteria desaturase and to build models of their regulatory activity in low temperature stress [9]. Temperature lowering to 15 °C results in stoppage of cyanobacteria growth and the synthesis of fatty acids for 10 hours. During this period, they desaturate and when the level of unsaturation reaches a critical level, the cells begin to grow again to synthesize fatty acids [10]. The subsequent rise in temperature again inhibits the synthesis of enzymes and activates the synthesis of fatty acids de novo. It has been demonstrated that changes in temperature may regulate the expression of desaturases [11, 12].

In higher plants, the ability of cells to survive in low temperatures, which depends on genes coding desaturases, also correlates in membranes with their composition of PUFA. Membrane lipids of higher plants are characterized by a high degree of unsaturation. Thus, trienoic fatty acids, such as 18:3 and 16:3 constitute up to 70 % of total fatty acid composition. While transferring plants in conditions of low temperatures, preferential transition is observed in 18:2 and 18:3.

Method of Estimation of Fatty Acid Composition in Yakutian Plants

Green sprouts, growing in autumn and those staying green under the snow at the beginning of winter, annual and perennial grassy plants, growing in Central Yakutian and Yana-Indigirka floristic provinces were studied in this research. Oat plants (*Avena sativa* L.), which were sown late in summer (July 15-17) and wild growing creeping couch grass (*Elytrigia repens* L. Nevski) leaves were picked up for analyses in Central Yakutia (62° N, 129° E), and the plant species of variegated horse-tail (*Equisetum variegatum* **Schleich. ex Web.)** and cane horse-tail (*Equisetum scirpoides* Michx.) in the North-East of Yakutia (67° N, 137° E) were also collected, in 2009.

The leaves and sprouts of fodder grasses were fixed in liquid nitrogen and then lyophilized in the VirTis lyophilizer (United States). For lipid extraction, 1 ml of methylating reagent (14% BCl_3 in methanol, the reagent Supelco no. 3-3033) was added to 10 mg of lyophilized material with the internal standard (5 mg/g of tridecane $C_{13}H_{28}$) and kept at 80 °C for 8 h in the hermetic 2 ml vial [13]. After termination of reaction, the vial was cooled and the reaction mixture was neutralized with 5% NaOH. Chloroform (0.2 ml) was added, and FA methyl esters were extracted. The chloroform extract of FA methyl esters was taken with the microsyringe, evaporated to 50 μl, and the aliquot of 2 μl was injected into the Agilent Technology 6890 chromatograph (United States) with the mass-spectrometric 5973 detector and the Innowax column 30 m in length and 0.25 mm inner diameter. Chromatography was conditioned by programmed thermostating from 50 to 240 °C at the rate of 5 °C/min and the temperature of evaporator of 250 °C. Component identification was performed by comparison with the NIST 0.5 mass spectral library.

To characterize the extent of lipid saturation, we used the double bond index (DBI) and unsaturation coefficient (UC) [14]. DBI – was estimated using the formula:

$$DBI = (M\,\% + 2\cdot D\% + 3\cdot Tr\% + 4\cdot Tt\%)\cdot 100,$$

where M – monoenic, D – dienic, Tr – trienic, Tt – tetraenic FA,% from the sum of FA. UC was calculated as the ratio of the total of unsaturated of fatty acids to the sum of saturated fatty acids.

The activity of acyl-lipid membrane ω9, ω6, and ω3 desaturases responsible for insertion double bonds in the carbon skeleton of oleic (C18:1), linoleic (C18:2), and linolenic (C18:3) FAs were calculated as stearoyl-, oleoyl-, and linoleoyl-desaturase ratios (SDR, ODR, LDR, respectively) [15]:

$$SDR = C18{:}1/\,C18{:}0 + C18{:}1,$$

$$ODR = C18{:}2 + C18{:}3/\,C18{:}1 + C18{:}2 + C18{:}3,$$

$$LDR = C18{:}3\,/\,C18{:}2 + C18{:}3,$$

where C18:0 – stearic, C18:1 – oleinic, C18:2 – linoleic and C18:3 – linolenic acids, % from the sum of fatty acids.

These relationships characterize the ability of organisms to support their fatty acid balance by way of changing the degree of saturation and unsaturation of fatty acid lipids during adaptation to the changing conditions of the environment. Each experiment was performed in three parallel biological replicates. All data were processed with Microsoft Excel 2002 software using the macrocomplement XLSTAT-Pro. Values were expressed as means with standard error of means (SEM).

Fatty Acid Composition of Yakutian Plant Lipids

Lipids of wintergreen variegated and cane horse-tails differed greatly from the plants growing in summer, in their content of unsaturated fatty acids (Tables 1 and 2). Emergence of a new row of complex of new fatty acids was observed. If in summer and in spring (autumn) we had identified 10-12 individual fatty acids, then in winter we identified 14-15 fatty acids. On the whole, the absolute content of all fatty acids in horse-tails fluctuates slightly seasonally and constitutes 11-14 mg/g absolute dry substance (ADS).

Table 1. Seasonal changes in the fatty acids composition of lipids of *E. variegatum* sprouts

Fatty acids	Summer mg/g ADS	wt % of total FAs	Autumn mg/g ADS	wt % of total FAs	Winter mg/g ADS	wt % of total FAs
C12:0	-	-	0.12±0.01	0.8±0.1	-	-
C14:0	0.14±0.03	1.2±0.3	0.42±0.04	3.0±0.4	0.12±0.02	1.0±0.2
C15:0	-	-	0.07±0.01	0.5±0.1	0.01±0.01	0.1±0.1
C16:0	4.60±0.30	40.7±5.7	5.61±0.60	40.5±0.6	3.88±0.27	33.5±3.0
C16:2ω4	0.07±0.04	0.6±0.3	-	-	-	-
C16:3ω3			0.34±0.02	2.5±0.4	0.36±0.04	3.1±0.3
C16:3ω1	0.57±0.15	5.1±0.9	-	-	-	-
C17:0	-	-	-	-	0.07±0.01	0.6±0.1
C18:0	0.41±0.10	3.7±1.0	0.73±0.02	5.2±0.7	0.28±0.01	2.4±0.2
C18:1ω9	1.31±0.26	11.6±1.1	0.95±0.09	6.9±1.0	0.44±0.09	3.8±0.9
C18:2ω6	1.30±0.29	11.5±1.3	2.11±0.17	15.2±0.2	1.79±0.12	15.4±0.4
C18:3ω3	2.62±0.54	23.2±2.3	2.83±0.51	20.4±2.0	3.75±0.60	32.4±3.9
C20:0	-	-	0.13±0.01	1.0±0.1	0.09±0.05	0.8±0.4
C20:1ω9	-	-	0.16±0.01	1.1±0.1	0.08±0.02	0.7±0.1
C20:4ω6	0.13±0.09	1.1±0.7	-	-	-	-
C20:4ω3	0.16±0.11	1.4±0.8	0.38±0.04	2.8±0.1	0.37±0.09	3.2±0.6
C22:0	-	-	-	-	0.05±0.01	0.4±0.1
C24:0	-	-	-	-	0.12±0.03	1.0±0.3
C24:1ω9	-	-	-	-	0.18±0.05	1.6±0.3
Σ:	11.31±1.30	100.0	13.86±1.30	100.0	11.57±0.67	100.0
Σ saturated:	5.15±0.43	46.9±6.8	7.08±0.62	51.2±0.7	4.61±0.30	40.0±3.0
Σ unsaturated:	6.16±1.41	53.1±6.8	6.78±0.68	48.8±0.7	6.96±0.69	60.0±3.0
Σ monounsaturated	1.31±0.26	11.3±1.1	1.11±0.09	8.2±1.1	0.70±0.07	6.1±0.7
Σ polyunsaturated	4.85±1.16	41.8±5.8	5.67±0.71	40.6±1.4	6.26±0.73	53.8±3.7
UC		1.13		0.95		1.50
DBI		1.31		1.18		1.56
SDR		0.76		0.57		0.62
ODR		0.75		0.84		0.93
LDR		0.67		0.57		0.68

A most interesting observation was an increase in the relative concentration of linoleic fatty acid: for *E. variegatum* it increased by 34%, *E. scirpoides* by 60%. This fatty acid was one of the most abundant unsaturated fatty acids in these plants, second only to linolenic acid. Such increase of the linoleic acid content, probably, depends on its important role in the adaptation of plants to the conditions of the extreme low temperatures of the polar regions. In contrast to grasses, horse-tails do not lose their over ground part, which stays green during the whole period of wintering under the snow. In connection with this, it is necessary to underscore the nutritive value of horse-tail plants in the capacity of fattening feed for animals, as was commonly thought by the native population, and also reported by researchers of the North [16, 17].

As can be seen from the foregoing data, the lipid composition of horse-tails sprouts consist mainly of unsaturated fatty acids (49-64%). The main portion is made up of the palmitic, oleinic, linoleic and linolenic acids. As earlier described, a reduction in atmospheric temperature causes a decrease in the viscosity of the lipid bilayer of membranes. Transition of membrane lipids from the liquid-crystalline into crystalline state distorts their transport functions in the photosynthetic process and thus interferes with energy production and also metabolism of the membrane protein. To counteract such negative events in the period of adaptation to low temperatures, fluidity of membranes increase. This is a result of an increase in the quantity of the unsaturated fatty acids in phospholipids.

Table 2. Seasonal changes in the fatty acid composition of lipids of *E. scirpoides* sprouts

Fatty acids	Summer mg/g ADS	wt % of total FAs	Autumn mg/g ADS	wt % of total FAs	Winter mg/g ADS	wt % of total FAs
C12:0	-	-	0.03±0.01	0.3±0.1	-	-
C14:0	0.11±0.01	0.9±0.1	0.12±0.01	1.1±0.1	0.10±0.02	0.7±0.1
C15:0	-	-	0.04±0.01	0.3±0.1	-	-
C16:0	4.43±0.47	36.2±4.1	3.60±0.45	32.7±1.1	3.92±0.27	30.7±2.0
C16:1ω7	0.17±0.01	3.6±0.1	0.07±0.02	1.7±0.2	-	-
C16:2ω4	0.13±0.02	1.1±0.1	-	-	-	-
C16:3ω3	-	-	0.47±0.02	4.3±0.3	0.59±0.16	4.6±1.1
C16:3ω1	0.62±0.09	5.1±0.7	-	-	-	-
C17:0	-	-	-	-	0.07±0.01	0.6±0.1
C18:0	0.31±0.08	2.6±0.7	0.25±0.04	2.3±0.2	0.23±0.01	1.8±0.1
C18:1ω9	0.41±0.04	3.3±0.3	0.67±0.07	6.1±0.3	0.60±0.01	4.7±0.4
C18:2ω6	1.40±0.21	11.5±1.4	2.19±0.17	20.0±0.5	2.35±0.01	18.4±1.1
C18:3ω3	4.34±0.33	35.4±1.8	3.13±0.37	28.5±1.3	3.89±0.23	30.4±0.1
C20:0	-	-	0.07±0.01	0.6±0.1	0.06±0.02	0.5±0.2
C20:1ω9	-	-	0.08±0.01	0.7±0.2	0.32±0.26	2.5±2.0
C20:4ω6	0.13±0.03	1.1±0.3	-	-	-	-
C20:4ω3	0.18±0.05	1.5±0.4	0.29±0.01	2.6±0.3	0.22±0.03	1.7±0.1
C22:0	-	-	-	-	0.06±0.01	0.5±0.1
C24:0	-	-	-	-	0.18±0.03	1.4±0.2
C24:1ω9	-	-	-	-	0.21±0.04	1.6±0.2
Σ:	12.24±0.44	100.0	10.99±1.11	100.0	12.79±0.72	100.0
Σ saturated:	4.85±0.56	39.7±4.8	4.10±0.52	37.1±1.4	4.62±0.28	36.2±1.9
Σ unsaturated:	7.39±0.75	60.3±4.8	6.89±0.60	62.9±1.4	8.17±0.59	63.8±1.9
Σ monounsaturated	0.58±0.05	4.8±0.3	0.82±0.08	7.5±0.6	1.12±0.29	8.7±2.0
Σ polyunsaturated	6.81±0.70	55.5±4.5	6.08±0.56	55.4±1.6	7.04±0.43	55.1±0.3
UC		1.52		1.70		1.76
DBI		1.64		1.57		1.57
SDR		0.57		0.73		0.73
ODR		0.93		0.89		0.91
LDR		0.76		0.59		0.62

As earlier noted, conversion of the saturated fatty acids into unsaturated ones in lipids, which is very distinctly observed in variegated horse-tail sprouts, is achieved by the action of desaturases. The activity of these enzymes, as well as the expression of the genes coding them, increases markedly in response to the effects of the hardening temperatures [9]. Furthermore, plants growing in the regions with cold and moderate climate, in adapting to the seasonal lowering of the temperature, experience severe water deprivation. Existence in the lipid matrix of the high unsaturated fatty acids helps to maintain fluid phase condition of the membranes, necessary for reducing water level in living cells, and thereby ensuring stability to low temperature effects.

Influence of Seasonal Variations on the Fatty Acid Composition of Yakutian Plants

The result of our investigation into the fatty acid composition of the forage plants, picked up during their vegetation and in the period of dying off of the over ground oats (taken by us as a forage standard) and creeping couch-grass (the latter is the most wide-spread and eaten grass in pastures) is shown in tables 3 and 4. In both species of plants 8 and 15 types of fatty acids were found, respectively, that is perennial wild growing grass turned out to be more diverse according to fatty acid composition. We associate this also with adaptive peculiarities of perennial plants, due to their ability to withstand low negative temperatures. Before the winter rest such grasses should support adequate amounts of cryoprotecting compounds, in order to be able to form underground supplying organs (roots, rhizomes, tubers). The total amount of fatty acids was considerably higher in oats – 1.72 times in comparison with the couch-grass, and 1.80 times when compared with horse tails.

Table 3. Seasonal changes in the fatty acid composition of lipids of *E. repens* leaves

Fatty acids	Summer mg/g ADS	wt % of total FAs	Autumn mg/g ADS	wt % of total FAs	Winter mg/g ADS	wt % of total FAs
o-C9:0	-	-	0.49±0.15	4.5±1.2	-	-
o-C10:1	-	-	0.92±0.15	8.6±1.0	-	-
C12:0	0.14±0.01	1.2±0.1	0.22±0.04	2.1±0.3	0.16±0.04	1.7±0.4
C14:0	0.35±0.01	2.9±0.1	0.26±0.03	2.5±0.2	0.26±0.03	2.9±0.3
C15:0	-	-	-	-	0.05±0.02	0.5±0.3
C16:0	2.60±0.20	21.6±1.4	3.35±0.53	31.4±3.7	2.95±0.22	32.0±2.0
C16:1ω9	0.28±0.03	2.3±0.3				
C16:1ω7	0.36±0.03	3.0±0.2	0.84±0.08	7.9±0.4	0.28±0.08	2.9±0.7
C18:0	0.20±0.03	1.6±0.3	0.36±0.06	3.4±0.4	0.29±0.04	3.1±0.5
C18:1ω9	0.25±0.02	2.1±0.2	0.07±0.01	0.7±0.1	0.30±0.04	3.2±0.2
C18:2ω6	1.26±0.06	10.4±0.4	1.05±0.26	10.1±2.8	0.77±0.24	8.7±3.1
C18:3ω3	6.62±0.12	54.9±1.5	2.59±0.30	24.8±3.9	3.86±0.56	41.3±4.5
C20:0	-	-	0.22±0.02	2.1±0.1	0.13±0.02	1.4±0.3
C22:0	-	-	0.20±0.03	2.0±0.4	0.13±0.03	1.5±0.3
C24:0	-	-	-	-	0.07±0.01	0.8±0.2
Σ:	12.06±0.18	100.0	10.57±0.46	100.0	9.25±0.48	100.0
Σ saturated:	3.29±0.23	27.3±1.6	5.10±0.79	47.8±5.4	4.05±0.22	43.9±2.6
Σ unsaturated:	8.76±0.15	72.7±1.6	5.47±0.35	52.2±5.4	5.21±0.44	56.1±2.6
Σ monounsaturated	0.89±0.01	7.4±0.1	1.83±0.22	17.2±1.4	0.58±0.11	6.1±0.9
Σ polyunsaturated	7.87±0.14	65.3±1.5	3.63±0.55	35.0±6.7	4.63±0.34	50.0±2.1
UC		2.67		1.09		1.28
DBI		1.93		1.12		1.47
SRD		0.56		0.17		0.51
ORD		0.97		0.98		0.94
LRD		0.84		0.71		0.83

More than 50% of all fatty acids consisted of polyunsaturated linolenic acid, followed by the saturated palmitic acid. Linoleic acid didn't constitute a major fraction, as noticed in horse-tails. Its relative amount constituted 9-14%; moreover, the fall in its index near winter was marked. Because of the large relative quantity of unsaturated fatty acids in oats, its indices of DBI and UC were higher than analogical indices in couch-grass: 1.08 and 1.21 times, respectively. Despite some background differences in the SDR index between plants, other desaturase relationships of ODR and LDR were almost equal, indicating the similarity of functioning of these desaturase systems.

Table 4. Seasonal changes in the fatty acid composition of lipids in *A. sativa* leaves

Fatty acids	Summer mg/g ADS	wt % of total FAs	Autumn mg/g ADS	wt % of total FAs	Winter mg/g ADS	wt % of total FAs
o-C10:1	-	-	0.45±0.10	2.7±0.8	-	-
C14:0	0.19±0.01	0.9±0.1	-	-	0.29±0.02	2.4±0.1
C16:0	4.32±0.25	20.9±1.0	4.30±0.38	24.7±0.8	3.06±0.30	24.9±0.8
C16:1ω7	0.70±0.13	3.4±0.7	0.88±0.03	5.1±0.4	0.37±0.04	3.0±0.1
C18:0	0.38±0.11	1.9±0.6	0.48±0.04	2.8±0.5	0.17±0.01	1.4±0.1
C18:1ω9	0.31±0.03	1.5±0.1	0.49±0.01	2.9±0.3	0.23±0.05	1.9±0.2
C18:2ω6	2.38±0.04	11.5±0.2	2.39±0.10	13.9±0.9	0.88±0.12	7.2±0.8
C18:3ω3	12.43±0.54	60.0±1.4	8.36±1.00	47.8±2.4	7.29±0.73	59.2±0.2
Σ:	20.70±0.47	100.0	17.36±1.26	100.0	12.30±1.19	100.0
Σ saturated:	4.89±0.29	23.6±1.4	4.78±0.35	27.6±0.8	3.52±0.33	28.7±0.9
Σ unsaturated:	15.81±0.52	76.4±1.4	12.58±0.96	72.4±0.8	8.78±0.89	71.3±0.9
Σ monounsaturated	1.01±0.13	4.9±0.7	1.82±0.10	10.7±1.4	0.61±0.09	4.9±0.3
Σ polyunsaturated	14.80±0.58	71.5±1.4	10.76±1.05	61.7±1.8	8.17±0.80	66.4±0.7
UC		3.23		2.63		2.49
DBI		2.08		1.82		1.97
SRD		0.44		0.50		0.57
ORD		0.98		0.96		0.97
LRD		0.84		0.77		0.89

Adaptive Mechanisms for Cryoresistance in Yakutian Plants

During autumn the growth and development of annual and perennial plants cease, and the plants undergo a period of transition with average daily temperatures of 0-5 °C. The duration of this transition in Central (from the 14th of September up to the 3rd of October) and North-East (from the 7th of September up to the 22nd of September) Yakutia is about two weeks. During this period the most favorable weather conditions for frost hardening of the plant organism are present. The predominant meteorological element is the presence of the large number of bright sunny days necessary for photosynthesis, and cool nights which decrease the expenditure of carbohydrates for breathing. Based on the meteorological data collected over several years, , the period with temperatures, optimal for the first phase of hardening (daylight temperatures of 10-15 °C, night time ones from -1 to 3 °C) falls between the second and the third ten-day periods of September. During this period, about 10-15% of annual quantity of sediments fall, and at the end of the season there is predominantly snowfall. A second period with weak (up to -5 °C) and moderate (up to -19-15 °C) frosts, suitable for the second phase of hardening, lasts 25-30 days. Grassy plants, growing in autumn, which undergo hardening, preserve their chlorophyll till the late autumn and stay under the snow in the same state. It is necessary to state that in the conditions of the cryolithic zone, during winter, unfavorable events as rotting and sticking out of the plants are reduced to the minimum; processes linked with the absence of recurrent frosts during this period. That's why, the conception evergreen grassy plants is widespread in Yakutia, because such plants are a source of food for many herbivorous animals in winter time. As previously stated, accumulation of the large quantity of sugar in plant organs during winter crop (being in the state of autumn vegetation) and of the woody plants (being in the state of physiological dormancy), is caused, first of all by the conditions of low temperatures [1, 6].

In a comparative study of the soluble sugar content in the leaves of grassy plants, growing in summer and in autumn in the cryolithic zone of Yakutia, the authors also observed considerable accumulation of mono and disaccharides in over-ground organs of fodder grasses, which remained green under the snow [16].

With increasing specific gravity of the anaerobic breathing, conditions which reduce the intensity of growth processes of the plant organism, the plants go into the state of physiological dormancy. During this period, the main source of getting of free energy is carbohydrate; while in aerobic conditions the main source of getting energy are fats.

The role of lipids in maintaining energetic balance of organisms is extremely vital. Lipids serve as the main reservoir of the reserve energy of organisms, storing it in the most advantageous form. Per unit of mass they contain twice as much quantity of potential energy than carbohydrates and protein. During oxidation of fats, a significantly large quantity of water is released. For example, during the complete oxidation of 100 grams of fats, the amount of the water will be 107.1, while from the protein – 41.3, and from the starch – 55.5 grams of water.

Effect of Cryoresistance on the Fatty Acid Composition of Yakutian Herbivorous Animals

The importance of water formation at the expense of fat burning is especially great under conditions of water deprivation, mainly in the period of winter and summer rest. Due to the specific climatic conditions in Yakutia, one of the main sources of meat and fat, and also of milk, is domestic horse-breeding. It is based on usage of wild-growing grassy plants (referred to as cereals), sedges, and horse-tails. The meat and fat of the horses differ in original consistency, and are a valuable source of unsaturated fatty acids. A unique ability of the native species of the horses is their ability to get food from the deep snow, digging it out with their hoofs – the so called «tebenevka». Wonderful winter pastures for horses are thickets of wintergreen variegated horse-tail and cane horse-tail, which are widely spread in the meadows of some small mountain rivers, flowing into Yana, Indigirka and Kolyma. In autumn, winter, under the snow, they are eaten with great pleasure by horses, domestic and wild reindeers, hares, geese and partridges.

According to several research reports, as well as narratives of the natives, variegated horse-tail possesses the unique ability in the course of a very short time (30-45 days) to restore the strength and fattiness of strongly exhausted horses (Figure 1). For this reason, in some areas of the Verkhoyansky district, horse-breeders in autumn and winter periods organize driving of herds of horses specially for fattening to the far mountain-taiga pastures, where they graze on species of horse-tails.

It is interesting to note, that the fat of the horse, which was fed on the horse-tail forage lands has a reddish-yellow tinge. The latter, according to our data, is due to accumulation of the secondary carotenoid by the sprouts of the variegated horse-tail – rhodoxanthin in the fat tissue of the herbivorous animal:

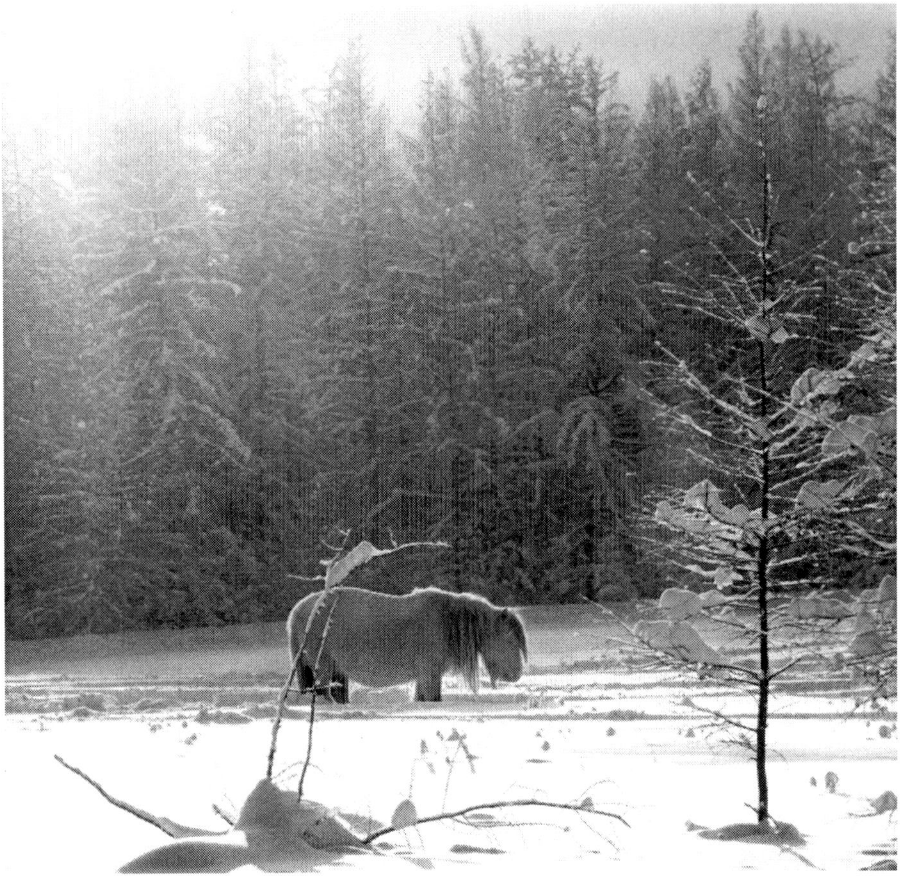

Figure 1. Putting on weight in autumn, the Yakut horse endures extreme low temperatures of the pole of cold quite easily. According to the archeological data, the horse inhabited Yakutia in Pleistocene period, about 35-37 thousand years ago, alongside with mammoths, bisons, saber-toothed tigers [18].

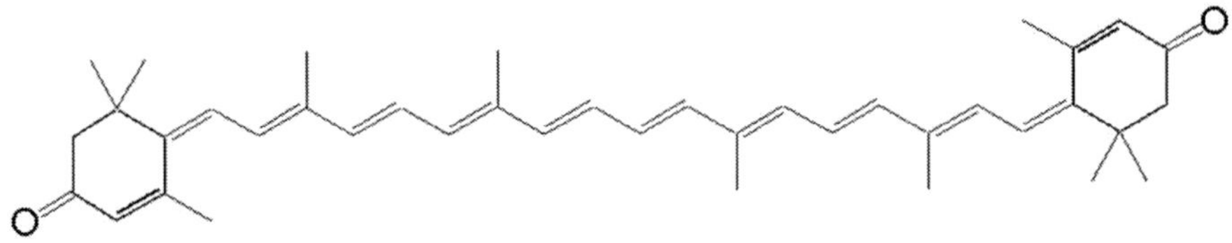

The ability to put on weight is wide-spread in many species of small animals. For example, in autumn, white hare accumulates large supplies of visceral and abdominal fat. Moreover, some hares are literally filled by fat. As is known, herbivorous animals have two main sources of fulfillment of fatty acids pool: biosynthesis of palmitic and stearic acids, and other various fatty acids which are ingested with food. From the mixture of triglycerides, which are in the liver, fatty acids are formed, the composition of which is peculiar to the given species of animal, though on the final fatty acid composition is to some extent influenced by the quality of the food. Saturated fatty acids increase the content of fat and cholesterol in blood of the animal. Thus, why from one side they are harmful, on the other hand they are useful if synthesized.

Table 5. Concentration of fatty acids in meat and fat tissues of agricultural animals (g/100 g)

Meat products	Fatty acids total	Fatty acid type *Saturated*	*Mono saturated*	*Poly saturated*	Polyunsaturated fatty acid content *Linoleic*	*Linolenic*	*Arachidonic and others* **
Beef, average [19]	15.10	7.12	7.42	0.56	0.40	0.14	0.02
Veal [19]	1.78	0.79	0.86	0.13	0.08	0.03	0.02
Meat of the Yakut cattle [17]	23.84	9.85	12.65	1.32	0.77	0.19	0.36
Pork [19]	30.74	11.82	15.38	3.64	3.28	0.22	0.14
Sucking-pig meat [19]	2.74	0.94	1.37	0.43	0.38	0.44	0.01
Horse-flesh [19]	7.84	2.81	3.79	1.24	0.90	0.17	0.02
Yakut foal [17]	17.24	6.50	8.40	2.34	1.90	0.16	0.28
Foal inner fat [17]	34.97	13.40	17.30	4.27	3.40	0.30	0.57
Abdominal fat [17]	21.73	8.20	10.30	3.23	2.70	0.18	0.35
Broilers [19]	11.98	3.70	6.02	2.26	2.04	0.17	0.04
Chicken meat [19]	16.20	4.44	8.59	3.17	2.96	0.17	0.04

**Eicosapentaenic and docosahexaenic acids

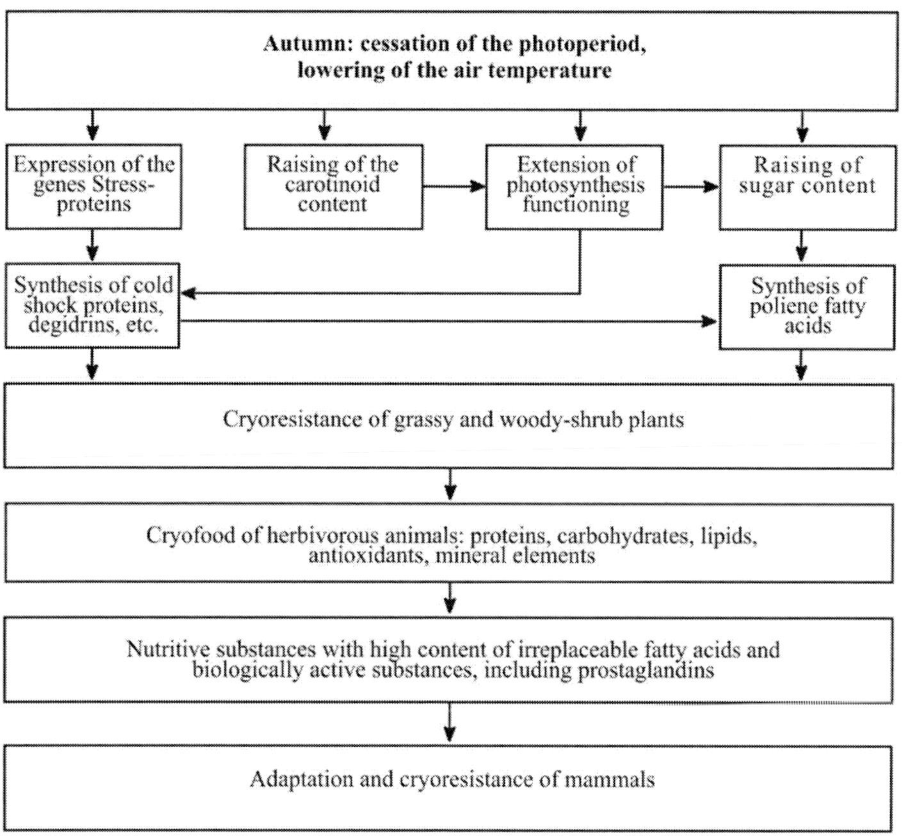

Figure 2. The influence of plant cryoresistance through their nutritive value on adaption and cryoresistance of animals in conditions of Yakutia.

Mono unsaturated fatty acids, primarily oleinic acid are synthesized via the following sequence: palmitic acid → stearic acid → oleinic acid. Of peculiar interest is the question about biosynthesis of PUFA: linoleic, linolenic, arachidonic, eicosapentaenic and docosahexaenic. Linoleic, linolenoic and arachidonic acids, being essential fatty acids, are not synthesized in the animal organism and enter into it with food.

As is seen from the data in table 5, the peculiarity of the Yakut cattle meat and foal's meat, is the high content of the linoleic, arachidonic, eicosapentaenic and docosahexaenic acids in their visceral and abdominal fat. They also confirm the fact, that herbivorous animals, inhabiting Yakutia, are capable of accumulating significant amounts of diet-fed unsaturated fatty acids (especially linoleic acid) in their body cells.

High concentration of arachidonic acid in tissues of the North Yakutian animals indicates active intake of linoleic and linolenic acids with food from grassy plants. In turn, arachidonic acid, being the precursor of prostaglandins, promotes the rise in concentration of these biologically active substances in the animal organism, which determines their adaptive metabolism in the conditions of low temperature stress.

The influence of plant cryoresistance through their nutritive value on adaptation and cryoresistance of animals can be depicted in form of a block diagram (Figure 2).

Effect of Dietary Changes on Fatty Acid Metabolism and Health in Yakutia

As earlier mentioned, in northern (polar) climate, special types of lipid exchange proteins were formed [17, 20]. The northerners' diet consisted predominantly of meat, milk and fish. Sugar, flour products and other carbohydrates were absent earlier in their menu. The natives of the circumpolar region were reputed for having lower risks of cardiovascular disease, bronchial asthma, and rheumatic arthritis. Because older generations ate natural products, they were healthy, gave birth to healthy children, and women were more fertile. But with the onset of civilization, their type of diet began to change. Metabolic changes were observed also in those who had lived in the North for a long time. During transition from one type of metabolism to the other as a result of the changes in diet, there is now an increased incidence of atherosclerosis, angina pectoris, arterial hypertension, diabetes and other diseases. The mortality rate due to these conditions has increased by 52-53%. Among these ailments, the most wide-spread among the inhabitants of modern Yakutia is cardiovascular disease [20]. At present, it is thought that the significant content in the Yakut horse fat of the PUFA (arachidonic and linoleic) promote the retention of the free cholesterol in suspended state in the form of esters. These cholesterol esters subsequently form atherosclerotic plaques in the walls of blood vessels, thereby impairing blood flow to vital organs including the brain and heart. Substances present in the foal fat also reportedly possess anticancer properties [21]. Under the influence of radiation in the human organism, oxidation of lipids is accompanied with an increased formation of free radicals, which promote violation of integrity and increase permeability of cell membranes, and thereby reducing life expectancy [22].

Conclusion

The cryolithic zone of Yakutia is characterized by climatic conditions present nowhere else on earth. Plants in this region undergo a series of changes including slowing down and stoppage of growth, and first and second stages of hardening, to cope with the extremes of temperature. The sharp changes in temperature influence the linoleic and other fatty acid composition of the lipids of plants. Meat of herbivorous animals in this region contains high concentrations of linoleic, linolenic and arachidonic fatty acids. Changes in the dietary habits of the inhabitants of the Yakutian region have resulted in alterations in the composition and metabolic pathway of fatty acids, with consequent detrimental effects on human health.

References

[1] Tumanov, II. Physiology of plant hardening and frost resistance. Moscow: Nauka; 1979 (in Russian).

[2] Levitt, J. Responses of plants to environmental stresses. N.Y.: Academic Press; 1980. Vol. 1.

[3] Petrov, KA; Sofronova, VE; Chepalov, VA; Perk, AA; Maksimov, TC. Seasonal changes in the content of photosynthetic pigments in perennial grasses of cryolithic zone, *Russian Journal of Plant Physiology*, 2010, vol. 57, N. 2, pp. 181-188.

[4] Petrov, KA; Sofronova, VE; Bubyakina, VV; Perk, AA; Tatarinova, TD; Ponomarev, AG; Chepalov, VA; Okhlopkova, ZhM; Vasilieva, IV; Maximov, TC. Woody plants of Yakutia and low-temperature stress, *Russian Journal of Plant Physiology*, 2011, vol. 58, N. 6, pp. 1011-1019.

[5] Petrov, KA; Perk AA; Osipova VV. *Cryo-resistance and formation of forage value of Yakutian grasses.* Yakutsk: Bichik; 2011 (in Russian).

[6] Trunova, TI. *Plant and low-temperature stress. The 64th Timiryazev Lecture. Moscow: Nauka*; 2007 (in Russian).

[7] Harwood, JL. Environmental factors which can alter lipid metabolism, *Prog. Lipid Res*, 1994, vol. 33, N 1/2, pp. 193-202.

[8] Smolenska, G.; Kuiper, PJ. Effect of low temperature upon lipid and fatty acid composition of roots and leaves of winter rape plants, *Phys. Plant.*, 1977, vol. 41, pp. 29-35.

[9] Los, DA. Molecular mechanisms of plant cold tolerance, *Vestn. Ross. Akad. Nauk*, 2005, vol. 75, pp. 338-345 (in Russian).

[10] Sato, N.; Murata, N. Temperature shift-induced responses in lipids in the blue-green alga Anabaena variabilis: the central rol of diacylmonogalatosylglycerol in thermo-adaptation, *Biochim. Biophys. Acta.*, 1980, vol. 619, pp. 353-366.

[11] Los, DA; Horwath, I; Vigh, L; Murata, N. The temperature-dependent expression of the desaturase gene desA in Synechocystis PCC6803, *FEBS Lett.*, 1993, vol. 318, pp. 57-60.

[12] Sakamoto, T; Los, DA; Higashi, S; Wada, H; Nishida, I; Ohmori, M; Murata, N. Cloning of □3 desaturase from cyanobacteria and its use in altering the degree of membrane-lipid unsaturation, *Plant Mol. Biol.*, 1994, vol. 26, pp. 249-263.

[13] Kates, M. *Techniques of lipidology: Isolation, analysis and identification of Lipids.* Amsterdam: Elsevier; 1972.

[14] Lyons, JM; Wheaton, TA; Pratt, HR. Relationship between the physical nature of mitochondrial membranes and chilling sensitivity in plants, *Plant Physiol.*, 1964, vol. 39, pp. 262-268.

[15] Jaworski, JG; Stumpf, PK. Fat metabolism in higher plants. Properties of a soluble stearyl_acyl carrier protein desaturase from maturing Carthamus tinctorius, *Arch. Biochem. Biophys.*, 1974, vol. 162, pp. 158-165.

[16] Potapov, VYa. *Carbon hydrates and lignin in forage grasses of Yakutia.* Moscow: Nauka; 1967 (in Russian).

[17] Abramov, AF. On food and health of the Northerners, *Nauka and technics in Yakutia*, 2007, vol. 13, N 2, pp. 92-96 (in Russian).

[18] Bravina, RI; Alexeeva; SG; Stepanova, NP. *The sacred horse sakha.* Yakutsk: Bichik; 2011 (in Russian).

[19] *Chemical composition of food products*. Moscow: Dely print; 2002 (in Russian).

[20] Timofeev LF; Krivoshapkin VG. *Public health service of the territories with low population density: On example of the Republic Sakha (Yakutia).* Novosibirsk: Nauka; 2006 (in Russian).

[21] Stepanov KM; Krivoshapkin VG; Timofeev GA. *The Yakut horse – the source, giving us health and long life: Prophylaxis of cardiac-vascular diseases.* Yakutsk, 2008 (in Russian).

[22] Harman, D. Aging: A theory based on free radical and radiation chemistry, *Journal of Gerontology*, 1956, vol. 11, N 3, pp. 298-300.

In: Linoleic Acids
Editor: Igho Onakpoya
ISBN: 978-1-62257-384-4
© 2012 Nova Science Publishers, Inc.

Chapter V

Influence of Variety, Geographical Site and Extraction System on Virgin Olive Oil (VOO) Linoleic ACID Composition and its Impact on Consumer Preference

Kaouther Ben Hassine[1,2,3], Amani Taamalli[4], Dhafer Malouche[5], Naziha Kammoun[2], Aida Lazzez[2], Cinzia Benincasa[6], Giovanni Sindona[6], Enzo Perri[6], Mohamed Hammami[7] and Mohamed Bouaziz[8]

[1]Biochemistry Laboratory - UR03/ES08 'Human Nutrition and Metabolic Disorders USCR 'Mass Spectrometry Lab of Monastir Medicine University', Tunisia
[2]Sfax Olive Institute, Tunisia
[3]National Institute for Applied Sciences and Technologies, Tunisia
[4]Centre of Biotechnology of Borj Cedria (CBBC), Tunisia
[5]School of Statistics and information Analysis, Tunisia
[6]CRA Experimental Institute for Olive Growing, C. da Li Rocchi, Rende (CS), Italy
[7]Dipartimento di Chimica, Università della Calabria, Italy
[8]Laboratory of Electrochemical and Environnement,
National Ingenier School of Sfax, Sfax, University, -Tunisia

Abstract

Virgin olive oil (VOO) is known for its unique taste and its effects on health due to its chemical composition. Fatty acid (FA) composition analysis is essential for the qualitative evaluation of VOO, as well as to ensure its authenticity and detect fraud. FA composition analysis is also useful for the classification of VOO and consequently for its commercialization. Studying the effects of the variety, climate, altitude and the degree of olive maturity is useful for improving VOO quality. The VOO FA composition differs from one cultivar to another depending on the region. This chapter aimed at evaluating the effect of the variety, geographical site, and the extraction system on the linoleic acid composition, sensory attributes and consumer preferences. Arbequina and Chemlali olives in same stage of maturity were harvested from various localities in Tunisia. The quality, FA composition, oxidative stability, sensory profile and consumer preferences were estimated using standardized methods. The percentage of linoleic acid ranged from 6.83% to 19.20% in Tunisian and foreign varieties (Coratina and Arbequina). The lowest concentration of linoleic acid was observed in the Italian Coratina variety. A significant effect of the extraction system was observed for major FFA (free fatty acids): oleic, linoleic, palmitic acids. Analysis of the effect of interaction between the extraction system and the geographical site on analytical parameters revealed significant statistical differences ($p<0.05$) in the FFA. Peroxide index, oxidative stability and extinction index K270 showed statistically significant differences ($p<0.005$) with respect to extraction system while extinction index K232 was significantly affected only by geographical site. FA composition revealed statistically significant differences ($p<0.005$) with respect to the interaction between the geographical site and the extraction system in palmitoleic, stearic and linoleic acid, whereas palmitic and oleic acids were affected only by geographical site. Arbequina olive oils extracted by pressure system (SP) showed defects principally musty, metallic and rancid. Other negative attributes such as rancidness and mustiness were the principals defects found in Chemlali olive oils extracted by SP system. In contrast, oils obtained by dual and triple-phase systems showed positive attributes of fruitiness, bitterness and pungency without defects. The consumer preference analysis revealed that Arbequina VOO obtained by 2P extraction system was the most preferred followed by oils obtained by 3P and SP systems respectively. Arbequina and Chemlali oils which are rich in linoleic acid were more preferred by consumers.

List of Abbreviations

2P	Dual-phase
3P	Triple-phase
FA	Fatty acid
FFA	Free fatty acids
VOO	Virgin olive oil
PI	Peroxide index
SP	Pressure system

Introduction

The Mediterranean area is the major international olive-growing area with 98% of the world's *Olea europaea* L. tree plantation [1]. In fact this tree is a typical one widely cultivated for oil production. Tunisia accounts for 57 million of such trees covering 12623 hectares. The most abundant olive variety is *O. europaea* L. cv. Chemlali, which represents more than 60% of the total olive trees [2].

Because of their natural bitterness, olives are rarely consumed as a natural fruit. They are commonly used for the extraction of oil and often as table olives. The decreased incidence of cardiovascular disease in the Mediterranean area is partly attributed to the consumption of olive products principally virgin olive oil (VOO) [3].

VOO possesses a characteristic aroma, taste and colour which distinguish it from other vegetable oils. VOO consumption is currently increasing thanks to its excellent organoleptic and nutritive qualities such as protection from cardiovascular disease and growing consumer preference for minimally processed foods. In fact, VOO is a valuable vegetable oil which is produced without any preliminary refining process [4]. It is extracted from fresh and healthy olive fruits by mechanical and other physical methods (washing, decantation, centrifugation or filtration). These technological procedures, if correctly adopted, are able to preserve the quality of VOO especially its delicate flavor which is highly regarded by the consumer.

The main VOO-producing countries have been particularly active in recent years at studying the chemical composition of VOO varieties or oil produced in a specific area and how this relates to oil quality [5]. VOO has a well-balanced composition of fatty acids (FA), mainly because of the high content of oleic acid, the high ratio of monounsaturated and polyunsaturated FA and the presence of minor compounds that makes it both fairly stable against oxidation, making it very suitable for human consumption. The FA composition analysis is essential for the qualitative evaluation of VOO. It is also one of the ways to ensure the authenticity of VOO and detect fraud. It is of great importance for the classification of VOO and consequently for its commercialization. However, several studies have reported that the quality of VOO depends on many factors: olive tree cultivation, harvesting, pedoclimatic conditions, olive cultivar and processing technique and number of steps required for it; mainly crushing, malaxation and centrifugation [5,6,7,8] . Thus, studying the effects of such factors on the chemical composition of VOO is of interest in order to improve VOO quality. This chapter aims at examining the effect of the variety, geographical site, and the extraction system on the linoleic acid composition, sensory attributes and consumer preferences.

Samples

Arbequina olives were harvested from six localities in Tunisia (Tastour, Fendek jdid, Tela, Grombalia, Sidi Bouzid and Zaghouan) and Chemlali olives were harvested from seven localities (Sawef, Moknine, Barone, Sidi Bouzid, Chaal, Chrarada and Taous) at the same ripeness stage. Olive fruits were processed in industrial olive mill by different extraction systems: pressure system (SP), dual-phase (2P) and triple-phase (3P) decanters. The obtained oils were directly transferred into dark glass bottles and stored for quick analysis.

Quality Indices

Free acidity, peroxide index (PI) and UV spectrophotometric indices (at 232 and 270 nm) were determined according to the European Communities official methods [9].

Fatty Acid Composition

Fatty acid methyl esters (FAMEs) from the oil samples were estimated as described by Issaoui et al. [10]. Individual FAMEs were separated and quantified by gas chromatography

(Hewelett-Packard Ca Palo Alto, Calif) equipped with a flame ionisation detector, and a fused silica capillary column CP-SIL (50m length x 0.25mm i.d. and 0.25µm of film thickness).

Oxidative Stability

Oxidation stability was evaluated by the Rancimat apparatus (Mod. 743, Metrohm Switzerland Ω) using an oil sample of 3g warmed to 120°C and an air flow of 20l/h. Stability was expressed as oxidative stability index (hours).

Sensory Analysis

Sensorial evaluation of the oils was performed according to the Panel test method (COI, 1996) by a fully trained analytical taste panel recognized by the International Olive Oil Council (IOOC). A panel test was established using a standard profile sheet method, (COI/T.20/Doc.15/Rev1, 1996).

Hedonic Study

A panel of 620 consumers (women and men) with an average age of 16 years to 60 years was assembled for this study. A specific investigation sheet was available for the consumers. The consumers were asked to fill out a form and give a grade ranging from 0 to 20.

Statistical Analysis

Statistical analyses were performed using the XLSTAT software v.2011 (Addinsoft). For consumer preference analysis we used SPSS 10.0 for windows.

Physicochemical Variations of VOO Based on Geographical Site and Extraction System

Based on the numerous parameters considered by regulation EC2568/91 for the merceological classification of olive oils, our results showed that all the mono varietal olive oil samples analysed were labelled as "extra virgin" (data not shown). Analysis of the effect of interaction between the extraction system and the geographical site for the two cultivars Chemlali and Arbequina revealed statistically significant differences ($p<0.05$) in few parameters mainly the free fatty acids (FFA). PI, oxidative stability and extinction index K270 showed significant difference ($p<0.005$) with respect to extraction system while extinction index K232 was significantly affected only by geographical site. The Principal component analysis (PCA) in figure 1 shows that acidity from Chemlali oils extracted by SP was higher than that from 2P and 3P systems irrespective of geographical site. A similar result was observed for Arbequina oils (figure 2). It is important to note that there was no significant difference between oils extracted by 2P and 3P systems.

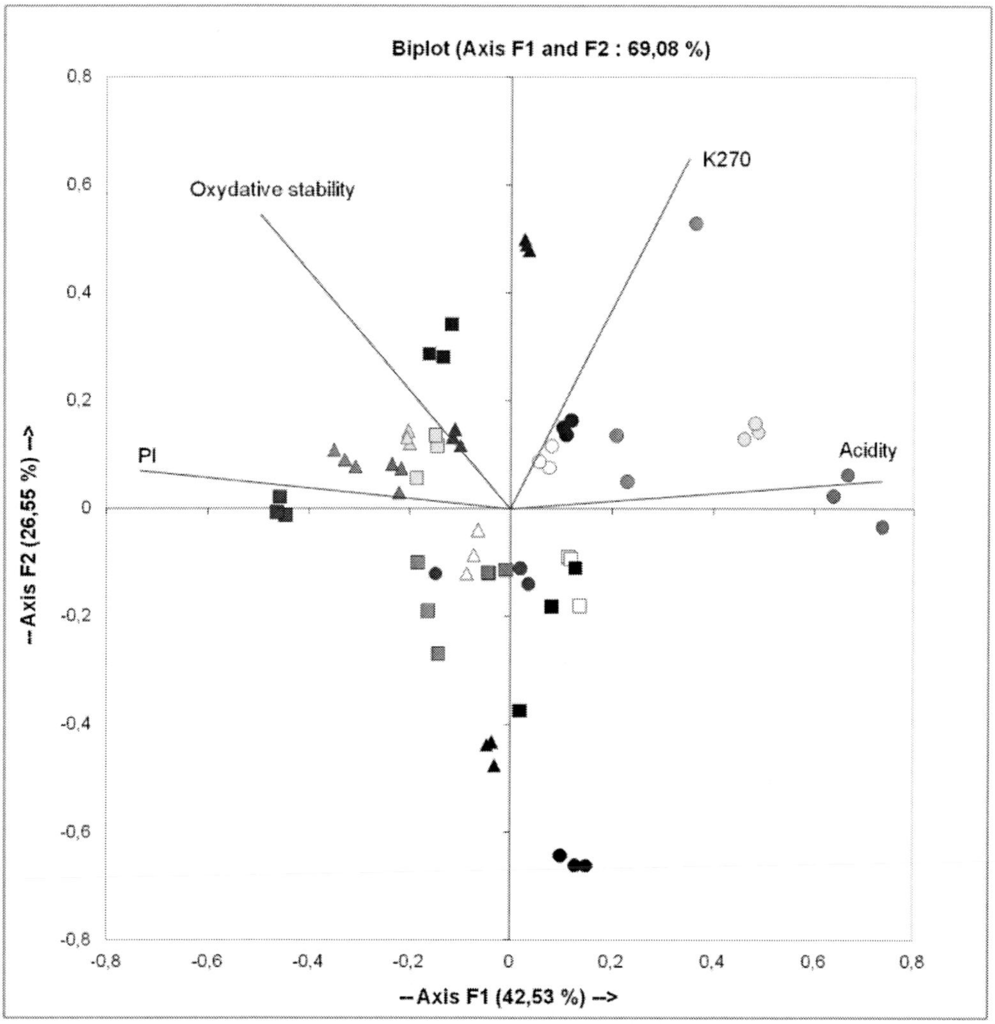

Figure 1. Principal Component Analysis of physicochemical parameters of virgin olive oil related to geographical site and extraction system for Chemlali cultivar. Circles correspond to oils extracted by SP system, squares to oils extracted by Dual-phase system and triangles to those extracted by Triple-phase system. Colours correspond to different geographical sites: Blue for Sawef, Red for Moknine, Yellow for Barone, Green for Sidi Bouzid, Black for Chaal, Orange for Chrarada and White for Taous.

These results corroborate those reported by Torres & Maestri [**Error! Bookmark not efined.,Error! Bookmark not defined.**]. In their study, they explained that in SP system, oil and the vegetable water are extracted and remain together until they are separated by decanting. This prolonged exposure of lipid phase to aqueous phase and solid wastes favour the hydrolysis of triglycerides, resulting in an increase of FFA level. Conjugated dienes (K232) and trienes (K270), and PI are indicators of oxidative deterioration of oils. The highest values of these two indicators are obtained for oils extracted with SP system.

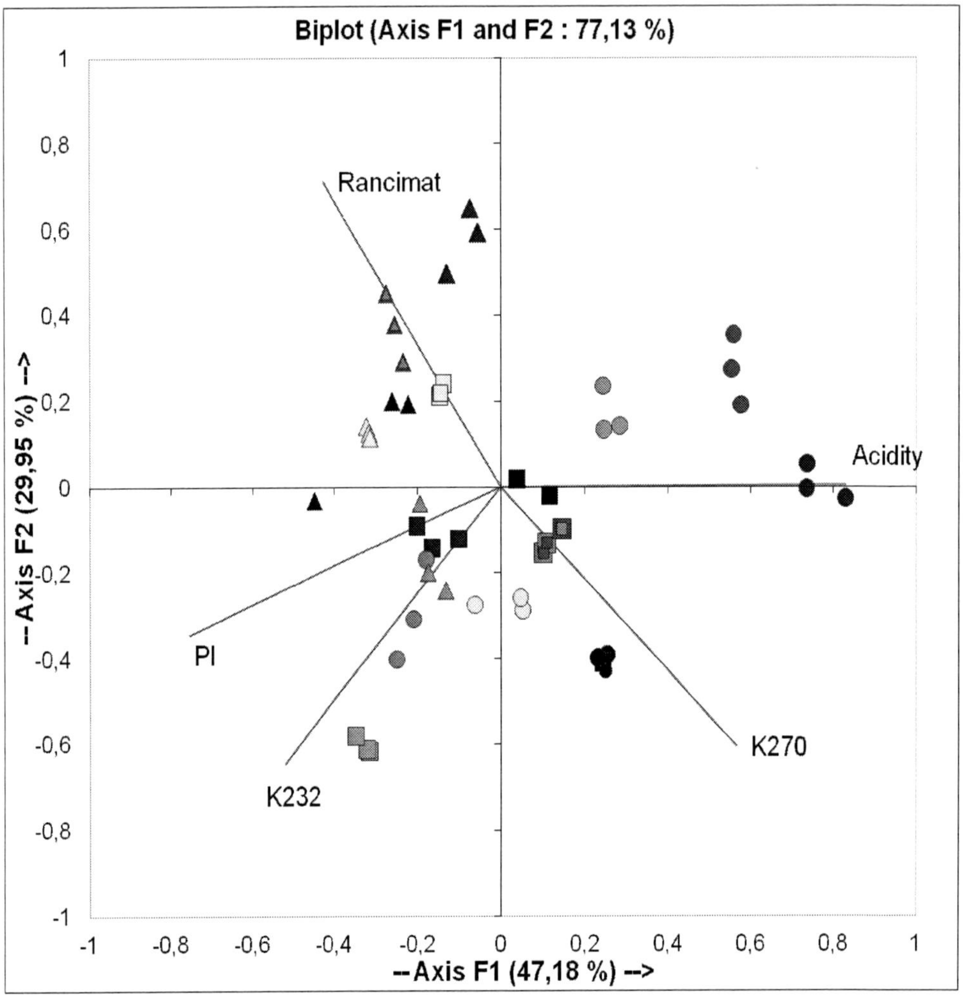

Figure 2. Principal Component Analysis of physicochemical parameters of virgin olive oil related to geographical site and extraction system for Arbequina cultivar. Circles correspond to oils extracted by SP system, squares to oils extracted by Dual-phase system and triangles to those extracted by Triple-phase system. Colours are correspond to different geographical sites: Blue for Tela, Red for Grombalia, Yellow for Tastour, Green for Sidi Bouzid, Black for Fendek Jdid and Orange for Zaghouan.

Fatty Acid Composition of VOO

Fatty acid composition revealed statistically significant differences ($p<0.005$) with respect to the interaction between the geographical site and the extraction system in palmitoleic, stearic and linoleic acids, whereas palmitic and oleic acids were affected only by geographical site. For multivariate analysis of VOO FA composition, PCA was used to assess characterize or classify the oils according to their geographical site and extraction system. The PCA (figures 3 and 4) revealed that VOO is classified by geographical site rather than by extraction system. Arbequina olive oils from Sidi bouzid were characterized by higher levels of linoleic acid whereas Arbequina olive oils from Tela were characterized by higher levels of oleic acid.

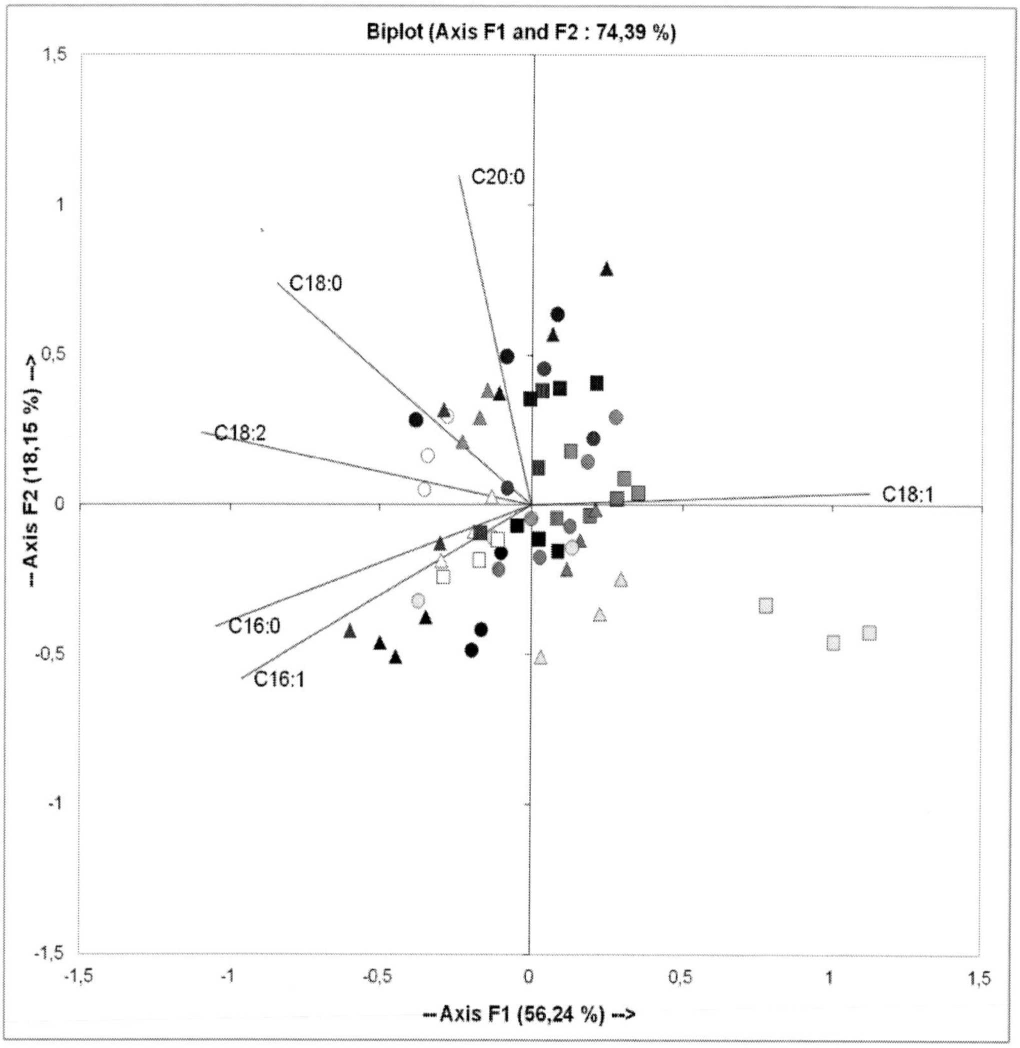

Figure 3. Principal Component Analysis of fatty acid composition of virgin olive oil related to geographical site and extraction system for Chemlali cultivar. Circles correspond to oils extracted by SP system, squares to oils extracted by Dual-phase system and triangles to those extracted by Triple-phase system. Colours correspond to different geographical sites: Blue for Sawef, Red for Moknine, Yellow for Barone, Green for Sidi Bouzid, Black for Chaal, Orange for Chrarada and White for Taous.

The percentage of linoleic acid ranged from 6.83% to 19.20% in Tunisian and foreign varieties (Coratina and Abequina). If we classify oil samples by geographical region into North, Center and South Tunisia, the study shows that there is a noticeable difference in palmitic acid moving from the North to the South. The lowest concentration of linoleic acid was observed in the Italian Coratina variety, one of the most important varieties of the Central region. The highest value of palmitic acid is observed in oils from the Southern regions while the lowest is observed in oils from the Northern regions. Many previous studies have shown that the higher the linoleic acid content of olive oil, the more rapid its oxidation occurs. This makes us conclude that the oils from the North are more resistant to oxidation than oils from the South.

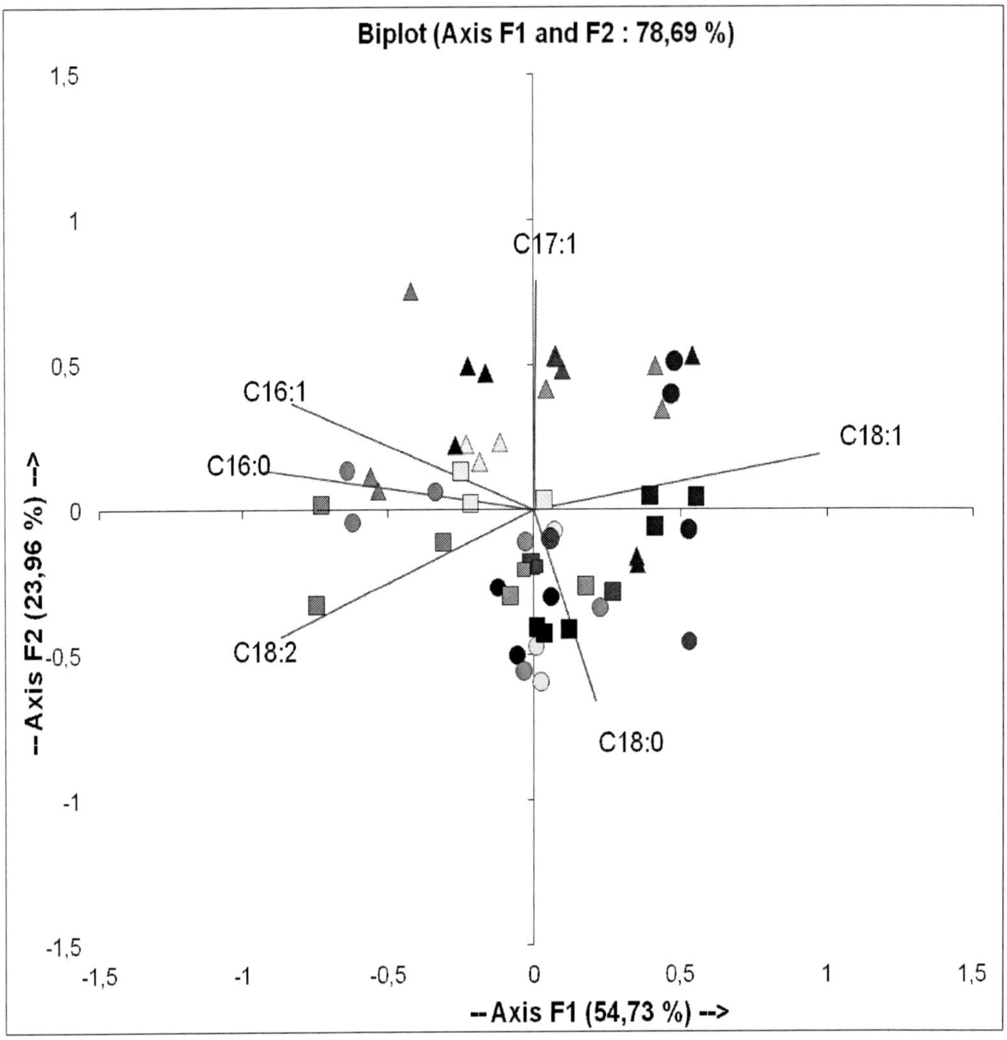

Figure 4. Principal Component Analysis of fatty acid composition of virgin olive oil related to geographical site and extraction system for Arbequina cultivar. Circles correspond to oils extracted by SP system, squares to oils extracted by Dual-phase system and triangles to those extracted by Triple-phase system. Colours correspond to different geographical sites: Blue for Tela, Red for Grombalia, Yellow for Tastour, Green for Sidi Bouzid, Black for Fendek Jdid and Orange for Zaghouan.

Sensory Profile of VOO

Statistical analysis showed that presence of defects detected by the panel was dependent principally on extraction system in Chemlali olive oils (figure 5). Oils extracted by continuous systems (2P and 3P) rarely showed negative attributes in Chemlali cultivar whereas for some localities, olive oils extracted by 2P and 3P systems revealed some defects in Arbequina cultivar (figure 6). This correlates with our statistical analysis which showed that sensory profile for Arbequina oils was related to the interaction between extraction system and geographical site, with a dominant effect of extraction system. We observed that all Arbequina olive oils extracted by SP system showed defects principally musty, metallic and rancid. Rancidness and mustiness were also the principals defects found in Chemlali olive oils extracted by SP system. These defects are related to the prolonged exposure of oil to aqueous phase that increase the apparition of these defects. In contrast to oils obtained by the SP system, those obtained by 2P and 3P systems showed positive attributes of fruitiness, bitterness and pungency without defects.

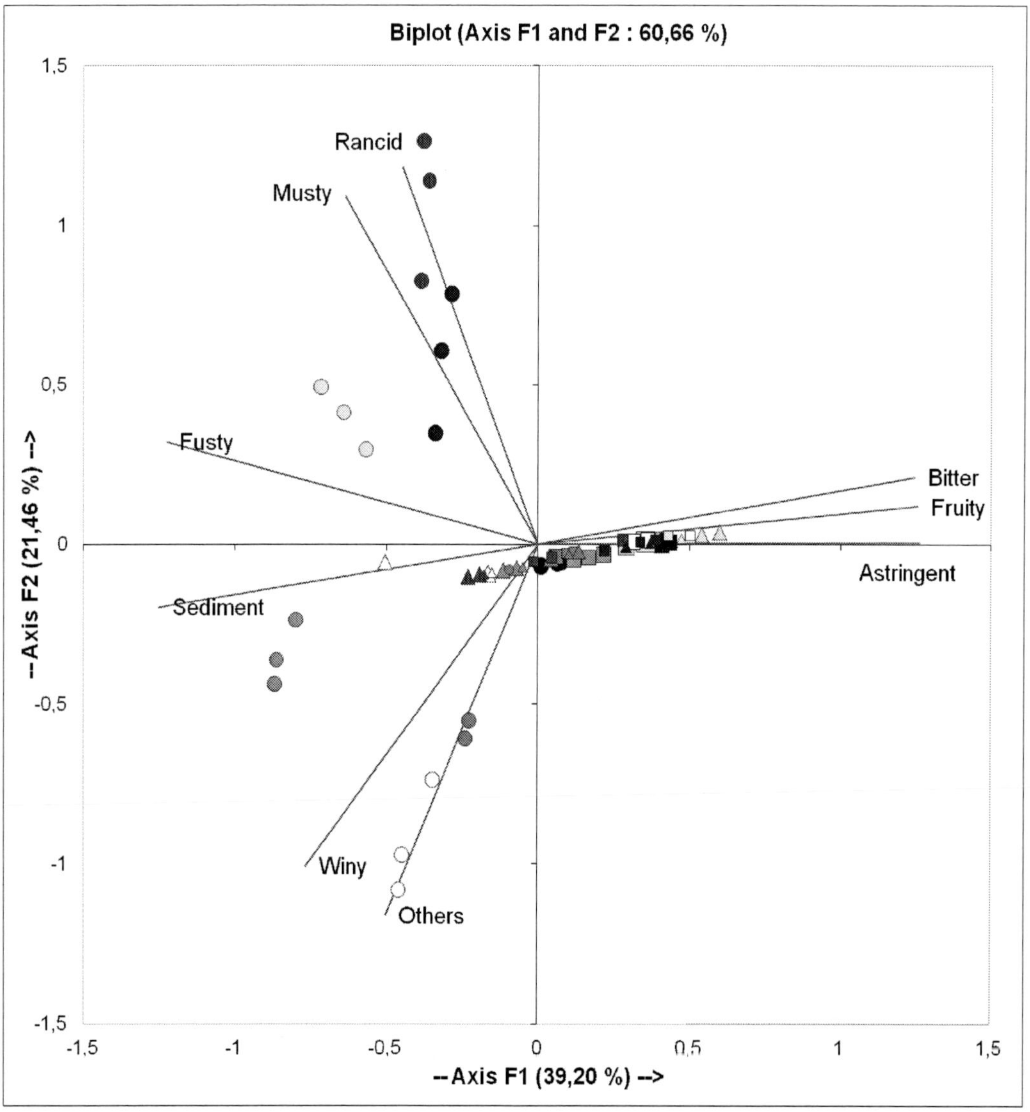

Figure 5. Principal Component Analysis of fatty acid composition of virgin olive oil related to geographical site and extraction system for Chemlali cultivar. Circles correspond to oils extracted by SP system, squares to oils extracted by Dual-phase system and triangles to those extracted by Triple-phase system. Colours correspond to different geographical sites: Blue for Sawef, Red for Moknine, Yellow for Barone, Green for Sidi Bouzid, Black for Chaal, Orange for Chrarada and White for Taous.

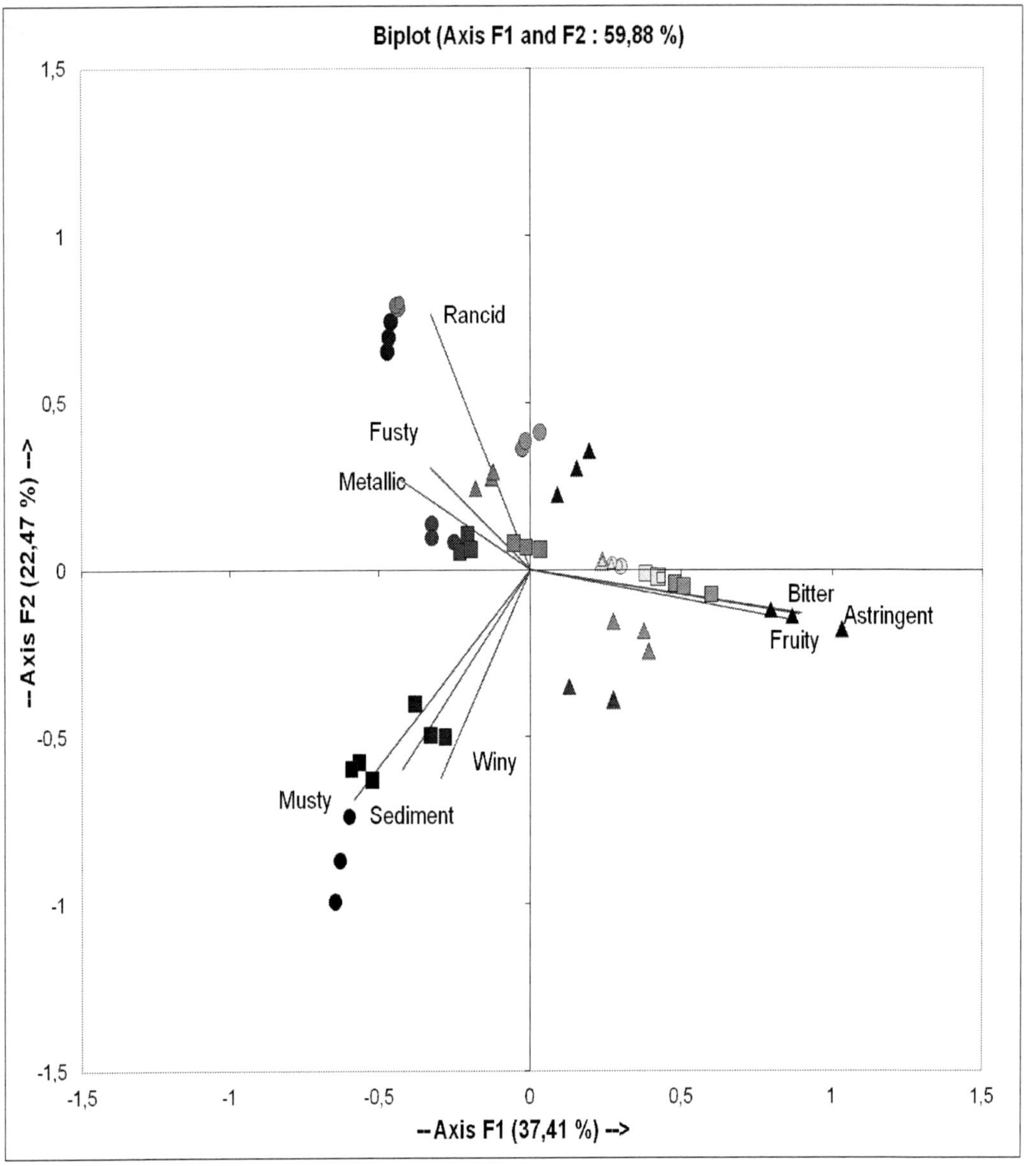

Figure 6. Principal Component Analysis of sensory attributes of virgin olive oil related to geographical site and extraction system for Arbequina cultivar. Circles correspond to oils extracted by SP system, squares to oils extracted by Dual-phase system and triangles to those extracted by Triple-phase system. Colours correspond to different geographical sites: Blue for Tela, Red for Grombalia, Yellow for Tastour, Green for Sidi Bouzid, Black for Fendek Jdid and Orange for Zaghouan.

Consumer Preferences

Consumers gave disgusted oil rating notes from 0 to 20. A Pearson test was used to determine if locality has an effect on consumer preferences.

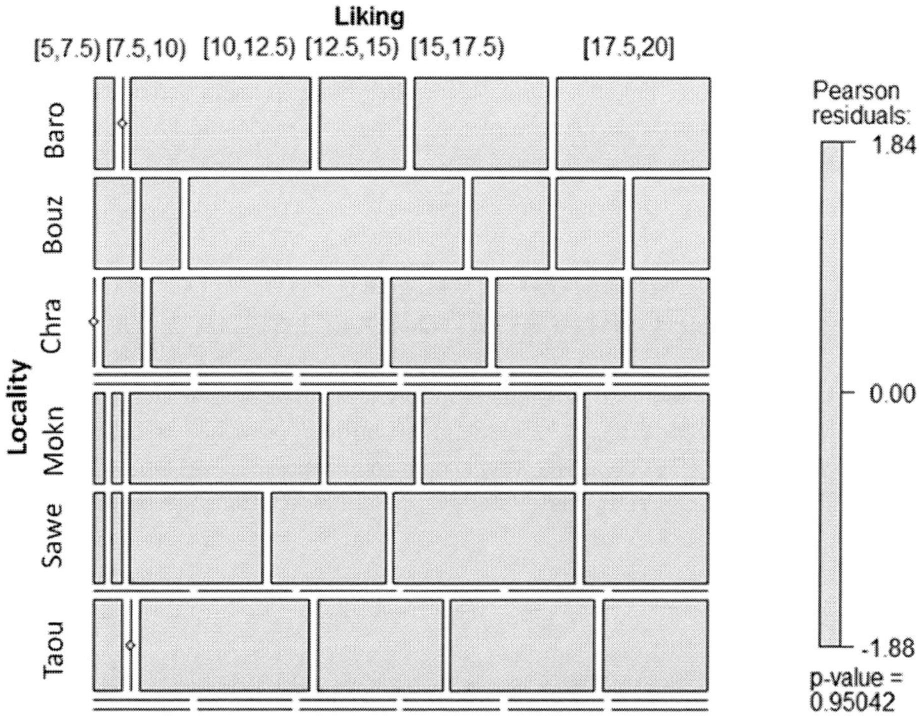

Figure 7. Pearson test for consumer preferences related to geographical site of Chemlali olive oils.

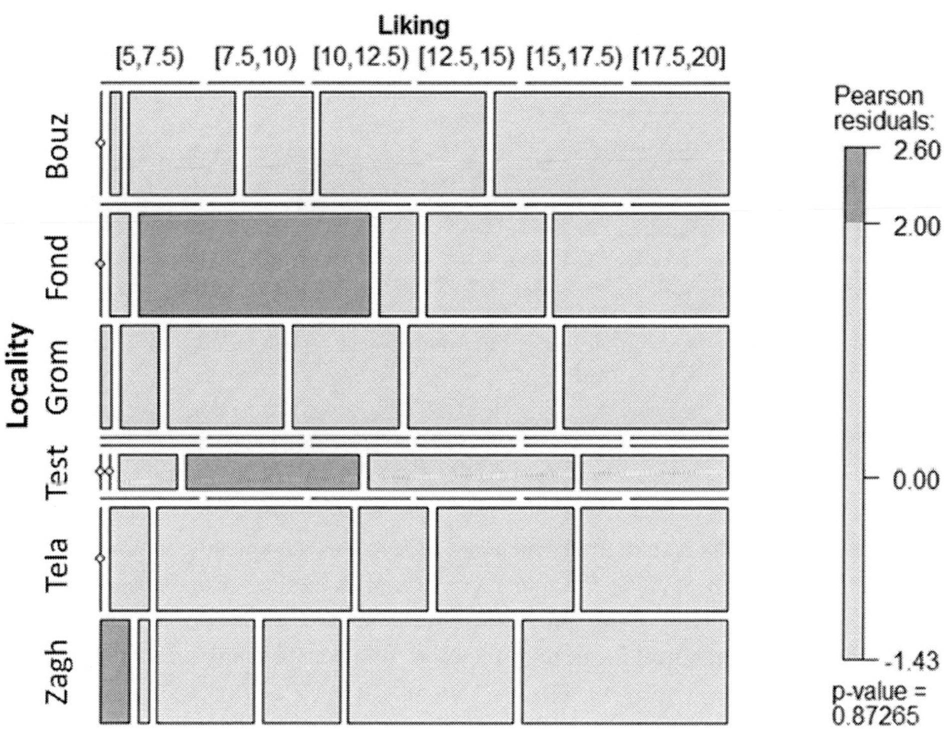

Figure 8. Pearson test for consumer preferences related to geographical site of Arbequina olive oils.

The results showed that the geographical site of Chemlali and Arbequina olive oils had no significant effect on the consumer preferences (figures 7 and 8). However, Arbequina olive oils from Fendek jdid, Zaghaoun and Tastour had more frequent bad and median scores compared to other samples. The absence of a significant effect could have been due to the choice of statistical test.

Linoleic Acid Content and Consumer Preference Related to Cultivar and Extraction System

For linoleic acid content and consumer preferences, there was a significant dominant effect of extraction system (figure 9). Arbequina cultivar presented a higher content of linoleic acid than Chemlali cultivar. However, consumers showed a preference for oils from Chemlali cultivar. This suggests that there's a potential relationship between consumer preferences and linoleic acid content.

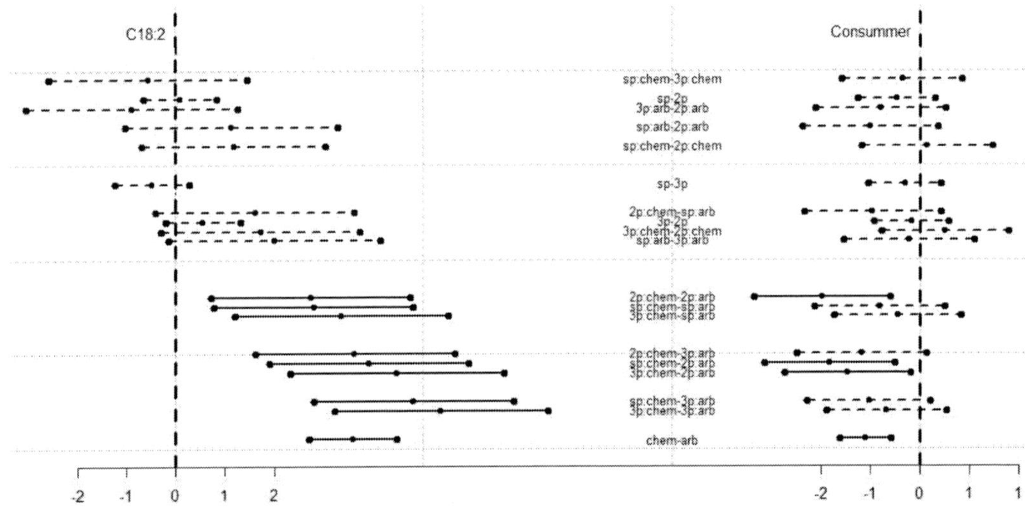

Figure 9. Pearson test for consumer preferences and Linoleic acid content in olive oils from Chemlali and Arbequina cultivars related to extraction system

Conclusion

VOO has unique characteristics which are due to its chemical composition. Its FA composition makes it very suitable for human consumption, and can also be used to classify it and ascertain its authenticity. The properties of VOO are influenced by the extraction methods as well as geographical location of the olive, and consequently affect the preferences of consumers. .

Regardless of the extraction system, oils from Arbequina showed higher content of linoleic acid. The extraction system also had a dominant effect on the sensory profile of Arbequina oil. Consumers showed a greater preference for oils from Chemlali cultivar.

References

[1] Ryan, D., Robards, K. (1998). Phenolic compounds in olive. *Analyst*, 123: 31R-44R

[2] Bouaziz, M., Chamkha, M., Sayadi. S. (2004). Comparative study on phenolic content and antioxidant activity during maturation of the olive cultivar Chemlali from Tunisia. *J. Agric. Food Chem.* 52: 5476 -5481.

[3] Visioli, F., Poli, A., Galli, C. (2002). Antioxidant and other biological activities of phenols from olives and olive oil. *Med. Res. Rev*, 22: 65-75

[4] Olias, J. M., Perèz, A. G., Rios, J. J., Sanz, L. C. (1993). Aroma of virgin olive oil: biogenesis of the "green" odor notes. *J. Agric. Food Chem.* 41: 2368–2373.

[5] Salvador, M.D., Aranda, F., Gómez-Alonso, S., Fregapane, G. (2003). Influence of extraction system, production year and area on Cornicabra virgin olive oil: a study of five crop seasons. *Food Chemistry*, 80: 359–366.

[6] Cerretani, L., Bendini, A., Rotondi, A., Lercker, G., Toschi, T.G. (2005). Analytical comparison of monovarietal virgin olive oils obtained by both a continuous industrial plant and a low-scale mill. *European Journal of Lipid Science and Technology*, 107: 93–100.

[7] Torres, M.M., Maestri, D.M. (2006). Chemical composition of Arbequina virgin olive oil in relation to extraction and storage conditions. *Journal of the Science of Food and Agriculture*, 86 : 2311–2317.

[8] Torres, M.M., Maestri, D.M. (2006). The effects of genotype and extraction methods on chemical composition of virgin olive oils from Traslasierra Valley (Cordoba, Argentina). *Food Chemistry*, 96: 507–511.

[9] EEC. 1991. Commission Regulation EC no 2568/91 July 11, 1991. *Official Journal of the European Communities*, L 248, 001–0082

[10] Issaoui, M., Dabbou, S., Brahmi, F., Ben Hassine, K., Hajaïj Ellouze, M., Hammami, M. (200)9. Effect of extraction systems and cultivar on the quality of virgin olive oils. *International Journal of Food Science and Technology,* 44: 1713–1720

In: Linoleic Acids
Editor: Igho Onakpoya
ISBN: 978-1-62257-384-4
© 2012 Nova Science Publishers, Inc.

Chapter VI

The Effect of Conjugated Linoleic Acid (CLA) Supplementation on Body Anthropometric Measures

Igho Onakpoya[1] and Edzard Ernst[2]
[1]Department of Primary Care Health Sciences, University of Oxford, UK
[2]Complementary Medicine, Peninsula Medical School, University of Exeter, UK

Abstract

Overweight and obesity are public health problems of immense concern, and a variety of management strategies are currently being employed to treat the condition. The use of dietary supplements to promote weight and fat loss has become popular, and the weight loss market is awash with hundreds of such supplements. Conjugated linoleic acid (CLA) is a group of positional and geometric isomers of linoleic acid which are linked by the presence of conjugated dienes. CLA occurs naturally, and can be found in ruminant and non-ruminant animals. CLA is present in moderate amounts in dairy products, and can also be synthesized commercially for dietary consumption. CLA has been reported to possess biologic properties, including anti-carcinogenic and anti-atherogenic functions, and is also thought to improve human immune response. There is some controversy regarding the benefits of CLA on human body composition. Results from animal studies have demonstrated beneficial effects of CLA on human body composition, but findings from human clinical trials have been less than convincing. Numerous clinical trials investigating the effects of CLA on body composition have been conducted, and systematic reviews reporting the effects of CLA on weight and fat loss have been published. This chapter briefly reviews the mechanism of action of CLA, and critically analyses the available evidence from systematic reviews evaluating the efficacy and safety of CLA on various body weight parameters.

Introduction

The prevalence of overweight and obesity have increased over the last two decades [1], and this has become a public health burden for governments across the world [2]. The economic consequences of obesity are enormous and continuous to increase; by one estimate Americans will spend $319 billion annually by 2020 on obesity treatment [3].

Overweight and obesity are defined as an excess in body weight. These excesses are usually defined in terms of the body mass index (BMI) in kg/m^2. Based on the World Health Organisation (WHO) criteria, a BMI range between 25 and 29.9kg/m^2 is defined as overweight, while a BMI $\geq$30kg/m^2 is defined as obesity. Obesity is also characterized by an excess of body fat accumulation with multiple organ-specific pathological consequences [4]. The WHO estimates that worldwide obesity has more than doubled since 1980, and that 65% of the world's population live in countries where overweight and obesity kills more people than underweight [5]. Overweight and obesity are risk factors for many diseases including diabetes, hypertension, osteoarthritis, and even some cancers [6]. Genetic, environmental, as well as lifestyle factors are thought to play a major part in the etiology of the condition [7].

Different management strategies are being employed to tackle this condition, and the use of weight loss supplements as anti-obesity treatments is quite popular. The dietary supplement industry is awash with hundreds of such supplements, yet the scientific evidence regarding the efficacy of most of these supplements is not convincing [8]. One such supplement which has generated much interest recently is conjugated linoleic acid (CLA).

Origin, Structure and Functions of CLA

CLA is a naturally occurring fatty acid which is produced by bio-hydrogenation in the rumen [9]. It is a group of 18-carbon positional and geometric isomers of linoleic acid which are linked by the presence of conjugated dienes [10]. These conjugated dienes could be in cis or trans configuration, are located at different points along the 18-carbon chain, but are usually found in the 7 and 9, 8 and 10, 9 and 11, or 10 and 12 positions [11]. Of all the isomers of CLA, the cis-9,trans-11 (c9,t11) and cis-10,trans-12 (c10,t12) have been reported to possess biologic activity [12]. The isomers are a component of the lipid fraction, and can be found in meat and dairy products [11]. CLA can also be synthesized by ruminants via the action of Δ9-desaturase on trans-11-octadecanoic acid [13]. The c9,t11, also known as rumenic acid is the most abundant isomer [14]. The CLA isomers can also be manufactured commercially by hydrogenation of linoleic acid or by heating linoleic acid in the presence of alkali [9]. CLA is also commonly available over-the-counter, either as a sole supplement, or in combination with other food supplements.

CLA has been reported to possess a variety of biologic functions which are beneficial to human health. It has been purported to have anti-carcinogenic, anti-atherogenic as well as anti-diabetic properties [15]. Dietary CLA is also been demonstrated to possess beneficial effects on the immune system [16]. Though animal studies have demonstrated beneficial effects of CLA on blood pressure [17], results from human studies have failed to report similar positive effects [18, 19].

Mechanisms of Anti-Obesity Effect

A number of mechanisms by which CLA supplementation causes changes in body composition have been proposed (Table 1). These mechanisms are largely based on research from animal models, as well as tissue cultures.

Increased Energy Expenditure

Animal models have demonstrated that CLA supplementation increases energy expenditure. Results from CLA-supplemented experimental animals fed a high or low-fat diet for 6 weeks showed significant reductions in growth rates, energy intake, adipose depot weight, and carcass lipid and protein content when compared with non-CLA supplemented controls [20]. The investigators postulated that CLA intake in the animals caused an increased stimulation of the autonomic nervous system, resulting in an alteration in energy utilisation via increased lipolysis.

Cellular mechanisms responsible for the increased energy expenditure caused by CLA have also been investigated. It has been reported that an uncoupling protein 2 (UCP2) plays a vital role in the energy expenditure caused by CLA [21]. CLA supplementation was reported to have increased UCP2 mRNA amounts. It has been speculated that the up-regulation of the mRNA in white adipose tissue of mice causes increased levels of energy expenditure [22].

The c10,t12 isomer of CLA, specifically, has been reported to increase oxygen consumption [23]. Human trials have also demonstrated that CLA supplementation resulted in increased resting metabolic rates when compared with placebo [24].

Increase in Fat Oxidation

Animal studies have shown that CLA supplementation results in increased carnitine palmitoyl- transferase activity, thereby resulting in increased oxidation of fatty acids [25]. The t10,c12-CLA isomer in particular was reported to increase hepatic and adipose carnitine palmitoyltransferase activity [26]. CLA supplementation has also been demonstrated to cause increased activity of hormone-sensitive lipase (HSL) and reduced activity of lipoprotein lipase (LPL) in adipose tissues [27, 28].

Human clinical trials have demonstrated that mixed CLA isomer supplementation positively altered fat oxidation as well as energy expenditure in the resting state [29]. The investigators postulated that the mechanism for the efficacy of CLA supplementation for fat loss was at least partly due to increased fat oxidation during sleep.

Inhibition of Lipid Synthesis

Experimental models and animal studies have shown that CLA supplementation inhibits the synthesis of lipids. A key enzyme in lipid metabolism is the adipocyte enzyme, lipoprotein lipase (LPL) which breaks down triacylglycerols, and thereby providing non-esterified fatty acids for tissue catabolism [30]. This enzyme breaks down fatty acids from circulating triacylglycerol, thereby enhancing fatty acid uptake and re-esterification by adipocytes [17]. *In vitro* studies have shown that the activity of LPL is reduced by CLA supplementation [25]. *In vitro* studies have also demonstrated that concentrations of intracellular triacylglycerols can be decreased by CLA [31]. CLA is also thought to inhibit the stimulation of peroxisome proliferators activated receptors (PPAR), thereby preventing the differentiation of preadipocytes into the adipocyte cells [32].

In vitro studies have demonstrated that when the t10,c12 CLA isomer is added to differentiating 3T3-L1 preadipocytes, there was a dose-dependent reduction in the expression of stearoyl-CoA desaturase 1, a vital enzyme in lipogenesis [33]. The t10,c12 isomer of CLA has also been reported to decrease the triacylglyceride content, as well as glucose incorporation into stromal vascular cells in human adipose tissues [34]. Some authors have reported that this reduction in fat synthesis is unrelated to the amount of fat ingested from diet, and the effect of CLA on reduced fat accumulation was unaffected by a reduction in daily caloric intakes [35].

Stimulation of Apoptosis

CLA has been reported to induce apoptosis in adipocytes. CLA is able to cross the cell membranes of adipocytes with the help of specific membrane-bound fatty acid transporters and binds to tissue-specific fatty acid binding protein (FABP) in the cytosol. CLA/FABP complex is able to stimulate specific PPAR. Stimulation of PPAR is thought to lead to adipocyte cell death.

CLA supplementation in animals has also been reported to increase the expression of the cytokine, tumor necrosis factor alpha (TNF α) [36]. *In vitro* studies have demonstrated that TNF α causes cell death in human adipose tissue [37].

Aside cell death, CLA has been reported to cause decreases in adipocyte size. Investigators have reported significant reductions in adipocyte cell size as well as reductions in triacylglyceol content due to CLA administration from *in vitro* studies [38].

Decreased Appetite

CLA has been reported to cause significant reductions in serum leptin levels [39, 40]. Animal studies have demonstrated that the reduction in serum leptin levels correlates with a reduction in appetite, and subsequent reduction in body weight and fat [40]. It has been hypothesized that CLA intake inhibits the synthesis of leptins from adipocytes, and thus reduces its serum concentrations [41].

The results from human studies investigating the effects of CLA supplementation on serum leptin have been inconsistent. In one study, while CLA supplementation resulted in a transient decrease in serum leptin levels, this decrease was not sufficient enough to alter appetite [42]. However, in another clinical study involving athletes, and lasting 6 months, the investigators reported that reduction in serum leptin concentrations correlated significantly with a decrease in body fat [43].

Table 1. Some proposed mechanisms of action of CLA*

Purported Action	Mechanism
Increased energy expenditure	a. Stimulation of the autonomic nervous system [21] b. Up-regulation of UCP2Mrna [22]
Increase in fat oxidation	a. Increased carnitine palmitoyl-transferase activity [25] b. Reduced activity of lipoprotein lipase [28]
Inhibition of lipid synthesis	a. Stimulation of PPAR [32] b. Reduction in the expression of stearoyl-CoA desaturase 1 [33]
Stimulation of apoptosis	a. Stimulation of PPAR [32, 36] b. Increased expresseion of TNF α [37]
Decreased appetite	a. Reduction in serum concentrations of leptin [39, 40, 41]

* these mechanisms have been largely described based on findings from animal studies

Table 2. Key details of systematic reviews of CLA supplementation on body anthropometric measures

First Author Year	Daily CLA dosage	No of trials (participants)	Quality of primary studies	Baseline BMI of participants	Study duration	Main Results	Other metabolic effects	Adverse Events	Adjustments for lifestyle factors	Authors' conclusions
Salas-Salvado 2006	0.7-6.8 g	21 (852)	Not reported	<25-35 kg/m²	12-104 weeks	20 trials reported no sig. effects on body weight	Possible negative effects on glucose metabolism	Lowering of HDL cholesterol	Not controlled for in most studies	"…not enough evidence to show that CLA has an effect on weight and body composition in humans"
Whigham 2007	Mean dose 3.2 g	18 (1258)	Not reported	24.5-40 kg/m²	≤12 weeks for most trials	3.2g/day of CLA caused a significant decrease in fat mass compared with placebo ($p<0.001$)	None reported	Increased WBC counts, increase in CRP	Not reported	"…CLA produces modest loss in body fat in humans"
Onakpoya 2011	2.4-6.0 g	7 (974)	Variable	≥25 kg/m²	6-12 mths	Small sig difference in weight loss and fat loss favoring CLA over placebo	Not reported	Constipation, diarrhea, muscle pain, MI	Dietary control, exercise	"..evidence from longer-term RCTs not convincing enough"

Abbreviations: CLA: conjugated linoleic acid; BMI: body mass index; HDL: high density lipoprotein; WBC: white blood cell; CRP: C-reative protein; MI: myocardial infarction; RCTs: randomized clinical trials.

Effect on Body Anthropometric Measures: Evidence from Systematic Reviews

A comprehensive search of the literature identified three systematic reviews analysing the effects of CLA supplementation on human body composition (Table 2). Two of these reviews [44, 45] included trials irrespective of study duration or body weight of participants; the third and more recent one included only longer-term trials involving overweight and obese individuals [46].

Effect on Body Weight

Salas-Salvado et al. [44] reported the effects of CLA on body weight from 21 trials. Of these, 20 reported no significant changes in body weight due to CLA intake.

In a meta-analysis of six studies lasting at least 6 months, Onakpoya et al. [46] reported a statistically significant difference in weight loss favouring CLA over placebo (MD: -0.70kg; 95% CI: -1.09, -0.32). This represented a weight loss of approximately 1% from baseline in comparison with placebo. A sensitivity analysis from the same review failed to reveal a statistically significant difference in weight reduction between CLA and placebo (MD: -0.66kg; 95% CI: -1.1, 0.21). The authors did not detect a significant relationship between CLA dosage and weight loss ($p > 0.05$).

Effect Waist Circumference and BMI

Increased waist circumference is a predictor of metabolic risk [4], thus a reduction in waist circumference is desirable in overweight and obese individuals. A BMI > 30kg/m^2 is usually reflected by an increase in waist circumference [4].

Onakpoya et al. [46] reported the effects of CLA supplementation on waist circumference and BMI. A meta-analysis of 3RCTs and involving 534 participants, the authors reported a non-significant difference in waist circumference between CLA and placebo (MD: -0.12cm; 95% CI: -0.82, 0.58). The same authors also reported a small significant decrease in BMI in the CLA group when compared with placebo (MD: -0.30kg/m^2; 95% CI: -0.44, -0.16).

Effect on Fat Mass

In a review by Salas-Salvado et al. [44] of 5 studies which measured body composition with DXA, significant reductions were found in fat mass in participants who took CLA in two studies; there was however no report on inter-group differences. The effect of CLA ingestion on fat mass was reported not to be significant in the 3 remaining studies. A significant increase in lean body mass was also noted in one of the studies.

In a meta-analysis of 18 studies, Whigham et al. [46] reported a significant difference in reduction in fat mass in the CLA group compared with placebo ($p = 0.03$). This result was based on an analysis of dose-effect. A further analysis based in the median dose of CLA revealed an even more significant effect of CLA intake in reducing fat mass when compared with placebo ($p < 0.001$). The measurement of body composition in the included studies was by validated methods such as Dual-energy X-ray absorptiometry (DXA), bioelectric impedance (BIA), hydrodensitometry and hydrostatic weighing. Most of the clinical trials in this review were less than 12 weeks in duration. The authors reported a significant dose-response effect relationship between CLA supplementation and loss of body fat.

In a more recent meta-analysis of 6 longer-term clinical trials, Onakpoya et al. [46] reported a small significant difference in fat loss favouring CLA over placebo (MD-1.33 kg; 95% CI: -1.79, -0.86). The studies included in the meta-analysis all determined body composition using DXA.

Effect on Other Metabolic Parameters

Salas-Salvado et al. [44] reviewed the effects of CLA on blood lipids in 6 trials. There was no significant effect of CLA on total or LDL-cholesterol observed in any study. Participants administered CLA in two studies had significant decreases in HDL-cholesterol, both with single and mixed isomers.

Salas-Salvado et al. [44] also reviewed the effects of CLA supplementation on glucose metabolism. Though the data was scarce, the authors reported that glucose metabolism may be negatively affected by CLA supplementation. The effects of CLA supplementation on insulin function were mixed, based on the findings from different trials included in the review.

Adverse Events

Salas-Salvado et al. [44] reported that CLA supplementation in obese individuals was associated with an increase in oxidative stress markers. The authors also drew attention to a possible link between CLA supplementation and lipid peroxidation. However, the findings from several studies in this review were contradictory in this respect.

Whigham et al. [45] reviewed the reports of adverse events from various other research. These included elevations in biomarkers of inflammatory disease, including C-reactive protein and WBC counts. The elevations of these biomarkers are in themselves regarded as indicators, rather than a cause of disease. Other adverse events include increased insulin resistance resulting in hyperinsulinemia; though this is controversial.

Onakpoya et al. [46] also reported on the adverse events of CLA consumption. These included diarrhea, soft stools, abdominal discomfort, musculoskeletal pain, as well as myocardial infarction.

Comments

Salas-Salvado et al. [44] and Whigham et al. [45] did not assess the methodological quality of included trials. The failure to account for the quality of the included trials casts doubts on the robustness of the meta-analytic results. Most of the trials included in both systematic reviews were ≤12 weeks, and this does not allow for an evaluation of CLA effects on body composition on the long-term.

Only 6 trials investigating the effects of CLA on body composition were included for meta-analysis by Onakpoya et al. [46]. In some of the outcomes, only 3 trials were included in the analysis. The small number of included trials, small sample sizes in included trials, as well as the poor reporting quality of the included trials limits the conclusion that can be drawn from the meta-analytic results.

Lifestyle modifications are an important component in the management of overweight and obesity [47]. There were large variations in how lifestyle changes were incorporated into the clinical trials included in the reviews. These included normal lifestyle, dietary control and dietary control with exercise. The extent to which these modifications influenced the outcome of the meta-analyses results does not seem to be accounted for.

The various mechanisms of actions by which CLA supplementation is purported to induce positive effects on body composition have largely been demonstrated only in animal studies. Unless such mechanisms are replicated in humans, similar significant effects may not be observed. The large variation in dosages also suggests that the minimum effective dose of CLA which could influence body weight and body fat is uncertain.

While animal studies seem to consistently indicate that CLA supplementation does have marked significant effects on body composition, results from systematic reviews of clinical trials have been less convincing. It has been suggested that this is possibly due to a variety of factors including discrepancies in experimental designs, gender factors as well as genetic predisposition to fat accumulation [14].

Almost all trials in the 3 systematic reviews had a mixture of both the c9,t11 and the c10,t12 isomers. While c9,t11 is more abundant, c10,t12 is reported to be the more active isomer metabolically [48]. Clinical trials involving single isomers may be of benefit in evaluating the effects of individual CLA isomers on human body composition.

Though CLA is reported to be generally safe, a number of adverse effects have been reportedly associated with its use. There has been an isolated case report of toxic hepatitis linked to CLA intake [49]. Significant impairments in endothelial function have also been reported with its usage [50]. Since CLA is reported to cause insulin resistance, there may be the possibility of interactions with anti-diabetic medications, and possibly with other types of medications. These issues suggest that CLA intake is not entirely risk-free, and longer-term surveillance may be needed to monitor its safety.

Conclusion

The findings from available systematic reviews fail to convincingly show that CLA supplementation results in any clinically relevant effects on body weight, waist circumference and BMI. The results from the systematic reviews all indicate that CLA supplementation results in statistically significant reductions in body fat mass; the clinical relevance of this effect is uncertain. CLA appears to be generally safe, but possible adverse effects linked to its usage have been reported.

References

[1] Jones-Smith JC, Gordon-Larsen P, Saddiqi A, Popkin BM. Is the burden of overweight shifting to the poor across the globe? Time trends among women in 39 low- and middle-income countries (1991–2008). *Int. J. Obes. (Lond.)*. 2011 Sep 13. doi: 10.1038/ijo.2011.179. [Epub ahead of print].

[2] Kelly T, Yang W, Chen C-S, Reynolds K, He J. Global burden of obesity in 2005 and projections to 2030. *Int. J. Obes*. 32, 1431-1437 (2008).

[3] Dor AF, Langwith C, Tan E. *A heavy burden: The individual costs of being overweightbese in the United* . The George Washington University School of Public Health and Health Services Department of Health Policy, 2010.

[4] Haslam D, Sattar N, Lean M. Obesity-time to wake up. In: Sattar N, Lean M (eds). *ABC of Obesity*. 2007, Blackwell, Malden, pp1.

[5] World Health Organisation, Mar. 2011. *Obesity and Overweight Fact sheet* No 311. Available from: *http://www.who.int/mediacentre/factsheet.* [Accessed 23 Jan, 2012].

[6] Kopelman P. Health risks associated with overweight and obesity. *Obes. Rev*. 8(Suppl 1), 13-17 (2007).

[7] Wadden, T.A., McGuckin, B.G., Rothman, R.A., Sargent, S.L. Lifestyle Modification in the Management of Obesity. *J. Gastro. Surg*. 7(4), 452-463 (2003).

[8] Onakpoya IJ, Wider B, Pittler MH, Ernst E. Food supplements for body weight reduction: a systematic review of systematic reviews. *Obes*. 19, 239-244 (2011).

[9] Banni S. Conjugated linoleic acid *Curr. Opin. Lipidol*. 13(3), 261-6 (2002).

[10] Belury M. Dietary conjugated linoleic acid in health:physiological effects and mechanisms of action. *Ann. Rev. Nutr*. 22, 505-531 (2002).

[11] Thomas M, Soren T, Arne A. Efficacy and safety of dietary supplements containing CLA for the treatment of obesity: evidence from animal and human studies. *J. Lipid. Res*. 44(12), 2234-2241 (2003).

[12] Silveira M-B, Carraro R, Monereo S, Tébar J. Conjugated linoleic acid (CLA) and obesity. *Public Health Nutr*. 10(10A), 1181–1186 (2007).

[13] Griinari JM, Corl BA, Lacy SH, Chouinard PY, Nurmela KV, Bauman DE. Conjugated linoleic acid is synthesized endogenously in lactating dairy cows by Delta(9)-desaturase. *J. Nutr*. 130, 2285-91 (2000).

[14] Plourde M, Jew S, Cunnane SC, Jones PJH. Conjugated linoleic acids: why the discrepancy between animal and human studies. *Nutr. Rev*. 66(7), 415-421 (2008).

[15] Aydin R. Conjugated Linoleic Acid: Chemical Structure, Sources and Biological Properties . *Turk. J. Vet. Anim. Sci*. 29, 189-195 (2005).

[16] Song HJ, Grant I, Rotondo D, Mohede I, Sattar N, Heys SD, Wahle KW. Effect of CLA supplementation on immune function in young healthy volunteers. *Eur. J. Clin. Nutr*. 59(4), 508-17 (2005).

[17] Declercq V, Taylor CG, Zahradka P. Isomer-specific effects of conjugated linoleic acid on blood pressure, adipocyte size and function. *Br. J. Nutr*. Sep 23,1-9 (2011). [Epub ahead of print].

[18] Raff M, Tholstrup T, Sejrsen K, Straarup EM, Wiinberg N. Diets Rich in Conjugated Linoleic Acid and Vaccenic Acid Have No Effect on Blood Pressure and Isobaric Arterial Elasticity in Healthy Young Men. *J. Nutr*. 136, 992-997 (2006).

[19] Engberink MF, Geleijnse JM, Wanders AJ, Brouwer IA. The effect of conjugated linoleic acid, a natural trans fat from milk and meat, on human blood pressure: results from a randomized crossover feeding study. *J. Human Hypertension* 26, 127-132 (2012).

[20] West DB, DeLany JP, Camet PM, Blohm F, Truett AA, Scimeca JA. Effects of conjugated linoleic acid on body fat and energy metabolism in the mouse. *Am. J. Physiol.* 275, 667-672 (1998).

[21] Tsuboyama-Kasaoka N, Takahashi M, Tanemura K, et al. Conjugated linoleic acid supplementation reduces adipose tissue by apoptosis and develops lipodystrophy in mice. *Diabetes* 49, 1534 – 42 (2000).

[22] Wang Y, Jones JPH. Conjugated linoleic acid and body composition. *Am. J. Clin. Nutr.* 79(suppl): 1153S– 8S (2004)

[23] Wang YM, Rahman SM, Nagao K, Han SY, Yanagita T. The comparative effects of triglyceride-type and free fatty acid-type conjugated linoleic acids on hepatic lipid content and metabolism in OLETF obese rats. *J. Oleo. Sci.* 52, 129-134 (2003).

[24] Kamphuis MMJW, Lejeune MPGM, Saris WHM, Westerterp-Plantenga MS. The effect of conjugated linoleic acid supplementation after weight loss on body weight regain, body composition, and resting metabolic rate in overweight subjects. *Int. J. Obes.* 27, 840-847 (2003).

[25] Park Y, Albright KJ, Liu W, Storkson JM, Cook ME, Pariza MW. Effect of conjugated linoleic acid on body composition in mice. *Lipids* 32, 853-858 (1997).

[26] Martin JC, Gregoire S, Siess MH, et al. Effects of conjugated linoleic acid isomers on lipid-metabolizing enzymes in male rats. *Lipids* 35, 91– 8 (2000).

[27] Park Y, Storkson JM, Albright KJ, Liu W, ParizaMW.Evidence that the *trans*-10,*cis*-12 isomer of conjugated linoleic acid induces body composition changes in mice. *Lipids* 34, 235– 41 (1999).

[28] Park Y, Storkson JM, Ntambi JM, Cook ME, Sih CJ, Pariza MW. Inhibition of hepatic stearoyl-CoA desaturase activity by *trans*-10,*cis*-12 conjugated linoleic acid and its derivatives. *Biochim. Biophys. Acta.* 1486, 285–92 (2000).

[29] Close RN, Schoeller DA, Watras AC, Nora EH. Conjugated linoleic acid supplementation alters the 6-mo change in fat oxidation during sleep. *Am. J. Clin. Nutr.* 86, 797-804 (2007).

[30] Mead JR, Irvine SA, Ramji DP. Lipoprotein lipase: structure, function, regulation, and role in disease. *J. Mol. Med. (Berl).* 80(12), 753-69 (2002).

[31] Park Y, Pariza MW. Lipoxygenase inhibitors inhibit heparin-releasable lipoprotein lipase activity in 3T3–L1 adipocytes and enhance body fat reduction in mice by conjugated linoleic acid. *Biochim. Biophys. Acta.* 1534, 27–33 (2001).

[32] Brown, J, Mclntosh M. Conjugated linoleic acid in humans: regulation of adiposity and insulin sensitivity. *J. Nutr.* 133: 3041–3046 (2003).

[33] Choi YJ. Kim YC, Han YB, Park Y, Pariza MW, Ntambi JM. The trans 10, cis-12 isomer of conjugated linoleic acid downregulates stearoyl- CoA desaturase gene expression in 3T3–L1 adipocytes. *J. Nutr.* 130, 1920 – 4 (2000).

[34] Brown JM, Halvorsen YD, Lea-Currie YR, Geigerman C, McIntosh M. Trans10cis12, but notcis9trans11, conjugated linoleic acid attenuates lipo-genesis in primary cultures of stromal vascular cells from human adipose tissue. *J. Nutr.* 131: 2316-2321 (2001).

[35] DeLany JP, West DB. Changes in body composition with conjugated linoleic acid. *J. Am. Coll. Nutr.* 19, 487-493 (2000).

[36] Tsuboyama-Kasaoka N, Takahashi M, Tanemura K, Kim HJ, Tange T, Okuyama H, Kasai M, Ikemoto S, Ezaki O. Conjugated linoleic acid supplementation reduces adipose tissue by apoptosis and develops lipodystrophy in mice. *Diabetes* 49, 1534–1542 (2000).

[37] Prins JB, Niesler CU, Winterford CM, Bright NA, Siddle K, O'Rahilly S, Walker NI, Cameron DP. Tumor necrosis factor alpha induces apoptosis of human adipose cells. *Diabetes* 46, 1939–1944 (1997).

[38] Evans M, Geigerman C, Cook J, Curtis L, Kuebler B, McIntosh M. Conjugated linoleic acid suppresses triglyceride accumulation and induces apoptosis in 3T3–L1 preadipocytes. *Lipids* 35, 899 –910 (2000).

[39] Rahman SM, Wang Y-M, Yotsumoto H, Cha J-Y, Han S-Y, Inone ,Yanagita T. Effects of Conjugated Linoleic Acid on Serum Leptin Concentration, Body-Fat Accumulation, and β-Oxidation of Fatty Acid in OLETF Rats. *Nutr.* 17, 385-390 (2001).

[40] Botelho AP, Santos-Zago LF, Costa de Oliveira A. Conjugated linoleic acid supplementation modified the body composition and serum leptin levels in weaning rats. *Arch. Latinoam. Nutr.* 58(2), 156-63 (2000).

[41] Yamasaki M, Ikeda A, Oji M, Hirao A, Kasai M, Iwata T, Tachibana H, Yamada K. Modulation of Body Fat and Serum Leptin Levels by Dietary Conjugated Linoleic Acid in Sprague-Dawley Rats Fed Various Fat-Level Diets. *Nutr.* 19, 30-35 (2003).

[42] Medina EA, Horn WF, Keim NL, Havel PJ, Benito P, Kelley DS, Nelson GJ, Erickson KL. Conjugated linoleic acid supplementation in humans: effects on circulating leptin concentrations and appetite. *Lipids*. 2000; 35(7): 783-8 (2000).

[43] von Loeffelholz C, Kratzsch J, Jahreis G. Influence of conjugated linoleic acids on body composition and selected serum and endocrine parameters in resistance-trained athletes. *Eur. J. Lipid Sci. Tech.* 105(6), 251-259 (2003).

[44] Salas-Salvadó J, Márquez-Sandoval F, Bulló M. Conjugated linoleic acid intake in humans: a systematic review focusing on its effect on body composition, glucose, and lipid metabolism. *Crit. Rev. Food. Sci.* Nutr. 46, 479–488 (2006).

[45] Whigham LD, Watras AC, Schoeller DA. Efficacy of conjugated linoleic acid for reducing fat mass: a meta-analysis in humans. *Am. J. Clin. Nutr.* 85, 1203–1211 (2007).

[46] Onakpoya IJ, Posadzki PP, Watson LK, Davies LA, Ernst E. The efficacy of long-term conjugated linoleic acid (CLA) supplementation on body composition in overweight and obese individuals: a systematic review and meta-analysis of randomized clinical trials. *Eur. J. Nutr.* 51(2), 127-34 (2012).

[47] Avenell A, Sattar N, Lean M. Management: part I-behaviour change, diet, and activity. In: Sattar N, Lean M (eds). *ABC of Obesity*. 2007. Blackwell, Malden, pp 8–11.

[48] Kang K, Liu W, Albright KJ, Park Y, Pariza MW. trans-10,cis-12 CLA inhibits differentiation of 3T3-L1 adipocytes and decreases PPAR gamma expression. *Biochem. Biophys. Res. Commun.* 303, 795–799 (2003).

[49] Ramos R, Duarte P, Vicente C, Casteleiro C. Conjugated linoleic acid-induced toxic hepatitis: first case report. *Dig. Dis. Sci.* 54(5): 1141-3 (2009).

[50] Taylor JS, Williams SR, Rhys R, James P, Frenneaux MP. Conjugated linoleic acid impairs endothelial function. *Arterioscler. Thromb. Vasc. Biol.* 26(2): 307-12 (2006).

In: Linoleic Acids
Editor: Igho Onakpoya

ISBN: 978-1-62257-384-4
© 2012 Nova Science Publishers, Inc.

Chapter VII

Conjugated Linoleic Acids in the Prevention of Ischemic Stroke

Yuri Clement
Pharmacology Unit, Faculty of Medical Sciences,
The University of the West Indies, St. Augustine,
Trinidad and Tobago

Abstract

Epidemiological and case-control studies show that high dietary intake of conjugated linoleic acids (CLA) is associated with a reduced risk of ischemic stroke. Atherosclerosis, a major risk factor for ischemic stroke, is precipitated by immune processes which involve the interplay between monocytes/ macrophages, pro-inflammatory and chemotactic mediators at the site of vascular injury. Sparse clinical evidence showed that CLA supplementation had no effect on a surrogate measure of atherosclerosis. However, animal models show significant CLA isomer-specific regression and resolution in established atherosclerosis.

Contrary to expectations, clinical trials found that linoleic acid supplementation actually increased plasma levels of pro-inflammatory markers, such as C-reactive protein, IL-6 and TNF- α. In contrast, *in vitro* studies show that linoleic acids inhibited the expression of pro-inflammatory mediators by modulating intracellular signaling pathways.

The results of *in vitro* studies are inconclusive regarding the effect of linoleic acids on chemotactic mediators which are critical in the initiation and progression of atherosclerosis. In conclusion, observational evidence points to an inverse relationship between dietary CLA intake and the risk of stroke.

However, the findings from clinical trials and laboratory studies are inconclusive and do not provide a clear understanding of the mechanisms underlying protection against ischemic stroke.

List of Abbreviations

CLA	Conjugated linoleic acid
COX-1	Cyclooxygenase-1
COX-2	Cyclooxygenase-2
CRP	C reactive protein
HUVEC	Human umbilical vein endothelial cells
ICAM-1	Intracellular adhesion molecule-1
IL-6	Interleukin-6
iNOS	Inducible nitric oxide synthase
LDL	Low density lipoprotein
LPS	Lipopolysaccharide
MCP-1	Monocyte chemotactic protein-1
NF-κB	Nuclear factor-κb
NO	Nitric oxide
PDGF	Platelet-derived growth factor
PECAM-1	Platelet/endothelial cell adhesion molecule-1
sVCAM-1	Soluble vascular cell adhesion molecule-1
TIA	Transient ischemic attack
TNF-α	Tumor necrosis factor-alpha

Introduction

Ischemic stroke occurs when there is a sudden diminution in the blood supply to the brain. Endothelial dysfunction and atherosclerotic plaque formation play major roles in the narrowing of arteries supplying cerebral tissue.

Observational studies suggest that linoleic acids may prevent the incidence of ischemic stroke. It has been hypothesized that these polyunsaturated fatty acids exert their effects by various mechanisms. In this paper the evidence regarding the probable role of conjugated linoleic acids in the prevention of ischemic stroke is presented based on the findings of observational studies, interventional studies in randomized, placebo-controlled clinical studies, *in vitro* cell cultures and animal models.

There is overwhelming clinical evidence which shows a direct correlation between saturated fatty acid intake and the incidence of cardiovascular and cerebrovascular diseases. Concurrently, there is much interest in the use of polyunsaturated fatty acids in the prevention of these conditions. Several studies have established an inverse relationship between polyunsaturated fatty acids intake, including linoleic acids, and the incidence of cardiovascular diseases.

However, the impact of dietary intake of linoleic acids and the incidence of cerebrovascular events, including ischemic stroke, has been less extensively investigated.

Observational Evidence

One of the earliest case-control studies which attempted to link linoleic acid levels in the blood to the incidence of ischemic stroke was reported by Ricci and colleagues [1]. In this study, the concentration of linoleic acid in red blood cell membranes was measured in 28 cases of recent ischemic events compared 56 age-matched controls. It was demonstrated that patients with ischemic stroke had significantly lower levels of linoleic acid compared with controls. Further evidence was provided by another case-control study which assessed linoleic acid content in subcutaneous adipose tissue in 10 recent cases of cerebral infarction and 10 matched controls [2]. These researchers showed that linoleic acid content in adipose tissue was 15% lower in ischemic stroke patients than in their matched controls.

A large prospective study screened and followed 7450 Japanese men and women between 40 and 85 years old for cardiovascular risk factors. After up to 9 years of follow-up, and 122 ischemic events, the study demonstrated that higher serum levels of linoleic acid was associated with a reduced risk of ischemic stroke [3]. It was postulated that this protection may be due to an effect of linoleic acid to lower blood pressure, reduce platelet aggregation and enhance erythrocyte deformation.

More recently, a study in Sweden followed 2313 middle-aged men for up to 32 years, with 412 cases of stroke or transient ischemic attacks during the period [4]. The investigators showed that a higher intake of linoleic acid protected against stroke and TIA. It was suggested that linoleic acid may be an appropriate long-term surrogate predictor for these cerebrovascular events.

Effects on Mediators of Inflammation

Besides being a lipid disorder, it is now well established that atherosclerosis is a chronic inflammatory disease. Several pro-inflammatory mediators, known as cytokines, are pivotal in the initiation and maintenance of the inflammatory atherosclerotic state [5]. It is hypothesized that linoleic acid has its protective effect by attenuating the inflammatory responses which lead to the series of events leading to atherosclerotic plaque formation, and subsequently ischemic stroke.

Smedman and colleagues [6] conducted a randomized double-blinded placebo controlled study which included 53 men and women to determine whether conjugated linoleic acids supplementation affected markers of inflammation associated with the initiation and progression of atherosclerosis. The investigators showed that a 3-month supplementation with 4.2g/day (containing equimolar concentrations of *cis*-9, *trans*-11 CLA and *trans*-10, *cis*-12 CLA isomers) significantly increased serum levels of the pro-inflammatory marker C-reactive protein. However, supplementation had no effect on levels of other inflammatory markers such as tumor necrosis factor- α (TNF-α) or sVCAM-1.

Another randomized, double-blind, parallel study by Tholstrup and colleagues [7] included 75 postmenopausal women who were given conjugated linoleic mixture, *cis*-9, *trans*-11 CLA or olive oil (placebo) over a 16-week period. Pro-inflammatory markers were measured at baseline and at the end of the study to determine the effects of the intervention. It was shown that the linoleic acid mixture significantly increased markers of inflammation including CRP, IL-6 and TNF-α; but had no effect on markers of endothelial reactivity such as ICAM-1, VCAM-1 and MCP-1. On the other hand, supplementation with *cis*-9, *trans*-11 CLA had similar effects on inflammatory markers as the olive oil control.

At the molecular level, tumor necrosis factor-α (TNF-α) is a potent pro-inflammatory cytokine which plays a pivotal role in augmenting the inflammatory response via the intracellular transcription factor NF-κB. De-Lima-Salgado and colleagues [8] showed that linoleic acid inhibited lipopolysaccharide (LPS)-induced TNF-α production in a mouse monocyte cell line. Cheng and colleagues [9] also demonstrated that conjugated linoleic acid inhibited the LPS-induced inflammatory response in a macrophage cell line (RAW 264.7). The decrease in inflammatory response was due in part to the significant decrease in NF-κB binding to promoter regions for inflammatory mediators. There was dose-dependent inhibition of the LPS-induced up-regulation of iNOS and COX-2 expression, with subsequent decreased production of NO and prostaglandin E2. These findings were corroborated by another *in vitro* study which showed that CLA inhibited the expression of COX-1 expression and production of prostaglandin E2 and thromboxane A2, by attenuating NF-κB nuclear translocation.

Anti-Atherosclerotic Effect of Linoleic Acids and Molecular Pathways

The initiation and propagation of atherosclerosis is a complex inflammatory process commencing with vascular injury, exposure of endothelium accompanied by adhesion and migration of monocytes into the intima. Oxidized LDL-cholesterol play a major role as macrophages are transformed into foam cells. The concerted interactions between transcription factors, intracellular signaling pathways and numerous pro-inflammatory cytokines, adhesion molecules and chemotactic molecules are vital to the formation of atherosclerotic plaques. The cascade of inflammatory events leading to initiation and progression of atherosclerosis involves the expression several mediators including intracellular adhesion molecule-1 (ICAM-1), soluble vascular cell adhesion molecule-1 (sVCAM-1) and monocyte chemotactic protein-1 (MCP-1). MCP-1 has an important role in the migration, adhesion and infiltration of monocytes to the site of vascular injury and plays a key role in medial thickening at the site of atherosclerotic lesions. These events further promote atherosclerotic progression resulting in endothelial dysfunction and plaque formation [10].

To date, the clinical evidence is sparse regarding the hypothesis that CLA supplementation inhibits the initiation and progression of atherosclerosis. However, a randomized, double-blinded, placebo-controlled trial was conducted which involved 401 overweight or obese, but otherwise healthy subjects, given either 4g CLA (2.5g *cis*-9,*trans*-11 CLA, 0.6g *trans*-10,*cis*-12 CLA) or placebo for six months [11]. In this trial aortic pulse wave velocity was used as a surrogate measure for atherosclerosis, and biochemical assays were performed, including CRP to assess the effect of supplementation. At the end of the study the researchers found that pulse wave velocity did not change from baseline values in both groups, indicating that supplementation at this dose over the 6-month period had no effect on either initiation or progression of atherosclerosis. An additional finding was that *cis*-9, *trans*-

12 conjugated linoleic acid had not effect of CRP levels; suggesting no anti-inflammatory effect.

On the other hand, several animal and *in vitro* studies were conducted to assess the effect of CLA and its isomers on established atherosclerosis, as well as to delineate the underlying molecular mechanisms involved. In an animal-based experiment by Kritchevsky and colleagues [12], rabbits were fed an atherogenic diet supplemented with CLA for 90 days. Compared to control animals, there was significant regression of established atherosclerosis in the arch and thoracic aorta by over 30% in CLA-treated animals. In yet another study, it was shown that apolipoprotein E knockout mice fed a high fat diet over 16 weeks, but given 1% ALA over the last 8 weeks, had not only regression of atherosclerotic plaque formation, but complete resolution compared with control animals [13]. It was also shown that there were significant decreases in aortic accumulation of macrophage and expression of macrophage scavenger receptor CD36 in CLA-fed animals.

Arbonés-Mainar and colleagues [14] conducted an *in vivo* study using apolipoprotein E knockout mice fed either *cis*-9, *trans*-11 CLA or *trans*-10, *cis*-12 CLA over 12 weeks. The investigators assessed atherosclerotic progression over the study period by measuring cross-sectional lesion and coverage area in the aortic root. It was demonstrated that *cis*-9, *trans*-11 CLA slowed the progression of atherosclerosis, whilst *trans*-10, *cis*-12 CLA accelerated progression.

In an *in vitro* experimental design using human macrophages incubated with *cis*-9, *trans*-11 CLA and linoleic acid for 48 hours there was significant increase in the expression of macrophage scavenger receptor CD36 [15]. This finding was in contrast to another *in vivo* study which showed otherwise13. A critical step in the initiation of atherosclerosis is the accumulation of lipids in macrophages, and Stachowska and colleagues [16] showed that *trans*-10, *cis*-12 CLA decreased lipid accumulation in macrophage and foam cell cultures.

Linoleic acid increased the platelet/endothelial cell adhesion molecule (PECAM)-1 and TNF-α-induced monocyte adhesion to human aortic endothelial cells [17]. These researchers also found that monocyte binding was enhanced by significant increase in E-selectin, vascular cell adhesion molecule (VCAM)-1, IL-8, MCP-1 and PGE2. In contrast, *cis*-9, *trans*-11 CLA reduced ICAM-1 and VCAM-1 expression on the surface of macrophages in culture [18]. It was also observed that this CLA isomer reduced the adhesion of macrophages to human umbilical vein endothelial cells (HUVEC). Similarly, using a HUVEC line, Lee and Vanden Heuvel [19] found that the less common *trans*-9, *trans*-11 isomer significantly reduced the expression of these atherogenic mediators, as well as E-selectin and P-selectin. These mediators are critically involved in the adhesion of monocytes to the site of vascular injury. Additionally, *trans*-9, *trans*-11 CLA decreased the adhesion of macrophages to the HUVEC cell line.

The complex pathways leading to arterial thickening, and subsequent occlusion, in atherosclerosis includes the incorporation of collagen into vascular intima-media. An *in vitro* experimental design using vascular smooth muscle cell lines from human aorta and coronary arteries showed that CLA isomers inhibited the platelet-derived growth factor (PDGF)-induced stimulation of collagen incorporation [20]. It was also shown that CLA inhibited the NF-κB nuclear translocation, which could lead to the down-regulation of inflammatory pathways in the gene expression of chemokines and cytokines.

Antithrombotic Effects of Linoleic Acids

The narrowing of the carotid artery by the formation of blood clots on ruptured plaques, which may break off and form emboli, also contribute to the dramatic reduction in cerebral blood supply and precipitate ischemic stroke. It has been hypothesized that linoleic acids may prevent cerebral infarction by modulating blood coagulation and fibrinolysis.

A clinical trial involving nine healthy young men, randomly assigned one of three diets enriched with stearic acid, oleic acid or linoleic acid, was conducted using a crossover design with 2-week intervention periods. There was at least 5 weeks washout between each intervention. In this study, by Hunter and colleagues [21], several factors for blood coagulation and fibrinolysis were measured at the start and end of each intervention period. The researchers found that fatty acid- enriched diets did not affect coagulability or fibrinolytic factors. However, it was shown that the linoleic-enriched diet significantly increased anti-aggregatory prostaglandin E1 binding to platelet membrane over the short-term.

In another clinical study [22], 17 healthy young women were randomly given either 3.9g/day conjugated linoleic acid supplement or sunflower oil (containing 72.6% linoleic acid, with no detectable CLA) for 63 days. The researchers found that short-term supplementation with CLA had no significant effect on platelet aggregation, prothrombin time, activated partial thromoplastin time or antithrombin III levels.

Antihypertensive Effects

Hypertension is a major risk factor for the development of ischemic stroke. Hypertension increases the likelihood of endothelial dysfunction and accelerates the events leading to atherosclerotic initiation and progression. The clinical evidence regarding the antihypertensive effects of linoleic acid is sparse. However, a randomized, placebo-controlled study involving 80 obese drug-naïve stage 1 hypertensive patients was conducted by Zhoa and colleagues [23] to determine the effect of add-on conjugated linoleic acid with ramipril (37.5mg/day) over 8 weeks. The supplement, containing equimolar concentrations of cis-9, *trans*-11 and *trans*-10, *cis*-12 isomers, was shown to significantly enhance the blood pressure lowering effect of ramipril over the study period.

Conclusion

The clinical evidence provided by epidemiological and case-control studies suggest that a diet high in CLA may protect against ischemic stroke. Many pathophysiological factors are predictors of ischemic stroke, and inflammation is a major player in the etiology of atherosclerosis. Interventional clinical studies showed that CLA supplementation over the short term actually increased the expression of inflammatory markers, which should enhance molecular events leading to atherosclerosis. On the contrary, *in vitro* studies show that CLA inhibited inflammation in stimulated cell cultures.

The single clinical trial showed that CLA supplementation had no effect on atherosclerotic progression over six months. However, animal studies show isomer-specific regression and complete resolution in established atherosclerosis. With regard to the involvement of monocytes/macrophages in the initiation of atherosclerosis, *in vitro* studies indicate that CLA modulates the expression of chemotactic mediators and adhesion molecules.

Observational evidence indicates that higher dietary intake of conjugated linoleic acids may reduce the risk of ischemic stroke. However, the findings from clinical trials and laboratory studies are mixed and do not clearly delineate mechanisms by which CLA may be acting to provide protection against ischemic stroke.

References

[1] Ricci S, Patoia L, Berrettini M, Binaglia L, Scarcella MG, Bucaneve G, Vecchini A, Carloni I, Agostini L, Parise P (1987) Fatty acid pattern of red blood cell membrances and risk if ischemic brain infarction: a case-control study. *Stroke* 18:575-578.

[2] Seidelin KN, Jensen B, Haugaard SB, Reith J, Olsen TS. (1997) Ischemic stroke and n-3 fatty acids. *J Stroke Cerebrovasc Dis* 6(6):405-409.

[3] Iso H, Sato S, Umemura U, Kudo M, Koile K, Kitamura A, Imano H, Okamura T, Naito Y, Shimamoto T (2002) Linoleic acid, other fatty acids, and the risk of stroke. *Stroke* 33:2086-2093.

[4] Wiberg B, Sundström J, Árnlöv J, Terént A, Vessby B, Björn Z, Lind L (2006) Metabolic risks factors for stroke and transient ischemic attacks in middle-aged men: A community-based study with long-term follow-up. Stroke 37:2898-2903.

[5] Kleemann R, Zadelaar S, Kooistra T. Cytokines and atherosclerosis: a comprehensive review of studies in mice. *Cardiovasc Res* 2008; 79:360-376.

[6] Smedman A, Basu S, Jovinge S, Fredrikson GN, Vessby B. Conjugated linoleic acid increased C-reactive protein in human subjects. *Br J Nutr* 2005; 94:791-795.

[7] Tholstrup T, Raff M, Straarup EM, Lund P, Basu S, Bruun JM. (2008) An oil mixture with *trans*-10, *cis*-12 conjugated linoleic acid increases markers of inflammation and in vivo lipid peroxidation compared with *cis*-9, *trans*-11 conjugated linoleic acid in postmenopausal women. *J Nutr* 138(8):1445-1451.

[8] de Lima-Salgado TM, Alba-Loureiro TC, do Nascimento CS, Nunes MT, Curi R. (2011) Molecular mechanism by which saturated fatty acids modulate TNF-α expression in mouse macrophage lineage. *Cell Biochem Biophys* 59(2):89-97.

[9] Cheng WL, Lii CK, Chen HW, Lin TH, Liu KL (2004) Contribution of conjugated linoleic acid to the suppression of inflammatory responses through the regulation of the NF-κB pathway. *J Agric Food Chem* 52:71-78.

[10] Marui N, Offermann MK, Swerlick R, Kunsch C, Rosen CA, Ahmad M, Alexander RW, Medford RM. Vascular cell adhesion molecule-1 (VCAM-1) gene transcription and expression are regulated through an antioxidant-sensitive mechanism in human vascular endothelial cells. *J Clin Invest* 1993; 92:1866-1874.

[11] Sluijs I, Plantinga Y, de Roos B, Mennen LI, Bots L (2010) Dietary supplementation with *cis*-9, *trans*-11 conjugated linoleic acid and aortic stiffness in overweight and obese adults. *Am J Clin Nutr* 91(1):175-183.

[12] Kritchevsky D, Tepper SA, Wright S, Tso P, Czarnecki SK (2000) Influence of conjugated linoleic acid (CLA) on establishment and progression of atherosclerosis in rabbits. *J Am Coll Nutr* 19:472S-477S.

[13] Toomey S, Harhen B, Roche HM, Fitzgerald D, Belton O (2006) Profound resolution of early atherosclerosis with conjugated linoleic acid. *Atherosclerosis* 187:40-49.

[14] Arbonés-Mainar, Navarro MA, Guzmán MA, Arnal C, Surra JC, Acín S, Carnicer R, Osada J, Roche HM. (2006) Selective effect of conjugated linoleic acid isomers on atherosclerotic lesion development in apolipoprotein E knockout mice. *Atherosclerosis* 189(2): 318-327.

[15] Stachowska E, Dolegowska, B. Dziedzieiko V, Rybicka M, Kaczmarczyk M. Bober J, Rac M, Machalinski B, Chlubek D (2009). Prostaglandin E (PGE2) and thromboxane A2 (TXA2) synthesis is regulated by conjugated linoleic acids (CLA) in human macrophages. *J Physiol Pharmacol* 60(1):77-85.

[16] Stachowska E, Baskiewicz M, Marhlewicz M, Czupryńska K, Kacmarczyk M, Wiszniewska B, Machaliński B, Chlubek D. (2010) Conjugated linoleic acids regulate triacylglycerol and cholesterol concentrations in macrophages/foam cells by the modulation of CD36 expression. *Acta Biochim Pol* 57(3):379-384.

[17] Matesanz N, Jewhurst V, Trimble ER, McGinty A. Owens D, Tomkin GH, Powell LA. (2011) Aug 11 Linoleic acid increases monocyte chemotaxis and adhesion to human aortic endothelial cell through protein kinase C- and cyclooxygenase-2-dependent mechanisms. *J Nutr Biochem*

[18] Stachowska E, Siennicka A, Baśkiewcz-Halasa M, Bober J, Machalinski B, Clubes D. (2012) Conjugated linoleic acid isomers may diminish human macrophages adhesion to endothelial surface. *Int J Food Sci Nutr* 63(1):30-35.

[19] Lee Y, Vanden Heuvel JP (2010) Inhibition of macrophage adhesion activity by 9-*trans*, 11-*trans* conjugated linoleic acid. *J Nutr Biochem* 21(6):490-497.

[20] Ringseis R, Gahler S, Eder K. (2008) Conjugated linoleic acid isomers inhibit platelet-derived growth factor-induced NF-κB transactivation and collegen formation in human vascular smooth muscle cells. *Eur J Nutr* 47:59-67.

[21] Hunter KA, Crosbie LC, Weir A, Miller GJ, Dutta-Roy AK (2000) A residential study comparing the effects of diets rich in stearic acid, oleic acid, and linoleic acid on fasting blood lipid, hemostatic variables and platelets in young healthy men. *J Nutr Biochem* 11(7-8):408-416.

[22] Benito P, Nelson GJ, Kelley DS, Bartolini G, Schmidt PC, Simon V (2001) The effect of conjugated linoleic acid on platelet function, platelet fatty acid composition, and blood coagulation in humans. *Lipids* 36:221-227.

[23] Zhoa WS, Zhai JJ, Wang YH, Xie PS, Yin XJ, Li LX, Cheng KL. (2009) Conjugated linoleic acid supplementation enhances antihypertensive effect ramipril in Chinese patients with obese-related hypertension. *Am J Hypertens* 22(6):680-686.

In: Linoleic Acids
Editor: Igho Onakpoya
ISBN: 978-1-62257-384-4
© 2012 Nova Science Publishers, Inc.

Chapter VIII

Gamma Linolenic Acid and Atopic Dermatitis

Igho Onakpoya[1] and James A. Taylor[2]
[1]Department of Primary Care Health Sciences, University of Oxford, UK
[2]Child Health Institute, University of Washington, Seattle, Washington, US

Abstract

Atopic dermatitis (AD) is a chronic inflammatory skin disorder, characterized by itching and scaling. Known more commonly as eczema, its precise etiology is unknown, but genetic, immunologic and epidermal barrier factors are believed to play a role in its pathogenesis. Environmental factors such as light, age, season, and temperature are also thought to be involved in the pathology of this condition. Its prevalence reaches 10 to 20% in the pediatric populations of some countries. Diagnosis is usually made clinically. Conventional management options include the use of steroids, tacrolimus ointment, and emollients. Dietary habits have been speculated to play a role in the development of AD, and results from cohort studies have suggested that eating foods rich in polyunsaturated fatty acids (PUFA) during pregnancy may decrease the risk of having AD in offspring of mothers. Dietary management with gamma (γ) linolenic acid (GLA) has been advocated for the treatment of AD. GLA is an omega 6 fatty acid which is present naturally in breast milk, beef, pork and poultry. It is commonly available as evening primrose oil (EPO), Borage oil (BO), and black currant seed oil (BCSO). Some authors have reported that a failure of conversion of linoleic acid (LA) to GLA is a factor causing AD; therefore increasing the amount of GLA through dietary supplementation, and thereby increasing the GLA/LA ratio may be beneficial in treating AD. Though several clinical trials investigating the effects of GLA on AD have been conducted, its use in the management of this condition remains controversial. This chapter investigates the purported mechanisms of actions of GLA in AD, and reviews the results of some clinical trials evaluating the efficacy of GLA in the prophylaxis and treatment of AD. We will also discuss the results of systematic reviews analysing the effects of GLA on AD.

List of Abbreviations

AA	Arachidonic acid
AD	Atopic dermatitis
ADASI	Atopic dermatitis area and severity index
AQP3	Aquaporin 3
BCSO	Black currant seed oil
BO	Borage oil
CLA	Conjugated linoleic acid
DGLA	Dihomo-gamma-linolenic acid
EFA	Essential fatty acids
EPO	Evening primrose oil
GLA	Gamma linolenic acid
HETE	Hydroxyeicosatetraenoic acid
HETrE	Hydroxyeicosatrienoic acid
IFN-γ	Interferon-gamma
IgE	Immunoglobulin E
IITA	Intensity item score aggregate
IS	Itch score
LA	Linoleic acid
LTB4	Leukotriene B4
PG	Prostaglandin
PGA	Patient Global Assessment
PUFA	Polyunsaturated fatty acids
RCT	Randomized clinical trial
SCORAD	Skin atopy score of atopic dermatitis
TEWL	Transepidermal water loss

Introduction

Atopic dermatitis (AD) is a chronic inflammatory skin disorder, characterized by itching and scaling [1]. Known more commonly as eczema, its precise aetiology is unknown, but genetic, immunologic and epidermal barrier factors are believed to play a role in its pathogenesis [2]. Environmental influences such as sodium lauryl sulphate (a detergent found in many skincare products), light, age, season, temperature as well as use of alcohol are also thought to be involved in the pathology of this condition [3,4,5,6]. Its prevalence reaches 10 to 20% in the pediatric populations of some countries [7, 8]. Diagnosis is usually made clinically. Conventional management options include the use of topical steroids, tacrolimus ointment, antihistamines, emollients, as well as avoidance of exacerbating factors [9].

Dietary habits have also been suggested to play a role in the development of AD [10], and the results of several cohort studies have suggested that eating foods rich in polyunsaturated fatty acids (PUFA) during pregnancy may decrease the risk of atopic dermatitis in offspring of mothers [11,12,13].

Dietary management with gamma (γ) linolenic acid (GLA) has been advocated for the treatment of AD. GLA (cis-6, cis-9, cis-12-octadecatrienoic acid) is an omega-6 fatty acid which is present naturally in breast milk, pork, beef, egg yolk and chicken [14]. It is a functional essential fatty acid (EFA) which can be synthesized endogenously from linoleic acid (LA) [15]. Some authors have speculated that a failure of conversion of LA to GLA is a factor causing AD, and therefore increasing the amount of GLA through dietary supplementation, and thereby increasing the GLA/LA ratio may be beneficial in the treatment of AD [16]. It has also been proposed that a defect of an enzyme, δ-6-desaturase, resulting in GLA deficiency is responsible for the dry skin seen in AD [17]. GLA is commonly available as evening primrose oil (EPO), Borage oil (BO), and Black Currant Seed Oil (BCSO). GLA constitutes approximately 9%, 23% and 18% of EPO, BO, and BCSO respectively [14, 18, 19].

Mechanisms of Action of GLA in Atopic Dermatitis

A number of mechanisms have been proposed by which GLA exerts its anti-atopic effect (Table 1).

Table 1. Purported mechanisms of action of GLA in atopic dermatitis

Proposed Mechanism	Suggested pathways
Change in membrane fluidity	• Bypassing δ-6-desaturase defect • Decrease in transepidermal water loss
Modulation of activity of membrane enzymes	• Conversion by cyclooxygenase to PGE_1 • Conversion by 15-lipoxygenase to 15-hydroxyeicosatrienoic acid (15-HETrE)
Production of immunoregulatory eicosanoids	• Stimulation of cyclic AMP • Reduction in LTB4 • Increase in IFN-γ • Reduction in IgE • Increase in PGE_2
Reduction of catecholamines	• Decreased expression of tyroxine hydroxylase • Overcoming defective feedback loop between catecholamine synthesis and induction

Change in Membrane Fluidity

AD is characterized by an increase in transepidermal water loss (TEWL) [20]. In normal skin, TEWL is increased when epidermal water content is high. However in AD, increased water loss occurs irrespective of epidermal water content [21]. Such losses result in a distortion of the integrity of the epidermal membrane. Genetic studies have also indicated that an increase in the expression, as well as an alteration in the cellular distribution of the gene, aquaporin 3 (AQP3), plays a role in the increased water loss observed in AD patients [22,23].

Studies in children have shown that increased TEWL is significantly correlated with deficiencies in GLA and dihomo-γ-linolenic acid (DGLA) [24, 25].Investigators have also reported that by administering GLA, the δ-6-desaturase defect observed in AD patients is bypassed, resulting in increased DLGA levels [26]. The increased DGLA levels are thought to help in restoring the integrity of the epidermal water barrier.

Modulation of the Activity of Epidermal Membrane-Associate Enzymes

GLA is converted by an elongase enzyme into DGLA [27, 28].When DGLA concentration is elevated in the epidermis, it is enzymatically converted by cyclooxygenase and 15-lipoxygenase into prostaglandin E1 (PGE1) and 15-hydroxyeicosatrienoic acid (15-HETrE) respectively [29]. PGE1 (an anti-inflammatory agent) is thought to be deficient in AD patients [30], but some authors have questioned this theory [31, 32].15-HETrE is thought to suppress epidermal hyperproliferation by its modulatory actions on a nuclear transcription factor (AP-1) and apoptosis [33]. 15-HETrE has also been reported to inhibit leukotriene B4 (LTB4) and 12-hydroxyeicosatetraenoic acid (HETE) which are proinflammatory agents [34].

Production of Immunoregulatory Eicosanoids

Decreased levels of the LA metabolites, DGLA and arachidonic acid (AA), have reportedly been observed in the breast milk of mothers with AD [35, 36].DGLA can be converted to PGE1, which could stimulate cyclic AMP, and thereby inhibit phospholipase [37]. In vitro studies have also shown that DGLA could also be metabolized to 15-hydroxy-DGLA, a potent inhibitor of lipoxygenases, resulting in a reduction in the production of LTB4 [38]. These processes result in a reduction of inflammation.

Investigators have suggested that GLA supplementation results in significant increases in interferon-γ (IFN- γ), with resultant decreases in immunoglobulin E (IgE) levels [39]. Furthermore, clinical trial results have demonstrated that long-term IFN- γ therapy is safe and efficacious for the treatment of AD [40].

Studies in humans have demonstrated that supplementation with GLA could lead to an alteration in response of the immune system, via significant reductions in the production of PGE2 [19]. It is thought that elevated DGLA concentration suppresses the production of PGE2 (a potent pro-inflammatory agent). The role of n-6 PUFA (including GLA and DGLA) in the development of AD has, however, been disputed by other authors [41].

Reduction of Catecholamines Concentration

Elevated plasma levels of norepinephrine have been reported in patients with AD when compared with controls [42, 43]. This is thought to be due to a pronounced expression of tyrosine hydroxylase, the rate-limiting enzyme in the synthesis of norepinephrine. It has also been postulated that a defective feedback loop between the catecholamine synthesis and induction causes accumulation of catecholamines in patients with AD [44]. Results of clinical trials in humans have suggested that administration of EPO results in significant reductions in the serum concentrations of catecholamines in patients when compared with controls [45].

Table 2. Summary of key details of RCTs evaluating GLA efficacy in atopic dermatitis

1st Author Year Country	Participants	Supplement	Daily GLA Dosage	Placebo	Co-treatment	Assessment of AD severity	Trial Duration	Main Results	Source of funding
Andreassi 1997 Italy	30 adults	GLA	548 mg	Unclear	Emollients	Linear scale	12 weeks	Significant improvements in GLA compared with placebo ($p < 0.001$)	Industry
Bahmer 1992 Germany	12 adults	BO	240 mg	Palm-kernel oil 500mg	Not specified	ADASI	16 weeks	GLA supplementation caused favourable effects on skin changes	Not specified
Bamford 1985 USA	154 adults and children	EPO	< 15 yrs 90-180 > 15 yrs 270-360 mg	Liquid paraffin 500 mg	Topical steroids Emollients Antihistamines	Need for steroid use	13 weeks	No significant effect of GLA on overall severity of AD	Industry
Berth-Jones 1993 UK	102 adults and children	EPO	270 mg	Liquid paraffin for adults; olive oil for children	Antihistamines	Leicester score Need for steroid	16 weeks	No significant difference between GLA and placebo ($p = 0.74$)	Charity
Biagi 1994 Italy	51 children	EPO	45 mg/kg	Olive oil	Steroids Emollients	Not specified	8 weeks	Significant improvement in overall severity of AD in GLA group.	Not specified
Borrek 1997 Germany	24 children	BO	360 mg	Maize seed oil	Corticosteroids Antihistamines	Costa Score	14 weeks	Significant improvement in AD in patients taking placebo	Not specified
Buslau 1996 Germany	50 adults	BO	320 mg	Palm-kernel oil 500mg	Emollients	ADASI	12	Significant improvements in AD patients taking GLA	Not specified
Hederos 1996 Sweden	58 Children	EPO	160 mg	Sunflower oil 500 mg	Emollients Antihistamines Antiasthmatics	Visual analogue scale	16 weeks	No significant differences between groups	Industry
Henz 1999 Germany	160 adults and children	BO	500 mg	Miglyol	Topical steroids	Costa Score	24 weeks	No significant difference in AD severity between GLA and placebo	Not specified
Humphrey 1994 UK	58 adults	EPO	540 mg	Liquid parrafin	Topical steroids	Mean Clinical Score	16 weeks	Significant effect of primrose oil on erythema	Industry

Table 2 (Continued)

1st Author Year Country	Participants	Supplement	Daily GLA Dosage	Placebo	Co-treatment	Assessment of AD severity	Trial Duration	Main Results	Source of funding
Kitz 2006 German	131at-risk infants	GLA in breastmilk	100 mg via mothers' breast-milk	Non-enriched whey formula	None	SCORAD	26 weeks	No detectable evidence of GLA influence on the development of AD	Not specified
Linnamaa 2010 Finland	313infants (256 at-risk)	BCSO	Not specified	Olive oil	None	SCORAD	24 months	No significant differences in prevalence of AD between groups at 24 months ($p = 0.18$)	Government
Lovell 1981 UK	32 adults and children	EPO	360 mg in adults 180 mg in children	Liquid paraffin	Topical steroids	Linear scale	3 weeks	GLA caused modest but significant improvements	Industry
Schalin-Karilla 1987 Finland	25 adults	EPO	90 mg	Liquid paraffin	Emollients Topical steroids	Linear scale	12 weeks	Significant decrease in inflammation in GLA group compared with placebo ($p < 0.001$)	Charity
Senapati 2008 India	53 adults and children	EPO	45-540 mg depending on age of patient	Sunflower oil 300 mg	Emollients	IITA	20 weeks	Significant improvement in GLA group compared with placebo ($p < 0.00001$)	Not specified
Valsecchi 1996 Italy	31 adults and children	BO	400 mg in adults 240 mg in children	Liquid paraffin	Emollients	Mean Clinical Score	14 weeks	No statistical difference in severity between GLA and placebo ($p = 0.165$)	Not specified
van Gool 2003 Netherlands	118 at-risk infants	BO	100 mg	Sunflower oil	None	SCORAD	26 weeks	GLA supplementation tended to alleviate the severity of AD in later infancy	Industry
Wright 1982 UK	99 adults and children	EPO	90-180 mg in children 180-540 mg in adults	Liquid paraffin	Emollients Topical steroids Antihistamines	Linear scale	12 weeks	Significant improvement in overall severity of AD in the GLA group compared with placebo ($p < 0.002$)	Industry

Abbreviations: EPO: Evening Primrose Oil; GLA: Gamma Linoleic Acid; BCSO: Black Currant Seed Oil; BO: Borage Oil; AD: Atopic Dermatitis; ADASI: Atopic Dermatitis Area and Severity Index; SCORAD: Skin Atopy Score of Atopic Dermatitis; IITA: Intensity Item Score Aggregate

Clinical Trials on Efficacy

A search of the literature identified several published reports of randomized, double-blind, placebo-controlled trials (RCTs) evaluating the efficacy of GLA in the prophylaxis and treatment of AD (Table 2).

Trials Involving Infants and Children Only

Biagi et al. [46] evaluated the efficacy of GLA in an RCT involving 51 children. They did not report how the severity of AD was assessed. The patients had topical steroids and emollients as co-treatments. They reported significant improvements in the overall severity of AD in the GLA group when compared with placebo ($p = 0.046$); this improvement was irrespective of whether or not, the children had IgE-mediated allergy. The trial duration was 8 weeks. The funding source was not specified.

Borrek et al. [47] evaluated the efficacy of GLA in a cross-over RCT involving 24 children aged 3 to 17 years. The severity of AD was assessed with the Costa-Score. Patients also received antihistamines and corticosteroids in the course of the trial. The authors did not observe any improvement in AD due to GLA; instead they reported significant improvements in patients administered placebo. The trial duration was 14 weeks. The funding source was not specified.

Hederos and Berg [48] evaluated the efficacy of GLA in an RCT involving 58 children who had AD and asthma. The severity of the AD was assessed using a visual analogue scale. The children also used emollients, antihistamines, as well as anti-asthmatic medications during the course of the trial. The authors reported a significant improvement in eczema symptoms in both the GLA and placebo groups, but there were no significant differences between groups. There was also a trend towards less steroid use in the GLA group. No serious adverse events were observed. The trial lasted 16 weeks. The study was industry-funded.

Kitz et al. [49] evaluated the prophylactic efficacy of GLA in preventing the expression of AD in an RCT involving 131 infants. Each infant had at least one first-degree relative with AD. The severity of atopic dermatitis was assessed using the skin atopy score of atopic dermatitis (SCORAD). Breast-fed infants received their GLA through supplementation of their mothers for six months. They reported a significant impact of GLA supplementation on IgE levels at one year ($p<0.05$). However, they concluded that GLA supplementation did not influence the development of AD in later life. The funding source was not specified.

Linnamaa et al. [50] evaluated the efficacy of GLA in preventing AD in an RCT involving 313 at-risk infants. The severity of AD was assessed using the SCORAD index. Doses were administered to mothers during the 8th to 16 weeks of pregnancy, and for the entire duration of the exclusive breastfeeding period. Infants then received the supplement as drops from the period after they stopped breastfeeding to 2 years of age. Subjects were assessed at 3, 12 and 24 months. There was a significant difference in the SCORAD index in favour of the GLA group compared with placebo at 12 months ($p = 0.035$). There was also a lower prevalence of AD in the GLA group compared with placebo at 12 months ($p = 0.035$); however, at 24 months, this difference was no longer significant ($p = 0.18$). The authors reported no significant differences in serum IgE levels or skin test results between the GLA and placebo groups. The study was government-funded.

van Gool et al. [51] evaluated the efficacy of GLA in the prophylaxis of AD in 118 at-risk infants, i.e., offspring of atopic pregnant women. The severity of AD was assessed using the SCORAD index. Infants in the GLA group showed a trend towards lower SCORAD values ($p = 0.06$), and a tendency towards higher IgE levels ($p = 0.06$). Adverse events were equally divided between groups. The investigators reported that supplementation with GLA did not prevent the expression of atopy, but it tended to alleviate the symptoms of AD in later infancy. The trial lasted 6 months. The study was funded by industry.

Trials Involving Both Children and Adults

Bamford et al. [52] evaluated the efficacy of GLA in a cross-over RCT ($n = 154$). The severity of AD was assessed by the need for use of topical steroids. The study patients also had emollients, topical steroids and oral antihistamines administered. They observed no significant effect on erythema, scale, excoriation, lichenification, or overall severity of AD in all patients at the end of the study. The trial lasted 13 weeks. The study was funded by industry.

Berth-Jones and Graham-Brown [53] evaluated the efficacy of GLA in an RCT involving 102 subjects. Disease activity was assessed using clinical severity scores (Leicester score), percentage of skin affected, topical steroid requirement, and patient diaries. Use of antihistamines was continued by patients if it was being used on entry. The authors observed no significant differences between GLA and placebo on any outcome indices. They concluded that essential fatty acid supplementation had no effect on AD. The trial lasted 16 weeks. The study was funded by charity.

Henz et al. [54] evaluated the efficacy of GLA in a multi-centre RCT involving 160 children and adults in Germany and Austria. Disease severity was assessed by use of the Costa-Score. The patients had topical steroids as co-treatment. The investigators did not observe any significant differences in the Costa-Score between GLA and placebo. They concluded that GLA has no overall efficacy in the treatment of AD, but a subgroup of patients may benefit from the treatment when combined with steroids. The duration of this trial was 24 weeks. The source of funding for the study was not specified.

Lovell et al. [55] evaluated the efficacy of GLA in an RCT involving 32 adults and children. Disease severity was assessed using a linear scale. Patients also used topical steroids as co-treatment during the trial. They reported modest but significant improvements in the severity of AD in the GLA group compared with placebo on both doctors and patients assessments ($p < 0.01$ and $p < 0.05$ respectively). No adverse effects were reported. The trial duration was 3 weeks. The study was in part supported by industry.

Senapati et al. [56] evaluated the efficacy of GLA in an RCT involving 53 participants. The investigators used an intensity item score aggregate (IITA) to assess the severity and activity of disease. The patients were also prescribed emollients for liberal application. The authors reported that compared to baseline values, there were significant reductions in the mean scores in the GLA group. The reductions in mean score observed for placebo were small, delayed, and inconsistent. The authors reported a significant improvement in outcome of treatment in the GLA group compared with placebo ($p < 0.00001$). They did not observe any significant adverse events. The trial lasted 5 months. The funding source for the study was not specified.

Valsecchi et al. [57] evaluated the efficacy of GLA in an RCT including 31 adults and children. A mean clinical score was used to assess disease severity. Patients also received unlimited emollient as co-treatment. They reported significant improvements in the severity of AD in both the GLA and placebo groups. There was no significant difference between groups. They also did not observe any significant difference in IgE levels. The trial lasted 14 weeks. The funding source for the study was not specified.

Wright and Burton [58] evaluated the efficacy of GLA in a cross-over RCT involving 99 patients (60 adults and 39 children). The severity of AD was assessed via a linear scale. GLA was administered as low and high doses to the intervention groups. Patients also used emollients, topical steroids and antihistamines throughout the duration of the trial. In the low-dose group, there was a significant improvement in itch symptoms compared with placebo ($p < 0.05$). In the high-dose group, there were significant improvements in itch, scaling and overall severity when compared with placebo ($p < 0.003$, $p < 0.002$, and $p < 0.01$ respectively). There was no description of any dose-response relationships. The authors concluded that administration of high dosages of GLA resulted in significant improvements in the symptoms of atopic dermatitis. They did not observe any adverse effects. The trial lasted 12 weeks. The study was industry-funded.

Trials Involving Adults Only

Andreassi et al. [59] evaluated the efficacy of GLA in an RCT involving 60 patients. Disease severity was assessed using a linear scale. They reported significant improvements in pruritus, erythema, vesiculation and oozing in the GLA group compared with placebo ($p < 0.001$). The trial duration was 12 weeks. The study was industry-funded.

Bahmer and Schafer [60] evaluated the efficacy of GLA in an RCT involving 12 patients. The severity of AD was assessed using the Atopic Dermatitis Area and Severity Index (ADASI) score. It was not specified whether the patients had any co-treatments. They reported favourable effects on the ADASI score in patients administered GLA. The trial duration was 16 weeks. The funding source was not specified.

Buslau and Thaci [61] evaluated the efficacy of GLA in an RCT involving 50 adults. Disease severity was assessed using the ADASI score. The patients had emollients as co-treatments. The authors reported that 78% of patients in the BO showed significant improvements, compared with 43% given placebo. There was no report on between-group differences. The duration of the study was 12 weeks. The funding source was not specified.

Humphrey et al. [62] evaluated the efficacy of GLA in treating AD in 58 patients. Disease severity was assessed using a mean clinical score. Patients also received topical steroids as co-treatment. They reported a significant effect of GLA on erythema and surface damage when compared with placebo. They did not observe a significant effect on lichenification. They concluded that GLA administration resulted in significant improvements in overall severity of AD. The trial duration was 16 weeks. The study was funded by industry.

Schalin-Karrila et al. [63] evaluated the efficacy of GLA in an RCT involving 25 patients. All patients had a family history of atopy. The overall severity of eczema was assessed through a linear scale. The trial patients also used emollients and topical steroids in addition to GLA. The authors reported a statistically significant decrease in inflammation in the GLA group compared with placebo at the end of the study ($p < 0.001$). The trial duration was 12 weeks. No side effects were observed. The study was funded by charity.

Systematic Reviews

A search of the electronic literature identified a few systematic reviews examining the effects of GLA supplementation on AD (Table 3).

Table 3. Key details of systematic reviews evaluating the efficacy of GLA in atopic dermatitis

First Author Year	No. of RCTs	No. of participants	Quality of included RCTs	Main Findings
Hoares 2008	14	913	Poor reporting quality for most of the included studies	Best reported studies did not suggest any evidence of beneficial effect
Morse 2006	26 clinical studies	1207	Variable; sensitivity analyses performed	EPO has some beneficial effects; magnitude is reduced with increased frequency of steroid use
Morse 1989	9	311	Not accounted for; 7RCTs unpublished	Highly significant improvement from baseline score due to EPO ($p < 0.0001$)
van Gool 2004	11	754	Variable; sensitivity analyses performed	No significant difference in severity between GLA and placebo ($p = 0.09$)

Hoare et al. [64] systematically reviewed the efficacy of GLA in AD. The review included fourteen RCTs ($n = 913$); nine of these trials used EPO, with five using BO. Several of the RCTs were of poor reporting quality. They could not pool the data from the trials because of discrepancies in dosages of GLA, as well as differences between study participants and outcomes. The authors concluded that the largest and best conducted trials did not show any convincing effects of GLA supplementation.

Morse and Clough [65] in a meta-analysis of 26 clinical studies ($n = 1207$) evaluated the effects of EPO on AD. There were variations in the reporting quality of the included RCTs. They reported that EPO supplementation results in beneficial effects on itch/pruritus, crusting, oedema and redness (erythema) that becomes apparent between 4 and 8 weeks after treatment is initiated. However, the magnitude of this effect is reduced in association with increasing frequency of potent steroid use. The authors suggested that further research is needed to understand the physiology of AD, as well as the beneficial role fatty acids play in the development and management of this condition.

Morse et al. [66] conducted a meta-analysis involving nine RCTs ($n = 311$) evaluating the efficacy of GLA in AD. Four of these trials were parallel, and five were cross-over. The methodological quality of the individual trials included in the review was not accounted for, and seven of the included studies were unpublished. For the parallel-design studies and the first phase of cross-over studies, the authors reported significant improvements in patient global assessment (PGA), clinician global assessment (CGA) and itch score (IS) in the GLA group compared with placebo (p = 0.04, 0.01 and <0.0001 respectively). The authors excluded one trial from their analyses because felt there was some inconsistency in the administration of the active and placebo treatment; however, this allegation has reportedly been refuted by the investigators of that trial [64]. The authors concluded that GLA supplementation is associated with improvement in clinical score.

van Gool et al. [67] meta-analysed the results of 11 RCTs (n = 754) evaluating the efficacy of GLA. There were variations in the reporting quality of the included RCTs, and they performed sensitivity analyses. Statistical analysis did not show a significant effect of GLA on the severity of GLA on AD when compared with placebo (pooled effect size =0.15; 95% confidence limits (CL) - 0.02, 0.32). They concluded that supplementation with EFA had no significant effect on the overall severity of AD.

Short Commentary

Evening primrose oil has a long history of being used for several different disorders. Based on the in vitro and in vivo biologic evaluations of its pharmacologic effects, there is both a biologic plausibility and rationale for EPO (and other sources of GLA) use to prevent or treat AD. It has been shown that neonates born to mothers with high dietary intake of PUFAs are less likely to have AD than those with lower intake, and GLA has been shown to modify processes that may be important in the pathogenesis of AD through several possible pathways. Given this, clinical trials on the effectiveness of GLA in preventing or treating AD are warranted, and several have been done. Unfortunately, the results of these trials have had decidedly mixed results. Although some positive effects have been observed in many trials, and in systematic reviews, there are seemingly an equal number of studies demonstrating no benefit over placebo.

There are several possible explanations for these contradictory results. The outcomes of the different trials tend to be related, but are not identical. AD is chronic disease with multiple treatment modalities. It is possible that the variability in the results of various trials may be due, in large part, to which treatments in addition to GLA are allowed. Although there is no consistent pattern that is immediately obvious, there is a suggestion in reviewing various trials that GLA might work best as an adjunct to standard therapy including emollients and topical steroids.

The gestalt of the data also suggests that studies including adults with AD are more likely to have positive results than those in which only children are enrolled. This could be because the pathogenesis or severity of AD differs in these two age-groups. Alternatively, assessment of response to therapy might be easier in adults (who can easily articulate changes in nebulous symptoms such as itchiness) than in younger patients.

Clearly, more and more rigorous study on the effects on GLA on AD is needed. Pending the results of these investigations, the evidence suggests that use of GLA is quite safe, at least for several months. Given this, a trial of GLA is a reasonable option in patients whose AD is not adequately controlled by frequent use of emollients and topical steroids.

Conclusion

The evidence from RCTs and systematic reviews are not consistent regarding the effectiveness of GLA for the prophylaxis and treatment of AD. GLA generally appears safe. Further rigorous clinical trials investigating its effects on AD are warranted.

References

[1] De Benedetto A, Agnihothri R, McGirt LY, Bankova LG, Beck LA (2009). "Atopic dermatitis: a disease caused by innate immune defects?". *The Journal of investigative dermatology* 129 (1): 14–30.

[2] Cooper KD. Atopic dermatitis: recent trends in pathogenesis and treatment. J Invest Dermatol. 1994;102:128–37.

[3] Heck DE, Gerecke DR, Vetrano AM, Laskin JD. Solar ultraviolet radiation as a trigger of cell signal transduction. *Toxicol Appl Pharmacol.* 2004;195:288–97.

[4] Rogers J, Harding C, Mayo A, Banks J, Rawlings A. Stratum corneum lipids: the effect of ageing and the seasons. *Arch Dermatol Res.* 1996;288:765–70.

[5] Beck HI, Bjerring P, Harving H. Atopic dermatitis and the indoor climate. The effect from preventive measures. *Acta Derm Venereol.* 1989;69(2):162-5

[6] Linneberg A, Petersen J, Grønbaek M, Benn CS. Alcohol during pregnancy and atopic dermatitis in the offspring. *Clin Exp Allergy.* 2004 Nov;34(11):1678-83.

[7] Shaw TE, Currie GP, Koudelka CW, Simpson EL Eczema prevalence in the United States: data from the 2003 National Survey of Children's Health. *J Invest Dermatol.* 2011 Jan;131(1):67-73. Epub 2010 Aug 26.

[8] Williams HC. Clinical practice. Atopic dermatitis. *N Engl J Med.* 2005 Jun 2;352(22):2314-24.

[9] Saeki H, Furue M, Furukawa F, Hide M, Ohtsuki M, Katayama I, Sasaki R, Suto H, Takehara K; Committee for Guidelines for the Management of Atopic Dermatitis of Japanese Dermatological Association. Guidelines for management of atopic dermatitis. *J Dermatol.* 2009 Oct;36(10):563-77

[10] Sakai K, Okuyama H, Shimazaki H, Katagiri M, Torii S, Matsushita T, et al. Fatty acid composition of plasma lipids in atopic dermatitis/asthma patients. *Arerugi.* 1994; 43:37–43.

[11] Sausenthaler S, Koletzko S, Schaaf B, Lehmann I, Borte M, Herbarth O, von Berg A, Wichmann HE, Heinrich J; LISA Study Group. Maternal diet during pregnancy in relation to eczema and allergic sensitization in the offspring at 2 y of age. *Am J Clin Nutr.* 2007 Feb;85(2):530-7

[12] Sausenthaler S, Koletzko S, Schaaf B, Lehmann I, Borte M, Herbarth O, von Berg A, Wichmann HE, Heinrich J; LISA Study Group. Maternal diet during pregnancy in relation to eczema and allergic sensitization in the offspring at 2 y of age. *Am J Clin Nutr.* 2007 Feb;85(2):530-7

[13] Businco L, Ioppi M, Morse NL, Nisini R, Wright S. Breast milk from mothers of children with newly developed atopic eczema has low levels of long chain polyunsaturated fatty acids. *J Allergy Clin Immunol.* 1993 Jun;91(6):1134-9.

[14] Horrobin DF. Nutritional and medical importance of gamma linoleic acid. *Prog Lipid Res* 1992; 31(2): 163-194

[15] Chen Q, Nimal J, Li W, Liu X, Cao W. Delta-6 desaturase from borage converts linoleic acid to gamma-linolenic acid in HEK293 cells. Delta-6 desaturase from borage converts linoleic acid to gamma-linolenic acid in HEK293 cells. *Biochem Biophys Res Commun.* 2011 Jul 8; 410(3):484-8.

[16] Horrobin DF. Essential fatty acid metabolism and its modification in atopic eczema. *Am J Clin Nutr* 2000; 71(Suppl 1): 367S-372S

[17] Manku MS, Horrobin DF, Morse N, Kyte V, Jenkins K, Wright S, Burton JL: Reduced levels of prostaglandin precursors in the blood of atopic patients: Defective delta-6-desaturase function as a biochemical basis for atopy. *Prostaglandins Leukotrienes Med* 1984;9:615–628.

[18] Chung S, Kong S, Seong K, Cho Y. Gamma-linolenic acid in borage oil reverses epidermal hyperproliferation in guinea pigs. *J Nutr.* 2002 Oct; 132(10):3090-7

[19] Wu D, Meydani M, Leka LS, Nightingale Z, Handelman GJ, Blubmerg JB,Meydani SM. Effect of dietary supplementation with black currant seed oil on the immune response of healthy elderly subjects. *Am J Clin Nutr* 1999; 70: 536-543

[20] Lee JH, Lee SJ, Kim D, Bang D. The effect of wet-wrap dressing on epidermal barrier in patients with atopic dermatitis. *J Eur Acad Dermatol Venereol.* 2007; 21(10): 1360-8

[21] Seidenari S, Giusti G. Objective assessment of the skin of children affected by atopic dermatitis: a study of pH, capacitance and TEWL in eczematous and clinically normal skin. *Acta Derm Venereol* (Stockh) 1995; 75: 429–433.

[22] Olsson M, Broberg A, Jernås M, Carlsson L, Rudemo M, Suurküla M, Svensson PA, Benson M. Increased expression of aquaporin 3 in atopic eczema. *Allergy* 2006; 61: 1132–1137

[23] [1] Nakahigashi K, Kabashima K, Ikoma A, Verkman AS, Miyachi Y, Hara-Chikuma M. Upregulation of aquaporin-3 is involved in keratinocyte proliferation and epidermal hyperplasia. *J Invest Dermatol.* 2011 Apr;131(4):865-73. Epub 2010 Dec 30

[24] Yen CH, Dai YS, Yang YH, Wang LC, Lee JH, Chiang BL. Linoleic Acid Metabolites and Transepidermal Water Loss in Children With Atopic Dermatitis. *Ann Allergy Asthma Immunol.* 2008;100(1):66–73

[25] Focke M, Sesztak-Greinecker G, Brannath W, Götz M, Jarisch R, Hemmer W. *Plasma levels of polyunsaturated fatty acids in children with atopic dermatitis and in atopic and nonatopic controls.* Wien Klin Wochenschr. 2005 Jul;117(13-14):485-91.

[26] Kanehara S, Ohtani T, Uede K, Furukawa F. Clinical effects of undershirts coated with borage oil on children with atopic dermatitis: A double-blind, placebo-controlled clinical trial. *J Dermatol* 2007; 34: 811-815

[27] Chilton-Lopez T, Surette ME, Swan DD, Fonteh AN, Johnson MM, Chilton FH. Metabolism of Gammalinolenic Acid in Human Neutrophils. *J Immunol* 1996; 156: 2941-2947

[28] Kerscher MJ, Korting HC. Treatment of atopic eczema with evening primrose oil: rationale and clinical results. Clin Investig 1992; 70: 167-171

[29] Ziboh VA, Miller CC, Cho Y. Metabolism of polyunsaturated fatty acids by skin epidermal enzymes: generation of antiinflammatory and antiproliferative metabolites. *Am J Clin Nutr* 2000; 71(Suppl): 361S-6S

[30] Melnik BC, Plewig G. Is the origin of atopy linked to deficient conversion of ω-6-fatty acids to prostaglandin E1? *J Am Acad Dermatol* 1989; 21(3) Part 1: 557-563.

[31] Leonhardt A, Krauss M, Gieler U, Schweer H, Happle R, Seyberth HW. In vivo formation of prostaglandin E1 and prostaglandin E2 in atopic dermatitis. *Br J Dermatol* 1997; 136(3): 337-340

[32] Levin G, Duffin KL, Obukowicz MG, Hummert SL, Hideji F, Needleman P, Raz A. Differential metabolism of dihomo-gamma-linolenic acid and arachidonic acid by cyclo-oxygenase-1 and cyclo-oxygenase-2: implications for cellular synthesis of prostaglandin E1 and prostaglandin E2. Biochem J 2002 July 15; 365(Pt 2): 489–496.

[33] Xi S, Pham H, Ziboh WA. 15-hydroxyeicosatrienoic acid (15-HETrE) suppresses epidermal hyperproliferation via the modulation of nuclear transcription factor (AP-1) and apoptosis. *Arch Dermatol Res.* 2000 Aug;292(8):397-403.

[34] Heitmann J, Iversen L, Kragballe K, Ziboh VA. Incorporation of 15-hydroxyeicosatrienoic acid in specific phospholipids of cultured human keratinocytes and psoriatic plaques. *Exp Dermatol* 1995; 4(2): 74-78

[35] Businco L, Ioppi M, Morse NL, et al. Breast milk from mothers of children with newly developed atopic eczema has low levels of long chain polyunsaturated fatty acids. *J Allergy Clin Immunol* 1993; 91:1134-1139.

[36] Thijs C, Houwelingen A, Poorterman I, Mordant A, van den Brandt P. Essential fatty acids in breast milk of atopic mothers: comparison with non-atopic mothers, and effect of borage oil supplementation. *Eur J Clin Nutr.* 2000 Mar;54(3):234-8

[37] Ziboh VA. Biochemical abnormalities in essential fatty acid deficiency. *Models Dermatol* 1987;3:106–11.

[38] Iversen L, Fogh K, Kragballe K. Effect of dihomogammalinolenic acid and its 15-lipoxygenase metabolite on eicosanoid metabolism by human mononuclear leukocytes in vitro: selective inhibition of the 5-lipoxygenase pathway. *Arch Dermatological Res* 1992; 284(4): 222-226

[39] Yoon S, Lee J, Lee S. The Therapeutic Effect of Evening Primrose Oil in Atopic Dermatitis Patients with Dry Scaly Skin Lesions Is Associated with the Normalization of Serum Gamma-Interferon Levels. *Skin Pharmacol Appl Skin Physiol* 2002;15:20–25

[40] Schneider LC, Baz Z, Zarcone C, Zurakowski D. Long-term therapy with recombinant interferon-gamma (rIFN-gamma) for atopic dermatitis. *Ann Allergy Asthma Immunol.* 1998 Mar;80(3):263-8

[41] Focke M, Sesztak-Greinecker G, Brannath W, Götz M, Jarisch R, Hemmer W. *Plasma levels of polyunsaturated fatty acids in children with atopic dermatitis and in atopic and nonatopic controls.* Wien Klin Wochenschr. 2005 Jul;117(13-14):485-91

[42] Schallreuter KU, Pittelkow MR, Swanson NN, Beazley WD, Körner C, Ehrke C, Büttner G. Altered catecholamine synthesis and degradation in the epidermisof patients with atopic eczema. *Arch Dermatol Res* 1997; 289: 663-666

[43] Ionescu G, Kiehl R. Plasma catecholamine levels in severe atopic eczema. *Allergy.* 1988 Nov;43(8):614-6

[44] Pochet R, Delaspesse G, DeManbuege J (1980) Characterization of beta adrenoceptors on intact circulating lymphocytes from patients with atopic dermatitis. *Acta Derm Venereol Suppl* (Stockh) 92:26–29

[45] Courage B, Nissen HP, Wehrmann W, Biltz H. *Influence of polyunsaturated fatty acids on the plasma catecholamines of patients with atopic eczema.* Z Hautkr 1991;66:509–10 (in German).

[46] Biagi PL, Bordoni A, Hrelia S, Celadon M, Ricci GP, Cannella V, *et al.* The effect of gamma-linolenic acid on clinical status, red cell fatty acid composition and membrane micro-viscosity in infants with atopic dermatitis. *Drugs Exp Clin Res* 1994; 20(2):77–84.

[47] Borrek S, Hildebrandt A, Forster J. Gammalinolenicacid- rich borage seed oil capsules in children with atopic dermatitis. A placebo-controlled doubleblind study. *Klin Padiatr* 1997;209(3)100–4.

[48] Hederos C-A, Berg A. Epogam evening primrose oil treatment in atopic dermatitis and asthma. *Archives of Disease in Childhood* 1996;75:494-497

[49] Kitz R, Rose MA, Scho¨ nborn H, Zielen S, Böhles HJ. Impact of early dietary gamma-linolenic acid supplementation on atopic eczema in infancy. *Pediatr Allergy Immunol* 2006: 17: 112–117

[50] Linnamaa P, Savolainen J, Koulu L, Tuomasjukka S, Kallio H, Yang B, Vahlberg T, Tahvonen R. Blackcurrant seed oil for prevention of atopic dermatitis in newborns: a randomized, double-blind, placebo-controlled trial. *Clin Exp Allergy* 2010; 40: 1247-1255

[51] van Gool CJAW, Thijs C, Henquet CJM, van Houwelingen AC, Dagnelie PC, Schrander J, Menheere PPCA, van den Brandt P. γ-Linolenic acid supplementation for prophylaxis of atopic dermatitis—a randomized controlled trial in infants at high familial risk. *Am J Clin Nutr* 2003; 77: 943-951

[52] Bamford JT, Gibson RW, Renier CM. Atopic eczema unresponsive to evening primrose oil (linoleic and gamma-linolenic acids). *J Am Acad Dermatol* 1985 Dec;13(6):959-65

[53] Berth-Jones J, Graham-Brown RAC. Placebo-controlled trial of essential fatty acid supplementation in atopic dermatitis. *Lancet* 1993; 341: 1557-60 atopic dermatitis

[54] Henz BM, Jablonska S, van de Kerkhof PCM, Stingl G, Blaszczyk M, Vandervalk PGM, *et al.* Doubleblind, multicentre analysis of the efficacy of borage oil in patients with atopic eczema. *Br J Dermatol* 1999;140:685–8.

[55] Lovell CR, Burton JL, Horrobin DF. Treatment of atopic eczema with evening primrose oil [letter]. *Lancet* 1981; 1(8214):278.

[56] Senapati S, Banerjee S, Gangopadhyay DN. Evening primrose oil is effective in atopic dermatitis: A randomized placebo-controlled trial. Indian *J Dermatol Venereol Leprol* 2008; 74: 447-52

[57] Valsecchi R, Di Landro A, Pansera B, Reseghetti A. Gammalinolenic acid in the treatment of atopic dermatitis [1]. *J Eur Acad Dermatol Venereol* 1996; 7(1):77–9.

[58] Wright S, Burton JL. Oral evening primrose oil improves atopic eczema. *Lancet* 1982; 2(8308): 1120-2

[59] Andreassi M, Forleo P, Di Lorio A, Masci S, Abate G, Amerio P. Efficacy of gamma-linolenic acid in the treatment of patients with atopic dermatitis. *J Int Med Res.* 1997 Sep-Oct;25(5):266-74

[60] Bahmer FA, Schafer J. [Treatment of atopic dermatitis with borage seed oil (glandol) – a time series analytic study]. [German*]. Kinderarztl Prax* 1992;60(7):199–202.

[61] Buslau M, Thaci D. Atopic dermatitis: borage oil for systemic therapy. *Z Dermatol* 1996; 182: 132–6.

[62] Humphreys F, Symons JA, Brown HK, Duff GW, Hunter JAA. The effects of gamolenic acid on adult atopic eczema and premenstrual exacerbation of eczema. *Eur J Dermatol* 1994;4(8):598–603.

[63] Schalin-Karrila M, Mattila L, Jansen CT, Uotila P. Evening primrose oil in the treatment of atopic eczema: effect on clinical status, plasma phospholipid fatty acids and circulating blood prostaglandins. *Br J Dermatol.* 1987 Jul;117(1):11-9

[64] Hoare C, Li Wan Po A, Williams H. Systematic review of treatments for atopic eczema. *Health Technol Assess* 2000; 4:37.

[65] Morse NL, Clough PM. A meta-analysis of randomized, placebo-controlled clinical trials of Efamol evening primrose oil in atopic eczema. Where do we go from here in light of more recent discoveries? *Curr Pharm Biotechnol.* 2006 Dec;7(6):503-24.

[66] Morse PF, Horrobin DF, Manku MS, Stewart JC, Allen R, Littlewood S, Wright S, Burton J, Gould DJ, Holt PJ, et al. Meta-analysis of placebo-controlled studies of the efficacy of Epogam in the treatment of atopic eczema. Relationship between plasma essential fatty acid changes and clinical response. *Br J Dermatol.* 1989 Jul;121(1):75-90.

[67] van Gool CJ, Zeegers MP, Thijs C. Oral essential fatty acid supplementation in atopic dermatitis-a meta-analysis of placebo-controlled trials. *Br J Dermatol.* 2004 Apr;150(4):728-40

In: Linoleic Acids
Editor: Igho Onakpoya

ISBN: 978-1-62257-384-4
© 2012 Nova Science Publishers, Inc.

Chapter IX

Modulation of Carcinogenesis and Inflammation by Linoleic Acid and its Derivatives

Túlio César Ferreira*[*] *and Élida Geralda Campos
Laboratório de Biologia Molecular- Departamento de Biologia Celular – Universidade de Brasilia - Campus Darcy Ribeiro - Brasília-DF, Brazil

Abstract

Fatty acids are bioactive organic nutrients important for human health. They are classified based on the number of carbon atoms present in their hydrocarbon chain (i.e. short-, medium- or long-chain) and also on the absence or presence of insaturations (i.e. saturated or unsaturated, respectively). Polyunsaturated fatty acids (PUFA) are represented by 3 major families: ω-3, ω-6, and ω-9, all of which are metabolized using the same group of enzymes. Humans can synthesize a number of different fatty acids; however, they are unable to synthesize two main PUFA: linoleic acid (LA, 18:2; ω-6) and α-linolenic acid (ALA, 18:3, ω-3). Therefore, these two fatty acids are essential to humans because they must be acquired from the diet. They are produced by plants and are the precursors of eicosapentanoic acid (EPA, 20:5, ω-3) and docosahexaenoic acid (DHA, 22:6, ω-3). LA, ALA and their derivatives are important in many physiologic processes and diseases, such as growth and development, diabetes, coronary disease and cancer. Though a well-established nutrient, the health benefits of LA are still controversial. LA is the major dietary PUFA but recent reports advocate for reduced LA intake based on the fact that it can be converted to AA, which leads to the synthesis of proinflamatory and prothrombotic eicosanoids. In addition, LA promotes cell invasion and cell growth in some cancer cell lines. Despite the undesired effects observed in cells treated with LA, its exact mechanism(s) of action is not clear, and even less clear are the effects of specific dietary ω-6 fatty acid deficiency. The different results obtained from experiments with LA supplementation may depend on cell line, cell differentiation status

* Laboratório de Biologia Molecular- Departamento de Biologia Celular - Universidade de Brasilia - Campus Darcy Ribeiro - Brasília-DF, CEP: 70910-900. Email: tulcesar@gmail.com.

and the dose of supplemented fatty acid. Our research group has reported that LA is toxic to yeast cell in a cell-density dependent manner causing cell death through oxidative stress. Yeast cells are considered suitable study models to characterize the biochemical mechanisms in response to nutrients, because yeast cells are quick and easy to grow, and their cell cycle is very similar to the cell cycle of human cells and is regulated by homologous proteins. Based on the various divergent results obtained from different studies on lipid metabolism, this chapter aims to give an overview about the latest studies on LA and its derivatives, mainly conjugated linoleic acids (CLA), with special emphasis on food sources, dietary recommendations, metabolism, and beneficial and non-beneficial properties of such compounds to human health.

List of Abbreviations

AA	Arachidonic acid
CLA	Conjugated linoleic acid
COX	Cyclooxygenases
DHA	Docosahexaenoic acid
EFA	Essential fatty acid
EFAD	Essential fatty acid deficiency
EPA	Eicosapentaenoic acid
IL	Interleukin
LA	Linoleic acid
LOX	Lipooxygenase
LT	Leukotriene
PUFA	Polyunsaturated fatty acid
TNF	Tumor necrosis factor
VEGF	Vascular endothelial growth factor

Introduction

In 1929 and 1930 the two first reports concerning the importance of fatty acids in human nutrition and disease were published [1, 2]. Prior to that time, the importance of fatty acids was mainly due to the fact that they were a source of calories in the diet and function as carriers of fat-soluble vitamins. These two studies showed that when rats received a diet depleted of fatty acids, they presented signs of illness due to fatty acid deficiency, which were reverted when linoleic acid (LA), a polyunsaturated fatty acid (PUFA), was included in the diet. Based on these results, the authors proposed that LA was an essential fatty acid (EFA) for mammals, and had some critical role in the metabolism. Nowadays, EFAs are recognized as an important nutrient for human growth, development, and other important physiologic functions.

Polyunsaturated fatty acids are constituted by 3 major families: ω-3, ω-6, and ω-9, all of which are metabolized by enzymes called desaturases and elongases [3], leading to the formation of products with longer carbon chain and increased levels of insaturation. Although humans can synthesize unsaturated fatty acids such as palmitoleic acid (PA, 16:1; ω-7) and oleic acid (OA, 18:1; ω-9), they are unable to synthesize the first two members of the ω-3 and ω-6 family, linoleic acid (LA, 18:2; ω-6) and α-linolenic acid (ALA, 18:3, ω-3). Therefore, humans must acquire them from the diet.

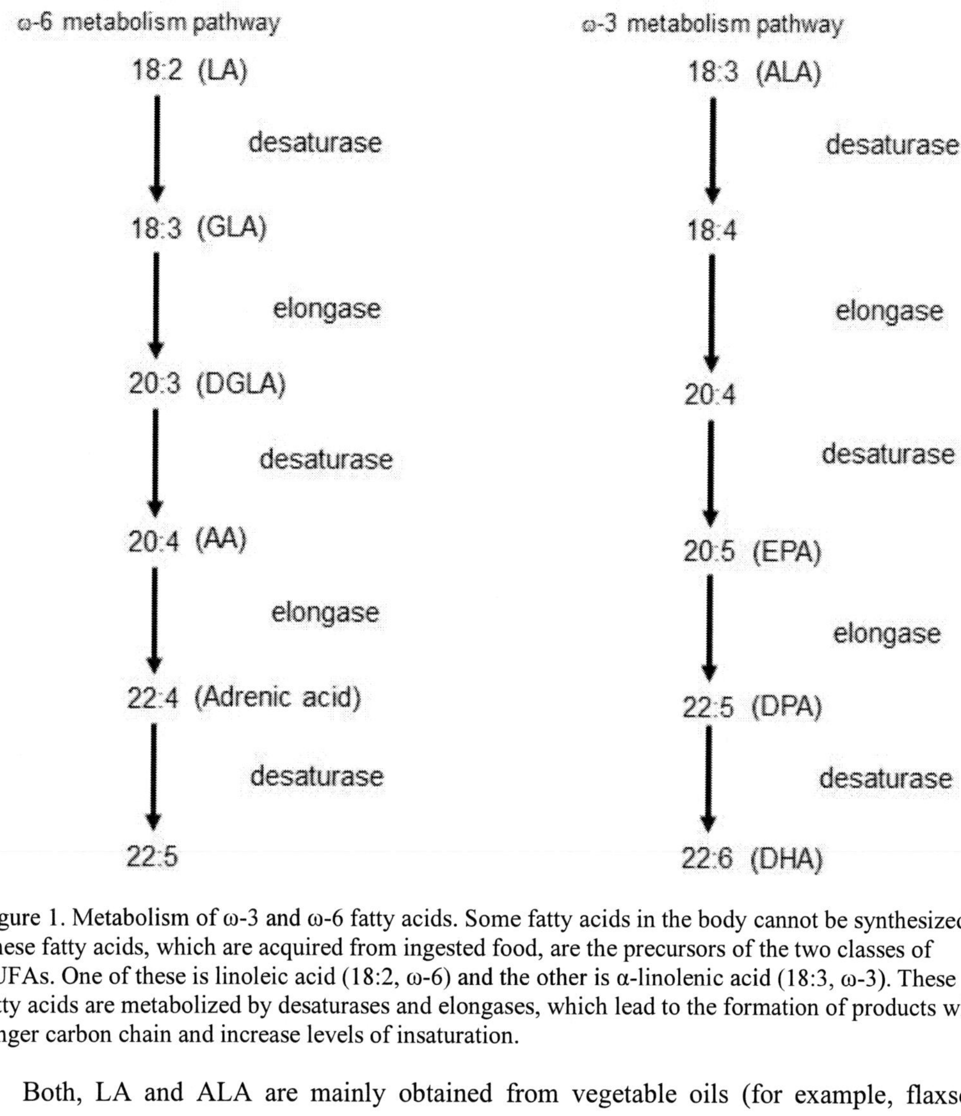

Figure 1. Metabolism of ω-3 and ω-6 fatty acids. Some fatty acids in the body cannot be synthesized. These fatty acids, which are acquired from ingested food, are the precursors of the two classes of PUFAs. One of these is linoleic acid (18:2, ω-6) and the other is α-linolenic acid (18:3, ω-3). These fatty acids are metabolized by desaturases and elongases, which lead to the formation of products with longer carbon chain and increase levels of insaturation.

Both, LA and ALA are mainly obtained from vegetable oils (for example, flaxseed, rapeseed and soybean oils) and other plant sources (for example walnuts), because plants have the appropriate enzymes capable of inserting double bonds after carbon 9. They can also be obtained from animals that have ingested these EFAs from plant sources [4, 5]. In mammals, the downstream product of LA includes the arachidonic acid (AA; 20:4, ω-6), and ALA metabolism produces eicosapentaenoic acid (EPA; 20:5, ω-3) and docosahexaenoic acid (DHA; 22:6, ω-3). Initially LA is desaturated by Δ6-desaturase to form γ-linolenic acid (GLA, 18:3, ω-6) and subsequent transformations of GLA produces dihomo-γ-linolenic acid (DGLA, 20:3, ω-6) and AA, by means of elongation and desaturation reactions (Figure 1). The reaction catalyzed by Δ6-desaturases is not limited to LA metabolism. Both EPA and DHA are produced by the desaturation of ALA by these same enzymes. Finally, these PUFAs can be metabolized afterwards to produce a variety of essential intermediate compounds. Both, EPA and AA are considered critical metabolites, because they are precursors of eicosanoids, including prostaglandins (PG), thromboxanes (TX), prostacyclins (PGI2), and leukotrienes (LT), which mediate a variety of physiologic and biochemical processes [6] LA has also been reported to help diminish the concentration of low-density lipoprotein (LDL) cholesterol, triglycerides and the total/high-density lipoprotein (HDL) cholesterol ratio, as well as increase the level of HDL cholesterol [7] Aside being present in high amounts in membranes, DHA is functionally by far the most important ω-3 PUFA because of its importance in the growth and development of the brain in infants and in the maintenance of normal neural functions in adults [8, 9]. DHA has also been reported to decrease the risk of degenerative diseases of the brain and cardiovascular system [10, 11]. Therefore, DHA must be acquired from the diet as ω-6 fatty acids cannot fulfill these requirements.

Dietary PUFAs and Deficiency of EFA

When less than 1%–2% of the total calories in a diet are composed of EFAs, EFA deficiency (EFAD) can occur [12]. In general, plants are the main sources of LA and ALA, but they do not contain their distal elongation and desaturation products, such as AA, EPA, and DHA. However, a modest intake of plant oil, which provides at least 1% to 2% of total energy intake, normally is sufficient to provide an adequate amount of LA and ALA, which are metabolized in animals generating AA, EPA and DHA, thus preventing the development of EFAD [13]. In humans, ALA is converted to EPA and DHA, but the rate of conversion of ALA into DHA is extremely limited with rates generally lower than 0.1%, as observed in many reports reviewed by Plourde and Cunnane [14]. Therefore, directly providing EPA and DHA via diet is more effective in increasing the levels of EPA and DHA in plasma and tissues, compared to their *de novo* synthesis from ALA [15]. The primary dietary source of EPA and DHA in human diets is fish and other marine sources, which acquire the ω-3 fatty acids from unicellular phytoplanktonic protists, mostly algae, and marine zooplankton which are rich sources of EPA and DHA as well as a range of other lipids with 16- and 18-carbon chains [16, 17].

The recommended intakes of PUFA to prevent biochemical and physiological symptoms of deficiency and to optimize tissue PUFA content in rats and humans, are about 2 energy (en) % of the diet for LA and 0.5 en% for ALA [18]. Deficiencies of ω-6 and ω-3 PUFA in mammals can occur due to consumption of diets devoid of fat or those containing dietary fat derived exclusively from saturated fatty acids. Deficiency can manifest as a variety of symptoms, such as decrease in growth rate, skin scaliness, impaired water retention, impaired reproduction, and increase ratio of mead acid/AA, in the tissue [19, 20].

Cunnane and Anderson [21] studied the effect of pure LA deficiency on rat growth as well as changes in the metabolism and oxidation of ω-6 PUFAs. These authors analyzed the fatty acid profiles of liver through neutral lipid thin-layer chromatography and observed that the concentration of total fatty acids in liver phospholipids was not significantly affected by LA deficiency, but there were marked decreases on accumulation of ω-6 PUFAs. Pure LA deficiency induced milder symptoms, particularly regarding growth retardation, when compared to symptoms due to classical (LA plus ALA) EFAD. The authors suggested that the presence of ALA and possibly oleic acid (OA, 18:1, ω-9) in the used diet may have spared LA in body stores of oxidation.

In recent years, many reports concerning the real requirement of EFA, especially LA, in the human diet, have been published, and many of them show controversial results. This controversy is due to the fact that some requirements were based on studies in which both LA and ALA were omitted from the diet. The ALA deficiency was not taken into consideration in such studies. In addition the oils that were given to correct the deficiency contained trace amounts of ALA. Thus the recommended LA intake levels may be overestimated [22].

PUFA in Carcinogenesis and Pro-Inflammatory Processes

In the last few years, many studies have suggested that excessive levels of ω-6 fatty acids, relative to ω3 fatty acids, may increase the risk of acquiring a number of human diseases. This may occur because ω-6 and ω-3 fatty acids compete for the same rate-limiting enzymes. A high proportion of ω-6 to ω-3 fatty acids in the diet may shift the physiological state in the tissues toward carcinogenesis, cause an increase in gastroschisis (a congenital abdominal wall defect) risk, and exacerbate an inflammatory process [23, 24, 25, 26, 27, 28]. Byon et al. [29] studied the effect of LA (500 μM) in the invasive and metastatic MDA-MB-231 breast cancer cell line and showed that this fatty acid induced the expression of plasminogen activator inhibitor-1 (PAI-1), as well as *in vitro* migration of these cells after 24 hours exposure to LA. PAI-1 belongs to the family of serine protease inhibitors and is the primary inhibitor of urokinase-type (uPA) and tissue-type (tPA) plasminogen activators. It is also a key prognostic factor in breast cancer [29]. In contrast, other EFAs tested had little or no effect on PAI-1 expression or cell migration. Nishioka et al. [30] analyzed the effect of LA on OCUM-2MD3 gastric carcinoma cells and observed that LA does not affect cell growth when added to OCUM-2MD3 cell cultures, but increased dietary LA enhanced tumor growth in orthotopic tissue implanted with OCUM-2MD3 cells in nude mice. This study suggests that dietary LA impacts multiple steps in cancer invasion and angiogenesis. The findings in both studies mentioned above indicate that reduction of LA intake may help slow cancer progression [29, 30].

Inflammation is a critical process of tumor progression. A number of cancers appear first in sites of infection, chronic irritation and inflammation. Tumor cells' microenvironment, orchestrated by cells of the inflammatory system, seems to be crucial in the promotion of proliferation, survival and migration of tumors [31]. Inflammation is characterized by the access of liquid and cells to the interstice [32]. During the inflammatory process, inflammatory chemical mediators attract leukocytes with chemostatic activity to the lesion/infection site. These mediators can vary depending on the type of inflammatory process involved, and may be amines, such as histamine, lipid-derivatives such as, prostaglandins (PG), short peptides, such as bradykinin and longer peptides, such as interleukin-1. These inflammatory agents act on the cell membrane inducing phospholipase A2 activation, which acts on the membrane phospholipids of all nucleated cells releasing AA. Phospholipase A2 participates in the maintenance of the cell membrane but it is induced in processes that trigger the initiation and maintenance of inflammation. In the inflammatory process some enzymes convert AA released from the membrane into molecules that act as mediators in this process and that also participate in platelets aggregation (inhibiting or inducing), constriction and relaxation of blood vessels. These mediators are the PG, which are products of the cyclooxygenases (COX) reactions and the leukotrienes (LT), products of the lipoxygenases (LOX) reactions [33].

Cyclooxygenases, known as prostaglandin H sintases or PGHS are bifunctional enzymes with both cyclooxygenase and peroxidase activities. The cyclooxygenase component converts AA to hydroperoxy-endoperoxide (prostaglandin G2; PGG2) and the peroxide component reduces the endoperoxide to the corresponding alcohol (prostaglandin H2; PGH2) [33]. The PGs have a central role in the inflammatory process and pain and are synthesized by three human cyclooxygenase isoforms: COX-1 which is constitutively expressed in a variety of cell types, COX-2 which is induced in the inflammation site, and COX-3 which is similar to COX-1 and also referred to as COX1-b. COX-3 is encoded by the same gene as COX-1, with the difference being that COX-3 retains an intron that is not retained in COX-1 [34]. COX-2 is also constitutively expressed in the central nervous system and may play an important role in nociceptive processes [35].

Lipoxygenases (LOX) catalyse the oxygenation of PUFA, such as LA and AA. There are three mammalian isoforms of LOX that are involved in the pathway of leukotriene production, 5-LOX, 12-LOX and 15-LOX [36]. When LOX acts on AA during the inflammatory process, the distinct hydroperoxy-eicosatetraenoics (HPETE) such as 5-HPETE, 12-HPETE and 15-HPETE are formed. These are unstable peroxide derivatives and are converted into their corresponding hydroxylated derivatives or, depending on the tissue, to leukotrienes (LT) or lipoxins (LX). The biosynthesis of LT occurs mainly in granulocytes, monocytes/macrophages and mastocytes and is orchestrated by the activation of LOX [36].

Although some studies indicate that high intake of LA increases the levels of pro-inflammatory metabolites as a consequence of high LA conversion to AA, in a study with human volunteers supplemented daily with a high amount (27 en%) of AA for up to 7 weeks, the production of inflammatory cytokines TNF-α, IL-1β, or IL-6 by peripheral blood mononuclear cells stimulated *ex vivo* by bacterial endotoxin was not detected [37]. Thies et al. [38] also reported that the supplementation of individuals with encapsulated oil blends containing moderate amount of ω-3- and ω-6- PUFA, including AA, in their diet for 12 weeks failed to significantly increase the production of these same proinflammatory cytokines and neither affected inflammatory cell numbers or neutrophil and monocyte responses in humans. These results differ from a previous report in which the effects of increasing concentrations of AA in cell culture were analyzed and showed that a human monocytic cell line treated with AA was able to increase the release of IL-like activity [39]. Taken together, these findings suggest that ω6-PUFA, enhance inflammatory cell responses whereas the ω3-PUFA (EPA and DHA), diminish these responses.

Linoleic Acid Cytotoxicity

Several experimental studies, both *in vivo* and *in vitro*, have shown that some PUFA act by promoting inhibitory effects on tumor cell growth [40]. In addition, induction of apoptosis by these fatty acids may have a crucial protective effect at the first stage of carcinogenesis, as exemplified by colonocyte deletion as a mechanism of cancer prevention [41]. Individual PUFA have been proposed as chemotherapeutic agents, and as potential adjuvants to radio- or chemotherapy [42]. Their cytotoxicity is dose-dependent and is attributed to the carbon chain length and the number of insaturations. These cytotoxic or antiproliferative effects of PUFA depend on the cell type and culture conditions [43, 44, 45]Such effects are complex and may be associated with changes in membrane composition, oxidative stress and metabolism which produce active bioproducts [42].

Our research group has studied the effect of LA on the baker's yeast *Saccharomyces cerevisae* viability [46]. We hypothesized that treatment of yeast cells with LA may cause the fatty acid to be up taken, become incorporated into the membranes and make the cells more prone to oxidative stress. Our results showed that oxidative stress and cell death increase in yeast cells treated with 100 μM LA. Oxidative stress indicators were measured by lipid peroxidation levels, mitochondrial respiration and activity of specific antioxidant enzymes, such as catalase and cytochrome c peroxidase and enzymes that participate in the pentose phosphate pathway, such as glucose-6-phosphate dehydrogenase and 6-phosphogluconate dehydrogenase. We observed that there was an increase in the lipid peroxidation levels, antioxidant and metabolic enzymes activities and reduction in the cellular respiration in yeast cells treated with LA compared to untreated cells.

Multicellular organisms have two mechanisms to eliminate cells: necrosis and apoptosis [47]. Necrosis may be triggered by the rupture of the plasmatic membrane causing a linkage of the cellular content on the environment, which leads to an inflammatory process [48]. However, apoptosis is a controlled form of cell death that plays fundamental roles during embryonic development and in the maintenance of tissues, which is characterized by a "cleaner" type of death. In apoptosis the chromatin is condensed; the DNA becomes fragmented forming vesicles known as "apoptotic bodies", which are rapidly phagocytosed by the macrophages resulting in process without any inflammatory phenomena [49]. Apoptosis is the process of programmed cell death (PCD) that occurs in uni- and multicellular and organisms. Apoptotic markers have been described in *Saccharomyces cerevisiae,* and the mechanism of apoptosis has been conserved from unicellular to multicellular organisms [50]. In our study, yeast cells treated with LA showed reduction in cell formation unit (CFU), an increase in chromatin fragmentation and alterations in cell permeability indicating apoptosis induction [46]. In addition cell density and growth phase were relevant to explain LA toxicity to yeast cells. These results provide new possibilities for investigating PUFA effects on cell growth and apoptosis, using yeast as a model. Our studies on LA toxicity to cells are in accordance with previous studies [43, 44, 45] which showed that different cell types (Jurkat and Raji cell culture and isolated human lymphocytes) undergo apoptosis when treated with 25 μM to 200 μM. The study of the effects of LA in different cell types can increase our understanding of its antiproliferative activity and modulatory effect relevant to cell growth. Therefore, yeast may be used to study the selective cytotoxic effect of LA and other PUFA, and to uncover new effects of their toxicity. Because several biochemical mechanisms are conserved between this unicellular eukaryotic cell and higher eukaryotes, in response to many chemicals such as drugs and supplements, the findings described by this approach may be valid for some mammalian cells.

Conjugated Linoleic Acid (CLA) and its Sources

Another naturally occurring PUFA that is implicated in a large number of beneficial properties to human health is a derivative from LA metabolism, known as conjugated linoleic acid (CLA, 18:2). CLA consists of a family of 28 members with different positional and geometric isomers of LA. This variation of isomers are possible due to the conjugated double bonds that range from 6,8 to 12,14. For every positional isomer there are four possible geometric pairs of isomers (*cis,trans*; *trans,cis*; *cis,cis*; and *trans,trans*) [51]. Despite the existence of a large number of LA isomers, they are found in nature mainly in cis-9, trans-11 and trans-10, cis-12 forms. Food products derived from ruminants (meat and milk) are the major source of CLA in human diets. In milk, for example, the *cis*-9, *trans*-11 isomer can represent 80% to 90% of the total CLA [52] while in meat this isomer is predominant and the amount varies depending on the cooking methods or the doneness [53].

CLA Synthesis

Conjugated linoleic acids are produced in ruminants by two pathways. One occurs through ruminal biohydrogenation of LA. This process is possible due to a large number of bacteria present in the rumen. The first step of rumen biohydrogenation occurs through the action of linoleate isomerase, an enzyme that hydrogenates the *cis*-12 double bound of LA, producing *cis*-9, *trans*-11 (18:2) CLA. However, this first product of biohydrogenation is rapidly converted to vaccenic acid (18:1; *trans*-11 octadecenoic acid) in an additional reduction reaction. Vaccenic acid can be converted to stearic acid (18:0) in a further reaction. This last reaction is significantly slower than the two first reactions, contributing to the accumulation of vaccenic acid in the rumen, which is absorbed and then accumulates in the tissues [51]. The second pathway is the desaturation of the vaccenic acid mediated by the Δ9-desaturase present in the animal's tissues. In the tissues, vaccenic acid, a major fatty acid produced in the rumen, is desaturated by the tissue/endogenous Δ9-desaturase producing *cis*-9, *trans*-11 CLA [54]. Several studies show that CLA milk content depends on a wide variety of dietary factors, such as, the plant species and the type of plant seeds ruminants ingest. It depends also on the lipid contents of the consumed plants and seeds and on the levels of food intake (for more details, see table 1 in Bauman et al., 2000 [51]).

Although CLA is generated from LA metabolism in ruminants, mammals are unable to synthesize LA and ALA by a "*de novo*" pathway, because they lack the fatty acyl-CoA desaturase activity able to insert double bounds beyond C-9. In ruminants, these fatty acids are acquired from the diet and then are immediately metabolized by anaerobic microbes in the rumen to produce trienoic, dienoic and monoenoic *trans* fatty acids, with major production of CLA [51]. CLA may also be synthesized during heat processing of animal-derived foods [55].

Anticarcinogenic Activity of CLA

An overview of the literature shows that CLA can have several beneficial properties important for human health. The numerous properties reported may be explained by different experimental protocols used to study CLA effects on biological systems that may result in different outcomes. Overall, these studies include the use of a mixture containing the *cis*-9,*trans*-11-CLA and *trans*-10,*cis*-12-CLA isomers, or only one isolated isomer, in addition to the use of different concentrations of CLA and treatment times and also different cell types or animal models [56, 57, 59]The majority of these reports show that dietary CLA prevents carcinogenesis in animal models [59] by the inhibition of the mechanisms involved in the initiation, promotion and progression of carcinogenesis or by inducing apoptosis in cancer cells. Although multiple mechanisms for the anticarconogenic effects of CLA have been proposed, the precise mechanism of action of CLA remains unclear.

Inhibition of Cell Growth

Vascular endothelial growth factor (VEGF) is a central regulator protein in angiogenesis, a primordial condition for solid tumor progression and which can contribute to metastasis [60]. The tumor associated angiogenesis occurs by the so called angiogenic switch [61]. This process is separated into two distinct phases. In the first phase, denominated as "avascular", the tumor reaches up to 1-2 mm in diameter. In this phase there is a balance between proliferation and apoptosis and in the second phase, denominated as "vascular phase", the tumor presents a potential for growth [61], where the expression of genes involved in angiogenesis are triggered, such as VEGF and matrix metalloproteinase (MMP)-9 [62], cyclooxygenase-2 [63] and hypoxia inducible factor 1 alpha (HIF-1) [64]. The latter is a heterodimeric transcriptor factor, involved in the control of a wide variety of genes involved in cell metabolism, iron homeostasis, oxygen supply, growth and cell death [65]. Therefore, it is plausible to consider inhibition of angiogenesis as an alternative for therapeutic applications, because the tumors mass could be arrested in a size about 1-2 mm and tumor progression could be avoided. A study by Wang et al. [66] exemplifies a possible mechanism for CLA inhibition of cell proliferation. These authors analyzed the effect of CLA on the expression of VEGF and showed that CLA down-regulate VEGF expression and induce the expression of the protein tyrosine phosphatase γ (PTPγ), an estrogen-regulated cancer suppressor gene in the human breast cancer cell line MCF-7. The reduced expression of these proteins leads to the suppression of tumor growth.

An approach that has also been exploited to investigate CLA inhibitory effect on cell proliferation is to verify if CLA interferes with cell metabolism. Donnelly et al. [57] have studied the effect of both CLA isomers, *cis*-9, *trans*-11- and *trans*-10, *cis*-12-CLA, on cancer cell lines viability and the expression of the fatty acid synthase (FAS) and Spot 14. The latter, is a nuclear protein involved in the regulation of genes required for fatty acid synthesis in normal and malignant mammary epithelial and adipose cells. They showed that in human breast cancer and liposarcoma cells, a mixture containing both CLA isomers significantly reduced the expression of Spot14 and FAS genes as well as cell growth, as did pure isomers. However, no change on cell growth was observed when LA was used on the cell culture. These authors support the hypothesis that the antiproliferative effect of CLA also relays on the blockage of lipid synthesis, which compromise the cell metabolism.

Induction of Apoptosis

Tumor mass formation is the net result of cell proliferation minus cell death. Consequently, deregulation of cell death can result in carcinogenesis [67]. CLA may inhibit clonal expansion by means of apoptosis modulation. Apoptosis is induced by a diverse range of cell signals, which may originate either extracellularly or intracellularly, and is regulated by various proteins, such as those encoded by the mammalian *Bcl-2* family of anti-apoptopic genes (Bcl-2, Bcl-XL, Bcl-w, Mcl-1 and A1), the pro-apoptotic Bax subfamily (Bax, Bak and Bok) and the pro-apoptotic BH3 subfamily (Bad, Bid, Bik, Blk, Hrk, BNIP3 and BimL) [68, 69]. Several reports show that CLA, mainly *cis*-9, *trans*-11-CLA and i-10, *cis*-12-CLA isomers, induce apoptosis in different human cell lines and tissues [70, 71], mainly through inhibition of Bcl-2, but not through changes in bax and bak expressions [72].

Anti-Inflammatory Effects of CLA

The attenuation of inflammation is an important approach in the prevention and progression of a large number of important human pathologies, including cancer. The anti-inflammatory properties of dietary CLA have been reported in studies with several animal models and the mechanisms that may explain how these fatty acids act include, (1) suppression of proinflammatory cytokines production, such as tumor necrosis factor-α (TNFα), interleukin (IL)-1β, IL-6, interferon-γ (IFNγ), and IL-12, from a variety of cell types, (2) binding to nuclear receptors and suppression of genes that participate in the inflammatory process and (3) inhibition of the generation of eicosanoid lipids.

Bassaganya-Riera et al. [73] studied the effect of CLA on the inflammatory response in pigs and demonstrated that dietary supplementation with increasing amounts of CLA (0%, 0.67%, 1.33%, and 2%) induced a linear increase in the percentages of cytotoxic T lymphocyte (CTL; CD8+ cells) (21.7%, 22.3%, 28.0, and 32.7%, respectively). These cells are also critical for the development of cellular immune responses involving the production of some cytokines and cytotoxins in viral and bacterial infections. The cytokine TNFα has an important role in the response against bacterial, and certain fungal, viral, and parasitic invasions. It is also involved in the necrosis of specific tumors and acts as a key mediator in the local inflammatory immune response. Kim et al. [74]studied the effect of *trans*-10,*cis*-12-CLA on TNFα production by lipopolysaccharide (LPS)-stimulated porcine peripheral blood mononuclear cells (PBMCs) and found that this CLA isomer was able to attenuate TNFα production through induction of IL-10.

The second mechanism that indicates how CLA attenuates inflammation concerns the role of CLA in binding to specific nuclear receptors that can act as transcription factors. CLA is known to bind to the steroid hormone receptors, peroxisome proliferator-activated receptor (PPARγ), and it is possible that its anti-inflammatory effects can be attributed to activation of this nuclear hormone receptor [75, 76]. PPARγ plays a crucial role in the regulation of adipocyte differentiation, fatty acid metabolism, and glucose homeostasis. It is also a negative regulator of macrophage differentiation and activation [77, 78]. Thus, CLA by binding to PPARγ leads to inhibition of the expression of genes implicated in the inflammatory response [73, 74].

The third mechanism that could be involved in the attenuation of an inflammatory response by CLA is the down-regulation of prostaglandin E2 (PGE2) and leukotriene B4 (LTB4) production. PGE2 and LTB4 are potent eicosanoid lipid mediators derived from phospholipase-released AA, involved in early micro-inflammatory events (endoplasmic). There are three supported theories that may explain the reduction of AA-derived eicosanoids, such as PGE2 and LTB4:

Theory 1

There is a competition between LA and CLA for the desaturase and elongase enzymes involved in the production of AA. AA is synthesized *in vivo* from dietary LA acid through two desaturations and one elongation reactions, mediated by Δ6-/Δ5-desaturase and elongase. Banni et al. [79] showed that supplementation with CLA in the diet of rats resulted in the suppression of the biosynthetic pathway of AA. The authors suggested that there is a parallel pathway of conjugated fatty acid biosynthesis when CLA is added to the diet. In this pathway CLA competes for the same set of desaturase and elongase enzymes used in the synthesis of AA, thus diminishing the availability of this fatty acid in the cell membrane as substrate for the COX and LOX enzymes.

Theory 2

There is a reduction in the expression of the COX, the rate-limiting enzyme, which catalyzes the conversion of AA into prostanoids. To exemplify the theory of downregulation of PGE2, Nakanishi et al. [80]conducted a study on the effect of CLA on cerebral PGE2. They fed mice from the age of 9 weeks until they mated, reproduced and lactated, with a diet containing 3% CLA. Biochemical analysis of the brain cells of the mice offspring, also fed with CLA, revealed a reduction in the production of PGE2 while COX mRNA expression was quantitatively increased by CLA supplementation. Their results indicate that brain PGE2 production can be reduced by dietary CLA without inhibition of COX gene expression in mice, which contrasts the second theory concerning PGE2 inhibition. This may be explained by the fact that CLA modulation of eicosanoid production is tissue specific [59].

Theory 3

The third theory postulates that CLA may act as substrates for COX, competing with AA for binding to this enzyme or CLA may have an antagonist effect inhibiting the COX activity, and thereby compromising the production of proinflammatory cytokines However, this mechanism is not well understood [59].

All these findings suggest that CLA may be useful as an immunomodulatory agent in the prevention or treatment of inflammatory and immune-mediated diseases, such as cancer. CLA improves certain aspects of the inflammatory response, particularly in cellular and animal models. However, the relevance of such effects has yet to be clarified within the context of human health.

Conclusion

Linoleic acid is a well-established nutrient. However, its benefits to human health and efficacy in disease prevention are still controversial. Recent reports advocate for reduced LA intake based on the fact that it can be converted to AA, which leads to production of proinflammatory and prothrombotic eicosanoids. Future research should consider the production of local and systemic inflammatory markers to extend the knowledge on LA effects. Little is known about the metabolism and mechanism of action of LA in humans, and even less is known about the effects of specific dietary ω-6 fatty acid deficiencies. Several of the reports concerning the effects of high amount of LA in human health are sometimes speculative because researchers are not completely aware of the possible methodological errors in this type of studies. In addition, supporting evidence from animal and *in vitro* studies is limited. Although some mechanisms of action of EFAs have been postulated, further studies are still necessary regarding LA requirements and its effects on human health.

Conjugated linoleic acid is an LA derivative much studied nowadays. This metabolite has been widely employed in studies that investigate anticancer and anti-inflammatory effects and several reports suggest that CLA is a promising nutrient that could be used to reduce or prevent carcinogenesis and the inflammatory events associated with it.

References

[1] Burr GO, Burr MM. (1929). A new deficiency disease produced by the rigid exclusion of fat from the diet. *J. Biol. Chem.* 82:345-367.

[2] Burr GO, Burr MM. (1930). On the nature and role of the fatty acids essential in nutrition. *J. Biol. Chem.* 86:587-621.

[3] Horrobin DF. (1993). Fatty acid metabolism in health and dis-ease: the role of delta-6-desaturase. *Am J Clin Nutr.* 57:732S-737S.

[4] Poulos A. (1995). Very long chain fatty acids in higher animals – a review. *Lipids.* 30:1-14.

[5] Spector AA. (1999). Essentiality of fatty acids. *Lipids.* 34:S1-S3.

[6] Bannenberg G, Serhan CN. (2010). Specialized pro-resolving lipid mediators in the inflammatory response: an update. *Biochim Biophys Acta.* 1801: 1260-1273.

[7] Mensink RP, Zock PL, Kester ADM, Katan MB. (2003). Effects of dietary fatty acids and carbohydrates on the ratio of serum total to HDL cholesterol and on serum lipids and apolipoproteins: a meta-analysis of 60 controlled trials. *Am. J. Clin. Nutr.* 77:1146–55.

[8] Salem N Jr., Wegher B, Mena P, Uauy R. (1996). Arachidonic and docosahexaenoic acids are biosynthesized from their 18-carbon precursors in human infants. *Proc. Natl. Acad. Sci. U S A.* 93(1):49-54.

[9] Horrocks LA, Yeo, YK. (1999). Health benefits of docosahexaenoic acid (DHA). *Pharmacological Research.* 40: 211-25.

[10] Freund-Levi Y, Eriksdotter-Jonhagen M, Cederholm T, Basun H, Faxen-Irving G, Garlind A, Vedin I, Vessby B, Wahlund LO, Palmblad J. (2006). Omega-3 fatty acid

treatment in 174 patients with mild to moderate Alzheimer disease: OmegAD study: a randomized double-blind trial. *Arch.Neurol.* 63(10):1402-8.

[11] Gebauer SK, Psota TL, Harris WS, Kris-Etherton PM. (2006). n-3 fatty acid dietary recommendations and food sources to achieve essentiality and cardiovascular benefits. *Am. J. Clin. Nutr.* 83(6 Suppl):1526S-1535S.

[12] Aaes-Jorgensen E, Leppik EE, Hayes HW, Holman RT. (1958). Essential fatty acid deficiency: II. In adult rats. *J. Nutr.* 66:245- 259.

[13] Institute of Medicine. *Dietary reference intakes for energy, carbohydrate, fiber, fat, fatty acids, cholesterol, protein and amino acids.* (2002/2005) Washington DC: National Academy Press.

[14] Plourde M, Cunnane SC. (2007). Extremely limited synthesis of long chain polyunsaturates in adults: implication for their dietary essentiality and use as supplements. *Appl. Physiol. Nutr. Metab.* 32: 619-634.

[15] Kris-Etherton PM, Grieger JA, Etherton TD. (2009) *Prostaglandins Leukot Essent Fatty Acids.* 81(2-3): 99-104. Epub 2009 Jun 13.

[16] Sargent JR, Henderson RJ. (1995). Marine (n-3) polyunsaturated fatty acids. In *Developments in Oils and Fats*, pp. 32-65 [R. J. Hamilton, editor]. London: Blackie Academic and Professional.

[17] Sargent JR. (1997). Fish oils and human diet. *Brit. J. of Nut.* 78(Suppl 1): S5-SI3.

[18] Simopoulos AP, Leaf A, Salem JrN. (2000). Workshop statement on the essentiality of and recommended dietary intakes for Omega-6 and Omega-3 fatty acids. *Prostaglandins Leukot Essent. Fatty Acids.* 63:119-121.

[19] Aaes-Jorgensen E. (1961). Essential fatty acids. *Physiol. Rev.* 41:1-51.

[20] Mohrhauer H, Holman RT. (1963). The effect of dose Ievel of EFA upon fatty acid composition of the rat liver. J *Lipid Res.* 4:151-159.

[21] Cunnane SC, Anderson MJ. (1997). Pure linoleate deficiency in the rat: influence on growth, accumulation of n-6 polyunsaturates, and [1-14C]linoleate oxidation. *Journal of Lipid Research.* 38:805-812.

[22] Cunnane SC. (2003). Problems with essential fatty acids: time for a new paradigm? Progress in Lipid Research. 42: 544-568.

[23] Calder PC. (2001). Polyunsaturated fatty acids, inflammation, and immunity. *Lipids.*36:1007-1024

[24] Simopoulos AP. (2003). Importance of the ratio of omega-6/omega-3 essential fatty acids: evolutionary aspects. World Review of Nutrition and Dietetics. 92:1-22.

[25] Hennig B, Lei W, Arzuaga X, Ghosh D, Saraswathi V, Toberek M. (2006). Linoleic acid induces proinflammatory events in endothelial cells via activation of PI3K/AKT and ERK1/2 signaling. *J Nutr Biochem* 17: 766-772

[26] Batlle J, Sauleda J, Balcells E, Gómez FP, Méndez M, Rodriguez E, Barreiro E, Ferrer JJ, Romieu I, Gea J, Antó JM, Garcia-Aymerich J, PAC-COPD (2011). Association between ω3 and ω 6 fatty acid intakes and serum inflammatory markers in COPD. *Journal of Nutritional Biochemistry.* In press.

[27] Espinosa-Neira R, Mejia-Rangel J, Cortes-Reynos P, Salazar EP. (2011). Linoleic acid induces an EMT like process in mammary epithelial cells MCF10A. *The International Journal of Biochemistry & Cell Biology.* 43:1782-1791.

[28] Weiss LA, Chambers CD, Gonzalez V, Hagey LR, Jones KL. (2012). The omega-6 fatty acid linoleic acid is associated with risk of gastroschisis: A novel dietary risk fact. *Am. J. Med. Genet.* A.158A(4):803-807.

[29] Byon CH, Hardy RW, Ren C, Ponnazhagan S, Welch DR, McDonald JM, Chen Y. (2009). Free fatty acids enhance breast cancer cell migration through plasminogen activator inhibitor1 and SMAD4. *Lab Invest.* 89:1221-1228.

[30] Nishioka TM, Yashiro M, Hirakawa K, Olden K, Roberts JD. (2011). Linoleic acid enhances angiogenesis through suppression of angiostatin induced by plasminogen activator inhibitor 1. *British Journal of Cancer.* 105: 1750-1758

[31] Coussens LM, Werb Z. (2002). Inflammation and câncer. *Nature.* 420(6917): 860–867.

[32] Lope ER, Chapadeiro E, Raso P, Tafuri WL. (1987). *Bogliolo - Patologia.* 4th. Edition. Belo Horizonte. Guanabara Koogan. p.67-112

[33] Funk CD. (2001). Prostaglandins and leukotrienes: advances in eicosanoid biology. *Science* 294:1871-1875

[34] Chandrasekharan NV, Dai H, Roos KL, Evanson NK, Tomsik J, Elton TS, Simmons DL. (2002). COX-3, a cyclooxygenase-1 variant inhibited by acetaminophen and other analgesic/antipyretic drugs: Cloning, structure, and expression. *Proc. Natl. Acad. Sci. U.S.A.* 99(21):13926–13931

[35] Martin F, Fletcher D, Chauvin M, Bouhassira D. (2007). Constitutive cyclooxygenase-2 is involved in central nociceptive processes in humans. *Anesthesiology.*106(5):1013-1018.

[36] Werz O, Bürkert E, Samuelsson B, Rådmark O, Steinhilber D. (2002). Activation of 5-lipoxygenase by cell stress is calcium independent in human polymorphonuclear leukocytes *Blood.* 99(3):1044-52.

[37] Kelley DS, Taylor PC, Nelson GJ, Mackey BE. (1998). Arachidonic acid supplementation enhances synthesis of eicosanoids without suppressing immune functions in young healthy men. *Lipids.* 33:125-130.

[38] Thies F, Miles EA, Nebe-von-Caron G, Powell JR, Hurst TL, Newsholme EA, Calder PC. (2001). Influence of dietary supplementation with long-chain n-3 or n-6 polyunsaturated fatty acids on blood inflammatory cell populations and functions and on plasma soluble adhesion molecules in healthy adults. *Lipids.* 36:1183-1193.

[39] Baldie G, Kaimakamis D, Rotondo D. (1993) Fatty Acid Modulation of Cytokine Release from Human Monocytic Cells. *Biochim. Biophys. Acta* 1179:125–133.

[40] Edwards IJ, O'Flaherty JT. (2008). Omega-3 Fatty Acids and PPARgamma in Cancer. *PPAR Res.* 2008:358052.

[41] Fan YY, Zhan Y, Aukema HM Davidson LA, Zhou L, Callaway E, Tian Y, Weeks BR, Lupton JR, Toyokuni S, Chapkin RS. (2009) Proapoptotic effects of dietary (n-3) fatty acids are enhanced in colonocytes of manganese-dependent superoxide dismutase knockout mice. *J. Nutr.* 139:1328–1332.

[42] Diggle CP. (2001). *In vitro* studies on the relationship between polyunsaturated fatty acids and cancer: tumour or tissue specific effects? *Prog. Lipid Res.* 41:240–253.

[43] Cury-Boaventura MF, Pompéia C, Curi R. (2004). Comparative toxicity of oleic acid and linoleic acid on Jurkat cells. *Clinical Nutrition.* 23:721–732.

[44] Cury-Boaventura MF, Pompéia C, Curi R. (2005). Comparative toxicity of oleic acid and linoleic acid on Raji cells. *Nutrition.* 21:395-405

[45] Cury-Boaventura MF, Gorjão R, de Lima TM, Newsholme P, Curi R. (2006). Comparative toxicity of oleic and linoleic acid on human lymphocytes. *Life Sciences*. 78:1448 – 1456

[46] Ferreira TC, de Moraes LMP, Campos EG. (2011). Cell density-dependent linoleic acid toxicity toSaccharomyces cerevisiae. *FEMS Yeast Res*. 5:408-417

[47] Jin S, DiPaola RS, Mathew R, White E. (2007). Metabolic catastrophe as a means to cancer cell death. *J Cell Sci*. 120:379–83.

[48] Brown GD. (2008). Sensing necrosis with Mincle. *Nat. Immunol.* 9:1099–1100

[49] Lauber K, Blumenthal SG, Waibel M, Wesselborg S. (2004). Clearance of apoptotic cells: getting rid of the corpses. *Mol Cell.*14:277–87.

[50] Madeo F, Fröhlich E, Ligr M, Grey M, Sigrist SJ, Wolf DH, Fröhlich KU. (1999). Oxygen stress: a regulator of apoptosis in yeast. *J Cell Biol*. 145(4):757-767.

[51] Bauman DE, Baumgard LH, Corl BA, Griinari JM. (2000) Biosynthesis of conjugated linoleic acid in ruminants. Proc. Am. Soc. Anim. Sci.,1999. Available at: *http://www.asas.org/jas/sympsia/proceedings/0937.pdf. Accessed {20/01/2012}*.

[52] Parodi PW. (1976). Distribution of isomeric octadecenoic fatty acids in milk fat. *J. Dairy Sci*. 59(11):1870-1873.

[53] Shantha NC, Crum AD, Decker EA. (1994). Evaluation of Conjugated Linoleic Acid Concentrations in Cooked Beef. *J. Agric. Food Chem.* 42: 1757-1760

[54] Corl BA, Chouinard PY, Bauman DE, Dwyer DA, Griinari JM, Nurmela KV. (1998). Conjugated linoleic acid in milk fat of dairy cows originates in part by endogenous synthesis from trans-11 octadecenoic acid. *J. Dairy. Sci*. 81(Suppl. 1):233 (Abstr.).

[55] Chin SF, Storkson JM, Liu W, Albright KJ, Pariza MW. (1994). Conjugated linoleic acid (9,11- and 10,12-octadecadienoic acid) is produced in conventional but not germ-free rats fed linoleic acid. *J. Nutr*. 124:694-701.

[56] Kim EJ, Jun JG, Park HS, Kim SM, Ha YL, Park JHY. (2002). Conjugated linoleic acid (CLA) inhibits growth of Caco-2 colon cancer cells - possible mediation by oleamide. *Anticancer Res*. 22:2193-2198.

[57] Donnelly C, Olsen AM, Lewis LD, Eisenberg BL, Eastman A, Kinlaw WB. (2009). Conjugated Linoleic Acid (CLA) inhibits expression of the Spot 14 (THRSP) and fatty acid synthase genes and impairs the growth of human breast cancer and liposarcoma cells *Nutr. Cancer*. 61(1):114–122.

[58] Muzio G, Maggiora M, Oraldi M, Trombetta A, Canuto RA. (2007). PPARα and PP2A are involved in the proapoptotic effect of conjugated linoleic acid on human hepatoma cell line SK-HEP-1. *Int. J. Cancer*. 121:2395–2401.

[59] Belury MA. (2002). Dietary conjugated linoleic acid in health: physiological effects and mechanisms of action. *Annu. Rev. Nutr*. 22:505–531.

[60] Senger DR, Van de Water L, Brown LF, Nagy JA, Yeo KT, Yeo TK, Berse B, Jackman RW, Dvorak AM, Dvorak HF. (1993). Vascular permeability factor (VPF, VEGF) in tumor biology. *Cancer Metastasis Rev*. 12: 303-324.

[61] Bergers G, Benjamin LE. (2003). Tumorigenesis and the angiogenic switch. *Nat Rev Cancer* 3:401-410.

[62] Bergers G, Brekken R, McMahon G, Vu TH, Itoh T, Tamaki K, Tanzawa K, Thorpe P, Itohara S, Werb Z, Hanahan D. (2000). Matrix metalloproteinase-9 triggers the angiogenic switch during carcinogenesis. *Nature Cell Bio*. 2:737-744.

[63] Subbaramaiah K, Altorki N, Chung WJ, Mestre JR, Sampat A, Dannenberg AJ. (1999). Inhibition of cyclooxygenase-2 gene expression by p53. *J Biol Chem. 274*:10911-10915.

[64] Wang GL, Semenza GL. (1993). Characterization of hypoxia-inducible factor 1 and regulation of DNA binding activity by hypoxia. *J. Biol. Chem.* 268: 21513-21518.

[65] Wenger RH, Stiehl DP, Camenisch G. (2005). Integration of oxygen signaling at the consensus HRE. *Sci. Stke.* re12.

[66] Wang LS, Huang YW, Sugimoto Y, Liu S, Chang HL, Ye W, Shu S, Lin YC. (2005). Effects of breast stromal cells on conjugated linoleic acid (CLA) modulated vascular endothelial growth factor (VEGF) expression in MCF-7 cells. *Anticancer Res.* 25:4061-4068.

[67] Luna-More S, Weil B, Bautista D, Garrido E, Florez P, Martinez C. (2004). Bcl-2 protein in normal, hyperplastic and neoplastic breast tissues. A metabolite of the putative stem-cell subpopulationof the mammary gland. *Histol Histopathol.* 19:457-463.

[68] Hockenbery D, Nuñez G, Milliman C, Schreiber RD, Korsmeyer SJ. (1990). Bcl-2 is an inner mitochondrial membrane protein that blocks programmed cell death. *Nature* . 348:334-336.

[69] Sasi N, Hwang M, Jaboin J, Csiki I, Lu B. (2009). Regulated cell death pathways: new twists in modulation of BCL2 family function. *Mol. Cancer Ther.* 8:1421-1429.

[70] Ou L, Ip C, Lisafeld B, Ip MM. (2007). Conjugated linoleic acid induces apoptosis of murine mammary tumor cells via Bcl-2 loss. *Biochem. Biophys. Res. Commun.* 356(4):1044–1049.

[71] Wang L-W, Huang Y-W, Liu S, Yan P, Lin YC. (2008). Conjugated linoleic acid induces apoptosis through estrogen receptor alpha in human breast tissue. *BMC Cancer.* 8:208-221.

[72] Ip C, Ip MM, Loftus T, Shoemaker S, Shea-Eaton W. (2000). Induction of Apoptosis by Conjugated Linoleic Acid in Cultured. Mammary Tumor Cells and Premalignant Lesions of the Rat Mammary Gland. *Cancer Epidemiology, Biomarkers & Prevention.* 9: 689–696.

[73] Bassaganya-Riera J, Hontecillas-Magarzo R, Bregendahl K, Wannemuehler MJ, Zimmerman DR. (2001). Effects of dietary conjugated linoleic acid in nursery pigs of dirty and clean environments on growth, empty body composition, and immune competence. *J. Anim. Sci.* 79:714–721.

[74] Kim KH, Kim DI, Kim SH, Jung EM, Kang JH, Jeung EB, Yang MP.(2011).Trans-10, cis-12-conjugated linoleic acid attenuates tumor necrosis factor-α production by lipopolysaccharide-stimulated porcine peripheral blood mononuclear cells through induction of interleukin-10. *Cytokine.* 56(2):224-230.

[75] Yu Y, Correll PH, Vanden Heuvel JP. (2002). Conjugated linoleic acid decreases production of pro-inflammatory products in macrophages: evidence for a PPAR[gamma]-dependent mechanism. *Biochim Biophys Acta.* 1581:89–99.

[76] Reynolds CM, Draper E, Keogh B, Rahman A, Moloney AP, Mills KHG, Loscher CE, Roche HM. (2009). A Conjugated Linoleic Acid-Enriched Beef Diet Attenuates Lipopolysaccharide-Induced Inflammation in Mice in Part through PPARγ-Mediated Suppression of Toll-Like Receptor 41–3. *J. Nutr.* 139:2351–2357.

[77] Tontonoz P, Hu E, Spiegelman BM. (1995). Regulation of adipocyte gene expression and differentiation by peroxisome proliferator activated receptor gamma. *Curr. Opin. Genet. Dev.* 5:571-576.

[78] Huang JT, Welch JS, Ricote M, Binder CJ, Willson TM, Kelly C, Witztum JL, Funk CD, Conrad D, Glass CK. (1999). Interleukin-4-dependent production of PPAR-gamma ligands in macrophages by 12/15-lipoxygenase. *Nature.* 400:378-382.

[79] Banni S, Carta G, Angioni E, Murru E, Scanu P, Melis MP, Bauman DE, Fischer SM, Ip C. (2001). Distribution of conjugated linoleic acid and metabolites in different lipid fractions in the rat liver. *J. Lipid Res.* 42:1056-1061.

[80] Nakanishi T, Koutoku T, Kawahara S, Murai A, Furuse M. (2003). Dietary conjugated linoleic acid reduces cerebral prostaglandin E(2) in mice. *Neurosci Lett.* 341:135-138.

In: Linoleic Acids
Editor: Igho Onakpoya
ISBN: 978-1-62257-384-4
© 2012 Nova Science Publishers, Inc.

Chapter X

Linoleic Acid and Cancer

Gerard G. Dumancas*[*1]*, Raluca Mateescu*[2]*,
***Elmer-Rico E. Mojica*[3] *and Rachel Murphy*[4]**
[1]Department of Chemistry, Oklahoma State University,
Stillwater, Oklahoma, US
[2]Department of Animal Science, Oklahoma State University,
Stillwater, Oklahoma, US
[3]Department of Chemistry and Physical Sciences,
Pace University, New York, NY, US
[4]Department of Oncology, University of Alberta,
Edmonton, Alberta, Canada

Abstract

Linoleic acid (LA) is a polyunsaturated ω-6 fatty acid. It is found in the lipids of cell membranes and is abundant in many vegetable oils such as poppy seed, safflower, sunflower, and corn oils. Its deficiency together with other ω-6 fatty acids in the diet may cause dry hair, hair loss, and poor wound healing and the intake of such acid can be detected by dietary assessments and biological measurements. Several studies showed contradicting results regarding the effects of LA in cancer. LA appears to be pivotal in the spontaneous metastasis of experimental tumors. One study showed an increase in cancer incidence after consumption of diets with very high LA for several years. Another study showed that LA is associated with the proliferation of human breast cancer cells in culture. In contrast to these findings, another study indicated that high intake of LA has no significant risk of cancer as compared to its low intake. This chapter describes the methods of detection of dietary LA, and explores the reasons for discrepancies in studies linking LA with cancers. We will also investigate the association between LA and the different types of cancer, as well as the role of LA as ω-6 in relation to ω-3 and cancer risks.

[*] Corresponding author: Department of Chemistry, Oklahoma State University, Stillwater, OK US 74078, Email: gerard.dumancas@okstate.edu.

List of Abbreviations

13-HOA	13-Hydroxy-10-oxo-trans-11-octadecenoic acid
13-HODE	13-Hydroxy-9Z,11E-octadecadienoic acid
AA	Arachidonic acid
AIN	American Institute of Nutrition
ALA	α-Linolenic acid
Aza	Azaserine
BOP	*N*-nitrosobis(2-oxopropyl)amine
COX	Cyclooxygenase
COX-2	Cyclooxygenase-2
DGLA	Dihomo-γ-linolenic acid
DHA	Docosahexaenoic acid
DMBA	Dimethyl Benz (α)anthracene
EFA	Essential fatty acid
EPA	Eicosapentaenoic acid
ERK	Extracellular-signal-regulated kinase
FFQ	Frequency questionnaires
FISH-OIL	Diet rich in ω-3 polyunsaturated fatty acids
GC	Gas chromatography
GC-MS	Gas chromatography-mass spectrometry
GLA	γ-Linolenic acid
HF	High fat
ICR	Institute of Cancer Research
LA	Linoleic acid
LF	Low fat
MF	Medium fat
NMR	Nuclear magnetic resonance
ODC	Ornithine decarboxylase
Pdcd4	Programmed cell death 4
PGE	Prostaglandin E
PGE_2	Prostaglandin E2
PUFA	Polyunsaturated fatty acid
SENCAR	Sensitive to carcinogenesis
SHF	Standard high fat
SMOF	Standard mixture of fatty acids (ω-3, ω-6, ω-9)
TPA	12-*O*-tetradecanoylphorbol-13-acetate
TPK	Tyrosine-specific protein kinase

Introduction

Cancer risk in humans may be linked to the composition of the diet [1]. An increased intake of polyunsaturated fat is considered beneficial because of its beneficial effects on blood cholesterol concentrations. It is also, however, possible to have adverse effect of a high polyunsaturated fat, thus, requiring keen investigation [2]. In most diets, the major polyunsaturated fatty acid (PUFA) is the LA (*cis, cis*-18:2n26). It is the major fatty acid in safflower, sunflower, corn, soy bean, and cottonseed oils, accounting for more than 50% of the total fatty acid content in these oils [3]. In the United States and Western Europe, the average LA acid intake has risen from ≈ 3% of energy in the 1950s to 6-7% in the 1990s [4-6].

Methods of Detection

Dietary Assessments

There are several tools that can be used to assess dietary LA. Diet records, food frequency questionnaires (FFQ) and 24-hour recalls are commonly used to estimate dietary LA [7-9] and all of these methods have been shown to correlate well with adipose tissue levels of LA [10-12]. A comprehensive overview on dietary assessment methods including strengths and weaknesses of each methodology can be found in Thompson *et al.* [13]. Diet records involve participants detailing the type and amount of food and beverages consumed over one or more days. FFQ's assess the habitual consumption of food and beverages in the previous months or previous year. With 24-hour recalls, participants are asked to recall the amount and type of everything they ate in the previous day. Records are then inputted into databases (i.e. Food Processor SQL) with analytical information on the fatty acid content of foods.

Over the past decades, interest in the potential health benefits of long chain ω-3 and ω-6 fatty acids has increased, creating a demand for specific measures of intake. In response several FFQ's focused on ω-3 and ω-6 fatty acid intake have been developed and validated against ω-3 and ω-6 fatty acid intake from diet and biological samples [14, 15]. These FFQ's include questions on the amount and frequency of consumption of the main food sources of linoleic and other ω-3 and ω-6 fatty acids, for example, vegetable oils, fats and eggs [14].

Biological Measurements

LA can be quantified in both tissue and blood. Adipose tissue is considered to be the best measure of long-term fatty acid intake because of its slow turnover [10, 16] but often studies measure LA in blood because it is less invasive. Blood levels of LA reflect dietary intake and indicate circulating levels of LA available for distribution to peripheral tissues. LA can be measured in whole blood, red blood cells, white blood cells, plasma and plasma fractions for example phospholipids, cholesterol and triacylglycerols. The fraction that is used to measure LA levels is dependent on several factors including, the study size, main study outcome, and availability of laboratory equipment. Whole blood requires less time to process, making it more expedient for large studies. Whole blood LA has been shown to correlate strongly with both adipose tissue linoleic and plasma LA [17]. Red blood cell LA can be used as an indicator of long-term LA levels. Neutrophils are involved in inflammation and their function can be modulated by the fatty acid content of their membrane [18]. Thus, the LA content of neutrophils in cancer is of interest [19]. The LA content of plasma phospholipids is commonly assessed [20, 21], as the phospholipid fraction contains the majority of ω-6 fatty acids in blood and is sensitive to short-term fluctuations (days, weeks). This also makes phospholipids attractive for measurements of LA over time [22].

There are several different methods for isolating fatty acids from blood and tissue. The Folch method was developed in the 1950's [23], and is still widely used for isolating fatty acids [20, 21, 24]. This method has multiple steps and requires 3 to 4 days to complete. Briefly, a solvent solution is used to extract lipids from biological material, extracted lipids are applied to thin layer chromatography plates which separate lipids into individual fatty acid classes: phospholipid, cholesterol, triglyceride, cholesterol esters, free fatty acids, phosphatidylethanolamine, phosphatidylcholine, sphingomyelin and lysophosphatidyl choline [25]. Following this, samples undergo a series of steps where they are heated with solvents to convert fatty acids to methyl esters. Methyl esters are then analyzed by gas chromatography (GC) or gas chromatography with mass spectroscopy (GC-MS) which enables quantification of individual fatty acids. GC with or without mass spectroscopy is the standard for quantifying fatty acids, due to its capacity to accurately quantify a dynamic range of fatty acids, repeatedly and reproducibly [26]. High performance liquid chromatography can also be used to quantify fatty acids, although it is mainly used to measure volatile short chain fatty acids, and not longer chain fatty acids like LA [27]. Nuclear magnetic resonance (NMR) spectroscopy is increasingly being used to quantify fatty acids as it does not require converting fatty acids to methyl esters. Thus, the sample often can be preserved with NMR analysis [28]. NMR analysis of LA has also shown to be in good agreement with gas chromatography measures of LA [28]. Although the methods described above can precisely measure linoleic and other fatty acids, they are time intensive and require skilled technicians. Thus, the development of cost-effective, high throughput methods for isolating and quantifying fatty acids in blood and tissue is an area of great interest. Alternative methods include preparation of fatty acid methyl esters (the form needed for analysis by GC) without performing lipid extraction [29] and fast GC [30], which cuts the time for running one sample from 76 minutes to 16 minutes while maintaining precision (difference of 3% between linoleic acid amounts determined with the two methods). Other methods currently being explored include microwave heating [31] and ultrasound energy [32] to decrease processing time. In summary, there are several dietary assessments and biological methods that can be used to provide an estimate of LA intake and LA content of tissues. Dietary assessments are useful in conjunction with biological measurements of LA or in large studies where biological measurements are not practical. Continued development of efficient methods for assessing fatty acid content of blood and tissue will encourage research on linoleic and other fatty acids in large populations and in clinical settings.

Linoleic Acid and Cancer Risks

Linoleic Acid and Breast Cancer

LA has been shown to influence experimental mammary tumorigenesis in rodents [33-36] and the growth and metastatic behavior of transplantable mammary carcinomas [37, 38]. However, there is still a high level of uncertainty about a similar effect in human breast cancer [39, 40]. While LA was found to increase the proliferation of human breast cancer cell lines *in vitro* [41], the role of LA in human tumorigenesis remains controversial due to conflicting results among case-control and prospective clinical studies [42, 43]. A recent meta-analysis of epidemiological studies focusing on the relationship of the LA and select sites of tumorigenesis found no increased relative risk from breast cancer [2].

Mechanism and Supporting Studies

The molecular mechanisms by which dietary fat in general, and LA in particular, might influence mammary tumors development are potentially numerous as dietary fat has been shown to have an effect on metabolism, cell differentiation, and proliferation through alteration of gene expression [44]. Most studies on the role played by LA in the development of mammary gland cancer have been conducted on animal models. In general, experimental data has now linked a high dietary intake of ω-6 PUFAs, such as LA, to an increased risk of mammary cancer. Studies on rodents point to a pivotal role played by LA in tumor induction and metastasis.

LA is an essential fatty acid required for normal development of mammary tissue [45, 46]. In rodents, LA has been shown to stimulate the proliferation *in vitro* of mammary epithelial cells when the epidermal growth factor was present [47, 48]. The effect of LA on human breast epithelial cells was investigated by several investigators using established cell lines [49, 50] or freshly isolated cells from tissue obtained from reduction mammoplasty [51]. These nontransformed human breast epithelial cells had a similar growth response as seen in the mouse mammary gland to LA in the presence of insulin or epidermal growth factor [51].

Prostaglandins. The effect of dietary LA on tumor development may also be indirect through alteration of hormonal [52] or growth factor mediated pathways [53]. The role of prostaglandins, fatty acid-derived metabolic products, in the developmental growth of rodent mammary tumors has been widely investigated, due to their active role in general cell proliferation processes. However, evidence was provided [54] that the enhanced the growth rate of a transplantable mammary tumor in mice on diet rich in LA was related to the arachidonate content rather than the linoleate content of the tumor. This evidence was further strengthened when high-fat diets and concurrent treatment with an inhibitor of prostaglandin synthesis, i.e. eicosa-5, 8-11, 14-tetraynoic acid, resulted in an inhibition of enhanced mouse mammary tumor growth [55]. This inhibitory effect of prostaglandin synthesis inhibitors on the development of both transplantable as well as autochthonous mammary tumors in rodents fed diets with high levels of unsaturated fatty acids has been reported in several studies [56, 57].

Oxidative DNA damage and lipid peroxidation. Another possible mechanism for the effect of dietary fat on tumor development is the oxidative stress due to generation of reactive oxygen species from fatty acids which may contribute to the promotional effect of dietary fat by lipid peroxidation and damage of DNA and protein [58, 59]. Oxidation of LA or AA results in *trans*-4-hydroxy-2-nonenal which is one of the major lipid peroxidation products and can form promutagenic exocyclic DNA adducts in human cells which may contribute to diet-related cancers [60, 61]. *Trans*-4-hydroxy-2-nonenal is readily oxidized by fatty acid peroxides to form 2,3-epoxy-4-hydroxynonasal, a bifunctional alkylating agent which can react with DNA to yield etheno and other base adducts. Etheno adducts are a new class of

DNA lesions with promutagenic potential capable of generating mainly base pair substitution mutations and are believed to initiate lesions in carcinogenesis [62, 63]. Analyses of white blood cell DNA in a controlled dietary study showed that a high intake of ω-6 PUFAs had a moderate effect on increasing the frequency of malonaldehyde-derived DNA adducts [64] while the frequency of etheno-DNA adducts in white blood cells was 40 times greater in women. While this study points out that a diet rich in ω-3 PUFA results in increased lipid peroxidation of membrane lipids, these results are inconclusive because of the great level of individual variation in etheno adduct levels in women on the high polyunsaturated fat diet. In addition, degradation of LA through the cytochrome-P450 pathway can also lead to formation of highly pro-oxidative and pro-inflamatory derivatives, such as epoxides and diol metabolites [65].

A possible link between exocyclic adducts formed through lipid oxidation of ω-6 PUFAs and breast cancer is supported by a 3-fold increase in the level of malondialdehyde-deoxyguanosine and malondialdehyde-deoxyadenosine adducts in breast tissue from breast cancer patients in comparison with cancer-free controls [66]. Several in *vivo* and *in vitro* studies provide additional data supporting a link between products derived from lipid peroxidation and oxidative DNA base damage and increased risk of breast cancer. Pre-menopausal women with mammographic dysplasia were found to have approximately double the amount of malonaldehyde in urine samples, a measure of lipid peroxidation [67]. Primary cultures of human mammary epithelial cells were examined for presence of DNA damage and the ability of lipid extracts of breast tissue to induce DNA strand breaks [68]. Pre-existing damage in human mammary epithelial cells was identified in untreated cells and lipid extracts from donors whose human mammary epithelial cells contained the most pre-existing DNA damage were the most active.

Dietary LA can also enhance the metastatic formation of mammary tumors through products of lipid peroxidation. The DNA damage induced by hydroxyl radicals has been linked to the progression of human breast cancer to the metastatic phase [69]. Although a detailed mechanism for how the dietary LA stimulates cancer metastasis is not fully understood, oxidative stress has been hypothesized to be one intermediary link. Oxidative stress can play a role in metastasis through the loss of cell adhesion which is the prerequisite for cellular detachment and invasion of host tissues. In particular, a diet with high levels of LA was shown to increase the rate of metastasis of mammary cancer in rats [70]. The mechanism proposed in this study was induction of genes coding for adhesion molecules or chemokines through an oxidative stress-related mechanism. Analysis of DNA from metastatic breast tumors when compared to the DNA from non-metastatic tumors showed an approximately 2-fold increase in oxidative base damage, suggesting a metastatic potential for cells with hydroxyl radical-induced DNA damage [69].

Hormonal effects. A series of studies staring in mid-1970s suggested that stimulation of secretion of mammogenic hormones, in particular ovarian steroids and prolactin resulting in enhanced rodent mammary tumorigenesis occurs in the presence of high levels of dietary fat. Plasma sex steroids are regulated by the sex hormone-binding globulin and decreased globulin levels associated with increased concentrations of unbound estrogen have been reported in high risk groups. High fat intake resulting in higher levels of free fatty acids in serum may affect the bioavailability of estrogen so that more estrogen is displaced from the serum globulin and available for uptake by the estrogen receptors. However, epidemiological studies in women have not provided any consistent results regarding the role played by increased levels of circulation estrogen hormones in breast cancer.

In mice, there is evidence for increased hormone-induced growth of the mammary gland as a function of the dietary fat content [71]. This increased responsiveness of the mammary gland to hormone-induced growth during increased levels of dietary fat could be explained through activation of protein kinase C, a lipid-dependent enzyme system [72]. Diacylglycerol is produced from phosphatidylinositol in response to extracellular signals such as hormones or other growth factors. However, diacylglycerols containing unsaturated fatty acids are more effective in activating protein kinase C than diacylglyerols containing saturated fatty acids. This could translate in the increased efficacy of diets rich in unsaturated fatty acids to enhance mammary tumorigenesis, through an enriched composition of the membrane lipid composition with critical unsaturated fatty acids which would increase the activity of this enzyme system. High intake of LA and AA was shown to inhibit the detoxification of estrogen by 2-hydroxylation [73] and to increase 16-αhydroxylation and the formation of metabolites that can generate hydroxyl radicals. The accumulation of 4-hydroyxyestradiol in target organs could mediate damage to cellular DNA and other macromolecules; furthermore the estradiol and its locally formed hormonally active 4–hydroxylated metabolite may stimulate the growth of transformed cells, a necessary step for the full development of estrogen-induced tumorigenesis [74]. Although high estradiol 4-hydroxylase activity has also been observed in human breast cancer tissue compared to normal breast tissue [75], more studies are needed to confirm a high level of 4-hydroxylestradiol in human breast tissues.

Linoleic Acid and Colorectal Cancer

Colorectal cancer is the third most common cancer in men (663,000 new cases in 2008) and the second in women (571,000 cases new cases in 2008) worldwide [76]. It is the fourth most common cause of death from cancer with an estimated 608,000 deaths in 2008 [76].

The consumption of PUFA particularly ω-6 LA has been related to an increased risk of colorectal cancer. A review on the epidemiological literature on LA utilization and cancer risk based on the meta-analysis of various case-control and prospective cohort studies concluded that it is doubtful that a high intake of LA substantially raises the risk of colorectal cancer in humans although a small increase in risk could still be possible [77].

Animal studies have shown that LA can enhance the risk of colorectal carcinogenesis [78-82]. For instance, the effect of corn oil is most prevalent during the postinitiation phase where there is a significant increase in the azoxymethane-induced incidence and multiplicity of colon adenocarcinomas [81]. In another study, higher adenocarcinoma incidence and total ras expression were found in animals fed with corn oil [78]. Lastly, animals fed with high levels of corn oil had increases in colon and liver ornithine decarboxylase (ODC) and tyrosine-specific protein kinase (TPK) activities, which are usually enhanced when applied with carcinogens [80]. However, the type of relationship between the LA and colorectal cancer in human studies is not consistent with the animal studies. Inconsistent results ranging from direct association, indirect association [83, 84] and no association [85, 86] were obtained in various studies between the fatty acid and colorectal cancer. A direct association between the cyclooxygenase-2 (COX-2) gene polymorphism and colon cancer risk among high consumers of dietary ω-6 PUFAs was observed in one study[87]. One study [83] showed a significant and inverse association between LA intake and the risk of colorectal cancer. Patients diagnosed with colorectal cancer had lower intake of LA than the controls. In another study, colon cancer patients showed decreased LA in red blood cells [84]. Lastly no clear association between LA and colorectal cancer risk was found in one study [86] in Sweden confirming the finding of another earlier study [85] where LA showed neither strong nor consistent associations in relation to colon or rectal cancer risk.

Linoleic Acid and Prostate Cancer

Prostate cancer is the second most frequently diagnosed cancer of men (with an estimated 899,000 new cases in 2008) and the fifth most common cancer over-all [88]. It is the sixth leading cause of death from cancer in men with an estimated 258,000 deaths in 2008 [88].

LA consumption is positively associated with prostate cancer risk [89]. Different animal experiments have shown that dietary PUFAs generally stimulated tumor development [90]. The growth of Dunning transplantable prostate adenocarcinomas in rats was enhanced with the presence of various amounts of corn (main source of LA) on diet in comparison to the ones fed without corn oil, where a reduced growth of the tumor was observed [91]. In another animal study, reduction of dietary fat substantially slowed the growth of tumors established from human prostatic adenocarcinoma cells in a murine xenograft model[92]. *In vitro* studies showed mixed results of LA on different prostate cancer lines. The growth of the androgen-unresponsive PC-3 human prostate cancer cell line was found to be stimulated *in vitro* by the presence of LA [93]. However, another androgen-unresponsive human prostate cancer cell line (DU 145) showed no growth response to LA. In another study which utilized human metastatic PC3, LNCaP and TSU prostate cell lines, results demonstrated that LA has promotional effects at doses of 1-100 ng/ml in all cell lines[94]. Lastly, LA has a dose dependent inhibitory effect on LNCaP prostate cell line while it showed stimulatory dose-dependent effect at 5 and 50 uM concentrations against PC3 prostate cell line. However, at 200 uM, the LA is toxic to both cell lines (LNCaP and PC3) since the cells died after a few hours' treatment. LNCaP cells are considered less deviated than PC3 cells because they maintain sensitivity to androgen [95]. Results of human clinical trials are consistent with the animal studies where LA consumption was positively associated with prostate cancer risk [89, 96]. In one study, men in the highest quartile of LA consumption had as much as a 5-fold increased risk of prostate cancer compared to men with low levels of consumption [96]. The trend toward increased risk was more evident using erythrocyte membrane samples than adipose tissue specimens. Another study utilizing blood samples from humans showed that there is a two-fold elevation in risk of prostate cancer associated with higher levels of LA and total ω-6 fatty acids [89].

Linoleic Acid and Skin Cancer

A diet deficient in LA is known to cause mild skin scaling and hair loss [97]. However, it is important to note that this ω-6 fatty acid must be balanced in the body in relation to ω-3s since ω-6s have pro-inflammatory properties [98].

Fischer *et al.* hypothesized that an increase in the consumption of LA would also cause an enhancement in mouse skin-tumor promotion on the basis of rat mammary and pancreas tumor models. In their study involving SENCAR mice placed on diets containing 0.8% to 8.4% LA, 1 week after initiation with carcinogen, 7,12-Dimethylbenz(a)anthracene, and 3 weeks before starting promotion with a tumor enhancer, 12-*O*-tetradecanoylphorbol-13-acetate, an inverse correlation was observed between papilloma number and level of LA. Tumor incidence, however, revealed little difference. A study was also done which involved the effect of dietary LA levels on the fatty acid composition of epidermal phospholipids. It was found out that 12-*O*-tetradecanoylphorbol-13-acetate (TPA)-induced prostaglandin E_2 levels generally decreased with increasing dietary LA. The study also found out that the effect of dietary LA on tumor development is target tissue specific rather than species specific. This was confirmed through a mammary carcinogenesis experiment involving SENCAR mice fed with 0.8%-8.4% LA diets and intragastric administration of up to 6 mg of 7,12-dimethylbenz(a)anthracene at 1 mg/week. Tumor appearance was delayed in the 0.8% LA diet group, and a positive dose-response relationship between dietary LA and mammary-tumor incidence was observed [99].

LA metabolite has also been investigated as with regards to its effect on the suppression of skin inflammation and tumor promotion. One of the lipoxygenase pathway metabolites of LA derived from corn germ called (±)-13-Hydroxy-10-oxo-trans-11-octadecenoic acid (13-HOA) was studied to determine its inhibitory effects on TPA-induced inflammation in ears and skin, as well as tumor promotion in female ICR mice. Results indicate that 13-HOA may be used as a novel anti-inflammatory and antitumor chemopreventive agent with a unique mode of action [100]. Pretreatment with 16 nmol of 13-HOA prevented the formation of ear edema by 95% in an inflammation test and reduced tumor incidence and the number of tumors per mouse by 40 and 64%, respectively, in a two-stage skin carcinogenesis model. Moreover, 13-HOA at 8-40 μM suppressed TPA-induced anchorage-independent growth of JB6 mouse epidermal cells by 70–100%, whereas LA was virtually inactive. At 40 μM of 13-HOA TPA-induced activator protein-1 transactivation was inhibited but not extracellular signal-regulated kinase1/2 activation. 13-HOA (40 mM and 1600 nmol in JB6 cells and mouse skin, respectively) induced expression of programmed cell death 4 (Pdcd4), a novel tumor suppressor protein [100].

Linoleic Acid and Pancreatic Cancer

Pancreatic cancer is the fourth most common cause of cancer-related mortality around the world, with incidence equaling mortality [101] and has often poor prognosis with survival rates of 25% and 6% for 1- and 5-year, respectively for all stages combined [102]. A number of studies have suggested that certain PUFAs can inhibit the growth of a variety of human cancer cell lines *in vitro* [103-107]. Although less studies have been done involving LA and pancreatic cancer directly, a study was reported which investigated whether fatty acids modify the growth of human pancreatic cancer. Several fatty acids consisting of lauric, stearic, palmitic, oleic, LA, α-linolenic, γ-linolenic, AA, docosahexaenoic (DHA) and eicosapentaenoic (EPA) acids were each incubated with the cells lines MIA PaCa-2, PANC-1 and CFPAC at concentrations ranging from 1.25 μM to 50 μM and the effect of each fatty acid on cell growth was examined. All the PUFAs including LA had an inhibitory effect suggesting that administration of such fatty acids may be of therapeutic benefit in patients with pancreatic cancer [108]. In another study, it was also shown that at a 200-μM concentration, both LA and DHA inhibited cell growth, while only DHA induced apoptosis in the human PaCa-44 pancreatic cell line [109].

While the above-mentioned study indicated that LA had an inhibitory effect on pancreatic cancer, several studies showed the opposite effect implicating that LA caused the tumor growth in several pancreatic cancer models [110-115]. Table 1 shows the summary of various studies showing the effect of LA on pancreatic cancer in various subjects.

Studies relating pancreatic cancer to individual fatty acid intakes are scarce. In human subjects, high consumption of PUFAs and more specifically LA has been associated with decreased risk in a few case-control studies [116-120] but not in cohort studies [121, 122]. A study by Thiébaut *et al.* suggested that no association between PUFA, total ω-6, or LA and cancer exists, and that only dietary AA from mostly animal foods, was statistically significantly associated with an increased risk of pancreatic cancer [123]. Besides the abovementioned subjects and studies, concentration-dependent promotion of pancreatic cancer cell growth by LA has been demonstrated both *in vivo* and *in vitro* [124, 125].

Linoleic Acid and Other Cancer Risks

Dietary LA is known to stimulate invasion and peritoneal metastasis of gastric carcinoma cells through cyclooxygenase (COX) – catalyzed metabolism and activation of extracellular-signal-regulated kinase (ERK), steps that are potentially amenable to therapeutic intervention [126]. In pulmonary metastasis, the occurrence and extent of such disease is known to be influenced by the level of LA present in diets which are isocaloric and contain the high (23%) level of total fat [127]. In general, studies involving the effect of LA on other cancer types are scarce since most studies conducted take into account the effect of total ω-6 fatty acids.

Zock *et al.* [2] provided a comprehensive review of LA intake and various cancer risks in their meta-analysis study. They reviewed the epidemiologic and experimental literature on LA intake and cancer risk and also did additional meta-analyses of risk estimates from case control and prospective cohort studies. Results showed that no combined estimates from within-population studies indicated a significantly increased risk of cancer with high compared with low intakes of LA or PUFA. Moreover, there seemed to be positive associations between cancer rates and per capita use of animal or saturated fat but to a lesser extent with per capita use of PUFA or vegetable oil.

Linoleic Acid and General Potent Cancer Mechanisms

Cancer is generally initiated by a primary genetic factor, followed by a series of genetic and/or epigenetic alterations leading to the development of precancerous cells and consequently, malignant tumors. High dietary levels of PUFA has been known to promote tumor growth in several animal models [35, 128, 129], including pancreatic cancer models. LA is known to cause this effect [110, 113, 114].

Table 1. Studies investigating the effects of LA (or as part of ω-6 PUFA) in animal pancreatic cancer models

Author(s)	Treatment Groups	Results
Roebuck *et al.* [110]	21-day-old male Wistar/Lewis rats 1. controls a. AIN(saline)/AIN (n=16) b. AIN (aza (azaserine))/AIN (n=17) 2. initiation phase a. saturated fat (aza)/AIN (n=18) b. unsaturated fat (aza)/AIN (n=19) c. low protein (aza)/AIN (n=19) d. AIN restricted (aza)/AIN (n=10) 3. postinitiation phase a. AIN (aza)/saturated fat (n=20) b. AIN (aza)/unsaturated fat (n=20) c. AIN (aza)/low protein (n=15) d. AIN (aza)/AIN restricted (n=9)	• suppression of pancreatic neoplasm in initiation phase in caloric-restricted diet • no effects of other diets in initiation phase on pancreatic cancer incidence • high unsaturated-fat diets but not the high-saturated-fat diets elevated pancreatic cancer incidence in postinitiation phase. No effects of other diets on the neoplasm incidence.
Birt *et al.* [111, 112]	Syrian golden hamsters 1. control (n=90 male, n=90 female) fed with corn oil at medium fat MF) level (9 g/385 kcal) for life 2. groups (n=60 male, n=60 female) fed with low fat (LF) and high fat (HF) diets in two different sequences. • first group: fed the LF and HF diets from 3-8 weeks of age and control diet (MF) for the rest of their lives. The second group • second group: fed the control diet up to 8 weeks of age and then received LF or HF diet • one half of animals of each sex from the 5 diet groups were given a single dose a single sc *N*-nitrosobis(2-oxopropyl)amine (BOP) (10 mg/kg body weight) at 8 weeks of age • animals changed from LF to HF diets to MF diet and from MF to LF and HF diets 2 days after BOP treatment	• ductular adenocarcinomas incidence increased in both males and females (LF diet 16%, HF diet, 34%) when the HF diet was fed after BOP treatment. • average number of carcinomas per carcinoma-bearing animal increased (LF diet, 1.3; HF diet, 3.0), but carcinoma incidence was not influenced by the diets being fed before carcinogen treatment. • incidence of ductular adenomas was high with all treatments and was not influenced by diet. However, adenomas increased in animal fed HF diets. • acinar cell nodules incidence elevated in animals fed the MF and HF diets after BOP administration.
Ip *et al.* [113, 114]	female rats treated with dimethylbenz(α)anthracene (DMBA) • different levels of linoleate: 0.5%, 1.1%, 1.7%, 2.2%, 3.5%, 4.4%, 8.5%, or 11.5% administered	• mammary tumorigenesis was very sensitive to linoleate intake and increased proportionately in the range of 0.5-4.4% of dietary linoleate. Tumor development leveled off at higher levels.
Appell *et al.* [115]	1-week pregnant female Wistar rats 1. control (n=5) treated with 0.9% NaCl solution 2. 5 groups (n=30/group) aza-treated with AIN diets containing 2, 4, 6, 10, 15 weight % LA. 4-week-old Syrian golden hamsters 1. control (n=5) treated with 0.9% NaCl solution 2. 5 groups (n=30/group) *N*-nitrosobis(2-oxopropyl)amine-treated with AIN diets containing 2, 4, 6, 10, 15 weight % LA	• 4 and 2 % weight dietary LA yielded the strongest enhancing effect on pancreatic (pre)neoplastic lesions, on rats and hamsters, respectively. • tumor response decreased at higher LA levels
Roebuck *et al.* [145]	male Lewis rats treated with aza (30 mg/kg) at 14 days of age • pups were weaned to test diets that contained 20% total dietary fat with essential fatty acid (EFA) compositions varying from 0.5 to 11.5% of the diet	• minimum dietary EFA required for enhancement of aza-induced, pancreatic carcinogenesis by a high fat diet lies in the range of 4 to 8%.

Table 1. (Continued)

Author(s)	Treatment Groups	Results
Gregor *et al.* [146]	male hamsters (n=15/group) and allocated to 3 main dietary categories: • groups 1, 2: standard high fat (SHF) diet rich in ω-6 PUFA • groups 3, 4: mixture of ω-3, ω-6, and ω-9 PUFA (SMOF) • groups 5, 6: diet rich in ω-3 PUFA (FISH-OIL) • groups 1, 3, 5: subcutaneous injections of 10 mg BOP/kg body weight • groups 2, 4, 6 (controls): 0.5 ml 0.9% NaCl	• different diets did not significantly alter the overall incidence of histologically proven pancreatic adenocarcinoma • number of macroscopically visible tumors was decreased in the FISH-OIL-group indicating the beneficial effects of ω-3 PUFA in attenuating tumor growth vs the ω-6 PUFA
Heukamp *et al.* [147]	male hamsters (n=15/group) randomized into 6 groups: • groups 1-3: healthy control • groups 4-6: subcutaneous injections of 10 mg BOP/kg body weight • group 1: SHF rich in ω-6 PUFAs • group 2: FISH-OIL • group 4: BOP + SHF • group 5: BOP + SMOF • group 6: BOP + FISH-OIL	• FISH-OIL decreased number of macroscopically visible pancreatic tumours (Gr. 4–6: 54.5% vs. 45.5% vs. 9.1%) as well as incidence of liver metastasis (Gr. 4–6: 90.9% vs. 72.7% vs. 36.4%) vs the other groups

While there are several mechanisms which could implicate LA as a cause of cancer, most studies don't take into account the total unsaturated fatty acids, rather than LA alone [130]. Regarding the association between LA and cancer, one hypothesized mechanism includes an accelerated prostaglandin synthesis, caused by the metabolism of LA-derived AA, in (pre)neoplastic tissue [131-133]. Such theory proposed by Karmali is supported by a frequently seen tumor growth inhibition concurrent with biochemical inhibition of the prostaglandin-synthesizing enzyme cyclooxygenase by indomethacin [38, 134] or by competitive inhibition by ω-3 fatty acids from fish oils [38, 135, 136].

The production of prostaglandin E2 (PGE_2), a primary product of AA metabolism synthesized via the COX and prostaglandin synthase pathways, appears to have a functional role for LA in supporting mammary tumor development. Since LA is converted to AA, and consequently to PGE_2, modulating LA limits the availability of AA and PGE_2 [99]. Abou-EI-Ela *et al.* found out a positive association among dietary LA, tumor PGE_2 levels, and incidence of chemically induced mammary tumors [137]. Moreover, it was also reported by several studies that the enhancement of mammary tumorigenesis by high dietary levels of unsaturated fatty acids is through increased synthesis of prostaglandins of series 1 or 2; prostaglandins of series 3 appear to be inhibitory to this tumorigenic process [130, 138]. Marnett *et al*, on the other hand, reported that the hydroperoxy and hyrdoxy antioxidation products of certain fatty acids such as AA and LA, stimulated colonic DNA synthesis and ornithine decarboxylase activity when instilled intrarectally into rats but not in the purified forms of such acids [139].

Diets rich in unsaturated fatty acids have been reported to increase cellular membrane fluidity [140]. Increased cellular membrane fluidity, on the other hand, is known to be associated with increased cell division [141]. That being said, increased concentrations of unsaturated fatty acids in the cell membrane is known to be associated with increased cell division [142]. This was confirmed when Kidwell *et al.* found out that more unsaturated fatty acids in particular LA were found in membranes of proliferating mammary cells [143].

Moreover, certain biologically active factors such as prolactin are known to enhance mammary tumor growth [144].

Despite the observations and conclusions about LA and its possible cancer mechanisms, more studies are necessary before recommendations can be made regarding alteration to human diet for cancer prevention.

Linoleic Acid as Ω-6 in Relation to Ω-3 and Cancer Risks

Although the focus of this chapter is LA, it has been suggested that it is important to consider not only the absolute amount of LA, but also the relative proportion of ω-6/ω-3 fatty acids [148-150]. LA is the main ω6 fatty acid in the human diet and is primarily found in vegetable oils. Due to increased use of vegetable oils and generally low fish consumption, it has been estimated that the ω-6/ω-3 ratio in Western diets is nearly 10:1 [151]. In contrast, the World Health Organization recommends 2.5-9% of energy from ω-6 fatty acids and 0.5-2% of energy from ω-3 fatty acids [152]. As populations continue to adopt more Westernized diets, the gap between ω-3 and ω-6 intakes is likely to become even more disparate.

LA is a precursor to arachidonic acid which is converted to proinflammatory eicosanoids. On the other hand, eicosanoids derived from ω-3 fatty acids are less inflammatory. Thus, it has been hypothesized that elevated ω-6/ω-3 ratios indicate inflammatory environments which may contribute to the development of some diseases including cancer [150].

The majority of evidence on the association between ω-6/ω-3 ratios and cancer risk is from breast cancer research. Experimental studies showed suppression of mammary tumors with a diet balanced in ω-6/ω-3 [153] or in diets with a low ω-6/ω-3 ratio [154]. Simonsen et al. [148] studied the ω-3 and ω-6 fatty acid content of adipose tissue in people with breast cancer and healthy controls from five European countries. They reported little association between individual fatty acids and breast cancer but when expressed as a ratio, there was a consistent association between elevated ω-6/ω-3 ratios and breast cancer. A second study of adipose tissue from women with breast cancer and women with benign breast disease found a similar relationship [155], the ratio of LA/ALA (α-linolenic acid) and ω-6/ω-3 fatty acids were both associated with breast cancer. This relationship appears to be stronger in premenopausal women than postmenopausal women, although the reasons are unclear [156].

These results have led some to suggest that dietary supplementation with ω-3 fatty acids with reductions of LA and overall dietary fat could substantially reduce the risk of developing breast cancer [157], and a review on ω-6 and ω-3 fatty acids and breast cancer risk concluded that a protective effect of ω-3 fatty acids on cancer development is dependent on background levels of ω-6 fatty acids [158].

Despite the promising findings in breast cancer, associations between ω-6/ω-3 ratios and the risk of developing other cancer types has not been shown consistently. A study of 47,866 US men found no relationship between the ratio of LA/ALA or LA/eicosapentaenoic acid plus docosahexaenoic acid on the risk of developing prostate cancer over a 14 year period [159]. Chajes et al. [160] also reported no effect of ω-6/ω-3 and an inverse relationship between LA/ALA and gastric cancer risk. The reasons for the inconsistencies are unclear but investigators suggest that it may be due in part to heterogeneity in evaluating fatty acid intake [161] (see Methods of detection for a review of common methods).

Although the evidence is inconclusive, as a whole, these studies suggest that the balance of ω-6 and ω-3 fatty acids is an important factor to consider when identifying cancer risk in relation to diet. The encouraging part is that the amount and balance of fatty acids is a modifiable risk factor and dietary changes can alter the ω-3 and ω-6 content in adipose tissue [162].

General Recommendations for Linoleic Acid Intake for Cancer Prevention

LA is the major dietary fatty acid present in high concentrations in corn, soy, sunflower, or safflower oils and it is estimated to provide approximately 7-8% of the average dietary energy intake [163]. It is hypothesized that LA is one of the most important dietary factors with the ability to activate the vascular epithelium, a process which is involved in induction of metastatic cancer among a variety of pathological conditions [2, 164, 165].

In animal models, diets rich in specific vegetable oils were found to enhance mammary gland tumorigenesis, while diets rich in specific animal fats were found to be less effective in stimulating tumorigensis [166-170]. A meta-analysis of data on mammary tumor incidence on rodents [171] indicated that ω-6 fatty acids in general have a strong effect on tumor enhancement when they represent less than 4% of total calories. LA in particular was demonstrated to have the ability to promote carcinogenesis. When the dietary content of LA is greater than 4%-5% of total calories, any additional fat tended to linearly increase chemically-induced tumorigenesis.

Although the hypothesis that increased levels of dietary fat promotes the development of breast cancer in post-menopausal women is supported when we take into account strong correlations between fat intake and rates of breast cancer, case-control studies offer only moderate associations with high fat diets. Moreover, because cohort studies fail to identify any association between dietary fat intake and breast cancer risk, it is difficult to make nutritional recommendations, including recommendations for dietary LA intake, for the prevention of breast cancer [172, 173].

In view of these conflicting findings, it might be beneficial to promote a dietary balance of ω-6 and ω-3 fatty acids, especially in women. This is supported by results from studies of oils with different ω-6/ω-3 ratio, in particular linoleic/ALA, on animal tumorigenesis. Diets rich in ALA (5%) or EPA (4%) and low in LA (0.3%) prevented tumorigenesis in mice [174].

Another important distinction needs to be made between the effect of high fat diets and diets rich in LA. In particular, results from *in vitro* experiments with cancer cell lines need to be interpreted carefully in terms of what is a biologically relevant concentration of LA. The results from *in vitro* experiments do not account for the interaction between the cancer cells and host tissue or the microenvironment therefore predictions of tumor response based on these observations may not be relevant *in vivo*. The cellular microenvironment is also important when evaluating the effects of different LA concentrations present in human diets on tumorigenesis. In human dietary studies where the total fat content was kept constant but the energy provided by LA varied from 8.4% to 2.5%, no change in plasma 20:4 ω-6 concentrations or in the urinary excretion of prostaglandin E (PGE) metabolites was observed [175, 176]. Therefore, although alterations of the relative proportions of ω-6/ω-3 or even LA and other unsaturated fatty acids may affect cancer progression and tumorigenesis, changes in dietary LA alone are unlikely to have these effects.

Conclusion

LA and its metabolites are known to be associated with various malignancies such as skin tumors, pancreatic, breast, colorectal, and prostate cancers. While several studies show a direct association between LA and cancer, some studies show an inhibitory effect of such fatty acid in human cancer cell lines. Few studies conducted relating LA and its inhibitory effects towards various cancer types limit the conclusive association between the two. When assessing LA it may be important to relate the levels of LA to ω-3 fatty acid levels as studies suggest that a high ω-6 to ω-3 fatty acid ratio may increase the risk of certain cancers. Thus, it appears that the relationship between LA and cancer may be more complex than considering only the absolute amount of LA. Despite the observations and conclusions about LA and its possible cancer mechanisms, more studies are necessary before recommendations are made to alter the human diet for cancer prevention.

References

[1] Doll, R. and R. Peto, The Causes of Cancer - Quantitative Estimates of Avoidable Risks of Cancer in the United-States Today. *Journal of the National Cancer Institute*, 1981. 66(6): p. 1191-&.

[2] Zock, P.L. and M.B. Katan, Linoleic acid intake and cancer risk: a review and meta-analysis. *American Journal of Clinical Nutrition*, 1998. 68(1): p. 142-153.

[3] Simopoulos, A.P.R.J., *The omega plan.* Vol. 41. 1998, New York: Harper-Collins.

[4] McDowell, M.A.B., R.R.; Alalmo, K.; et al., Energy and macronutrient intakes of persons ages 2 months and over in the United States: third National Health and Nutrition Examination Survey, phase 1, 1988–91. *Vital Health Stat,* 1994. 255: p. 1-21.

[5] Ministry of Health, W., and Sports, Ministry of Agriculture, Nature Management, and Fisheries. Zo eet Nederland, 1992., Resulaten van de Voedselconsumptiepeiling. (The second Dutch National Food Consumption Survey, 1992.). 1993: *The Hague: Dutch Bureau for Nutrition Education.*

[6] Gregory, J.F., K.; Tyler, H.; Wiseman M., *The dietary and nutritional survey of British adults. A survey of dietary behavior, nutritional status and blood pressure of adults aged 16 to 64 living in Great Britain.* London, M.o.A. Office of Population Censuses and Surveys, Fisheries and Food and the Department of Health, Editor. 1990.

[7] Willett, W.C., et al., Dietary fat and the risk of breast cancer. *N Engl J Med,* 1987. 316(1): p. 22-8.

[8] Giovannucci, E., et al., A prospective study of dietary fat and risk of prostate cancer. *J Natl Cancer Inst*, 1993. 85(19): p. 1571-9.

[9] Voorrips, L.E., et al., Intake of conjugated linoleic acid, fat, and other fatty acids in relation to postmenopausal breast cancer: the Netherlands Cohort Study on Diet and Cancer. *Am J Clin Nutr*, 2002. 76(4): p. 873-82.

[10] Baylin, A., et al., Adipose tissue biomarkers of fatty acid intake. *Am J Clin Nutr,* 2002. 76(4): p. 750-7.

[11] Kabagambe, E.K., et al., Application of the method of triads to evaluate the performance of food frequency questionnaires and biomarkers as indicators of long-term dietary intake. *Am J Epidemiol,* 2001. 154(12): p. 1126-35.

[12] Hunter, D.J., et al., Comparison of measures of fatty acid intake by subcutaneous fat aspirate, food frequency questionnaire, and diet records in a free-living population of US men. *Am J Epidemiol,* 1992. 135(4): p. 418-27.

[13] Thompson, F. and S. AF, Dietary assessment methodology. *Nutrition in the Prevention and Treatment of Disease.* 2001, San Diego, California: Academic Press. 3-30.

[14] Swierk, M., et al., Validation of an Australian electronic food frequency questionnaire to measure polyunsaturated fatty acid intake. *Nutrition*, 2011. 27(6): p. 641-6.

[15] McNaughton, S.A., M.C. Hughes, and G.C. Marks, Validation of a FFQ to estimate the intake of PUFA using plasma phospholipid fatty acids and weighed foods records. *Br J Nutr,* 2007. 97(3): p. 561-8.

[16] Katan, M.B., et al., Kinetics of the incorporation of dietary fatty acids into serum cholesteryl esters, erythrocyte membranes, and adipose tissue: an 18-month controlled study. *J Lipid Res*, 1997. 38(10): p. 2012-22.

[17] Baylin, A., et al., Fasting whole blood as a biomarker of essential fatty acid intake in epidemiologic studies: comparison with adipose tissue and plasma. *Am J Epidemiol*, 2005. 162(4): p. 373-81.

[18] de Pablo, M.A. and G. Alvarez de Cienfuegos, Modulatory effects of dietary lipids on immune system functions. *Immunol Cell Biol,* 2000. 78(1): p. 31-9.

[19] Pratt, V.C., et al., Plasma and neutrophil fatty acid composition in advanced cancer patients and response to fish oil supplementation. *Br J Cancer*, 2002. 87(12): p. 1370-8.

[20] Murphy, R.A., et al., Aberrations in Plasma Phospholipid Fatty Acids in Lung Cancer Patients. *Lipids*, 2011.

[21] Pratt, V.C., et al., Alterations in lymphocyte function and relation to phospholipid composition after burn injury in humans. *Crit Care Med,* 2002. 30(8): p. 1753-61.

[22] Vidgren, H.M., et al., Incorporation of n-3 fatty acids into plasma lipid fractions, and erythrocyte membranes and platelets during dietary supplementation with fish, fish oil, and docosahexaenoic acid-rich oil among healthy young men. *Lipids*, 1997. 32(7): p. 697-705.

[23] Folch, J., M. Lees, and G.H. Sloane Stanley, A simple method for the isolation and purification of total lipides from animal tissues. *J Biol Chem,* 1957. 226(1): p. 497-509.

[24] Denomme, J., K.D. Stark, and B.J. Holub, Directly quantitated dietary (n-3) fatty acid intakes of pregnant Canadian women are lower than current dietary recommendations. *J Nutr,* 2005. 135(2): p. 206-11.

[25] Touchstone, J.C., J.C. Chen, and K.M. Beaver, Improved separation of phospholipids in thin layer chromatography. *Lipids*, 1980. 15: p. 61.

[26] Kulig, C.C., T.P. Beresford, and G.T. Everson, Rapid, accurate, and sensitive fatty acid ethyl ester determination by gas chromatography-mass spectrometry. *J Lab Clin Med,* 2006. 147(3): p. 133-8.

[27] van Eijk, H.M., J.G. Bloemen, and C.H. Dejong, Application of liquid chromatography-mass spectrometry to measure short chain fatty acids in blood. *J Chromatogr B Analyt Technol Biomed Life Sci,* 2009. 877(8-9): p. 719-24.
[28] Knothe, G. and J. Kenar, Determination of the fatty acid profile by ^{1}H-NMR soectroscopy. *Eur J Lipid Sci Technol,* 2004. 106: p. 88-96.
[29] Kang, J.X. and J. Wang, A simplified method for analysis of polyunsaturated fatty acids. *BMC Biochem*, 2005. 6: p. 5.
[30] Masood, A., K.D. Stark, and N. Salem, Jr., A simplified and efficient method for the analysis of fatty acid methyl esters suitable for large clinical studies. *J Lipid Res,* 2005. 46(10): p. 2299-305.
[31] Armstrong, J.M., A.H. Metherel, and K.D. Stark, Direct microwave transesterification of fingertip prick blood samples for fatty acid determinations. *Lipids*, 2008. 43(2): p. 187-96.
[32] Metherel, A.H., et al., The application of ultrasound energy to increase lipid extraction throughput of solid matrix samples (flaxseed). *Prostaglandins Leukot Essent Fatty Acids,* 2009. 81(5-6): p. 417-23.
[33] Braden, L.M. and K.K. Carroll, Dietary Polyunsaturated Fat in Relation to Mammary Carcinogenesis in Rats. *Lipids*, 1986. 21(4): p. 285-288.
[34] Carroll, K.K.K., H. T., Dietary fat in relation to tumorigenesis. *Prog. Biochem. Pharmacol.*, 1975. 10: p. 308-353.
[35] Cohen, L.A., et al., Dietary-Fat and Mammary-Cancer .1. Promoting Effects of Different Dietary Fats on N-Nitrosomethylurea-Induced Rat Mammary Tumorigenesis. *Journal of the National Cancer Institute*, 1986. 77(1): p. 33-42.
[36] Kamano, K., et al., Effects of a High-Linoleate and a High-Alpha-Linolenate Diet on Spontaneous Mammary Tumorigenesis in Mice. *Anticancer Research*, 1989. 9(6): p. 1903-1908.
[37] Katz, E.B. and E.S. Boylan, Stimulatory Effect of High Polyunsaturated Fat Diet on Lung Metastasis from the 13762 Mammary Adenocarcinoma in Female Retired Breeder Rats. *Journal of the National Cancer Institute*, 1987. 79(2): p. 351-358.
[38] Kort, W.J., et al., Omega-3-Fatty-Acids Inhibiting the Growth of a Transplantable Rat Mammary Adenocarcinoma. *Journal of the National Cancer Institute,* 1987. 79(3): p. 593-599.
[39] Chlebowski, R.T., et al., Adjuvant Dietary-Fat Intake Reduction in Postmenopausal Breast-Cancer Patient-Management. *Breast Cancer Research and Treatment,* 1992. 20(2): p. 73-84.
[40] Rose, D.P., Dietary Factors and Breast-Cancer. *Cancer Surveys,* 1986. 5(3): p. 671-687.
[41] Rose, D.P., J.M. Connolly, and X.H. Liu, Effects of Linoleic-Acid on the Growth and Metastasis of 2 Human Breast-Cancer Cell-Lines in Nude-Mice and the Invasive Capacity of These Cell-Lines in-Vitro. *Cancer Research*, 1994. 54(24): p. 6557-6562.
[42] Lee, M.M. and S.S. Lin, Dietary fat and breast cancer. *Annual Review of Nutrition,* 2000. 20: p. 221-248.
[43] Noguchi, M.T., T.; Kumaki, T.; Ohta, O.; Kitagawa, H.; Kinoshita, K.; Earashi, M.; Yagasaki, R.; Minami, M.; Kawahara, F.; Tsuyama, H.; Miwa, K., Dietary Fat and Breast Cancer: A Controversial lssue. *Breast Cancer,* 1997. 4: p. 67-75.
[44] Jump, D.B. and S.D. Clarke, Regulation of gene expression by dietary fat. *Annual Review of Nutrition,* 1999. 19: p. 63-90.

[45] Knazek, R.A., et al., Requirement of Essential Fatty-Acids in the Diet for Development of the Mouse Mammary-Gland. *Journal of the National Cancer Institute*, 1980. 64(2): p. 377-382.

[46] Miyamototiaven, M.J., L.A. Hillyard, and S. Abraham, Influence of Dietary-Fat on the Growth of Mammary Ducts in Balb-C Mice. *Journal of the National Cancer Institute*, 1981. 67(1): p. 179-188.

[47] Bandyopadhyay, G.K., et al., Linoleate Metabolites Enhance the Invitro Proliferative Response of Mouse Mammary Epithelial-Cells to Epidermal Growth-Factor. *Journal of Biological Chemistry,* 1987. 262(6): p. 2750-2756.

[48] Bandyopadhyay, G.K., et al., Proliferative Effects of Insulin and Epidermal Growth-Factor on Mouse Mammary Epithelial-Cells in Primary Culture - Enhancement by Hydroxyeicosatetraenoic Acids and Synergism with Prostaglandin-E2. *Journal of Biological Chemistry*, 1988. 263(16): p. 7567-7573.

[49] Grammatikos, S.I., et al., Diversity in the Ability of Cultured-Cells to Elongate and Desaturate Essential (N-6 and N-3) Fatty-Acids. *Biochemical Engineering Viii,* 1994. 745: p. 92-105.

[50] Grammatikos, S.I., et al., N-3 and N-6 Fatty-Acid Processing and Growth Effects in Neoplastic and Non-Cancerous Human Mammary Epithelial-Cell Lines. *British Journal of Cancer*, 1994. 70(2): p. 219-227.

[51] Balakrishnan, A., et al., Differential Proliferative Response to Linoleate in Cultures of Epithelial-Cells from Normal Human-Breast and Fibroadenomas. *Cancer Research,* 1989. 49(4): p. 857-862.

[52] Chalbos, D., et al., Progestin-Induced Fatty-Acid Synthetase in Human Mammary-Tumors - from Molecular to Clinical-Studies. *Journal of Steroid Biochemistry and Molecular Biology,* 1992. 43(1-3): p. 223-228.

[53] Yu, H.B., H., Insulin-like growth factors and cancer. *J. La State Med. Soc.*, 1999. 151: p. 218-223.

[54] Rao, G.A. and S. Abraham, Enhanced Growth-Rate of Transplanted Mammary Adenocarcinoma Induced in C3h-Mice by Dietary Linoleate. *Journal of the National Cancer Institute,* 1976. 56(2): p. 431-432.

[55] Rao, G.A. and S. Abraham, Reduced Growth-Rate of Transplantable Mammary Adenocarcinoma in C3h Mice Fed Eicosa-5,8,11,14-Tetraynoic Acid. *Journal of the National Cancer Institute*, 1977. 58(2): p. 445-447.

[56] Carter, C.A., et al., Effect of the Prostaglandin Synthetase Inhibitor Indomethacin on 7,12-Dimethylbenz(a)Anthracene-Induced Mammary Tumorigenesis in Rats Fed Different Levels of Fat. *Cancer Research*, 1983. 43(8): p. 3559-3562.

[57] Kollmorgen, G.M., et al., Influence of Dietary-Fat and Indomethacin on the Growth of Transplantable Mammary-Tumors in Rats. *Cancer Research*, 1983. 43(10): p. 4714-4719.

[58] Bartsch, H., J. Nair, and R.W. Owen, Dietary polyunsaturated fatty acids and cancers of the breast and colorectum: emerging evidence for their role as risk modifiers. *Carcinogenesis*, 1999. 20(12): p. 2209-2218.

[59] Brown, N.S. and R. Bicknell, Hypoxia and oxidative stress in breast cancer - Oxidative stress: its effects on the growth, metastatic potential and response to therapy of breast cancer. *Breast Cancer Research,* 2001. 3(5): p. 323-327.

[60] Chung, F.L., H.J.C. Chen, and R.G. Nath, Lipid peroxidation as a potential endogenous source for the formation of exocyclic DNA adducts. *Carcinogenesis*, 1996. 17(10): p. 2105-2111.

[61] Vaca, C.E., J. Wilhelm, and M. Harmsringdahl, Interaction of Lipid-Peroxidation Products with DNA - a Review. *Mutation Research,* 1988. 195(2): p. 137-149.

[62] Barbin, A., Etheno-adduct-forming chemicals: from mutagenicity testing to tumor mutation spectra. *Mutation Research-Reviews in Mutation Research,* 2000. 462(2-3): p. 55-69.

[63] Bartsch, H., et al., Formation, Detection, and Role in Carcinogenesis of Ethenobases in DNA. *Drug Metabolism Reviews,* 1994. 26(1-2): p. 349-371.

[64] Nair, J., et al., High dietary omega-6 polyunsaturated fatty acids drastically increase the formation of etheno-DNA base adducts in white blood cells of female subjects. *Cancer Epidemiology Biomarkers & Prevention,* 1997. 6(8): p. 597-601.

[65] Weisz, J., Invitro Assays of Aromatase and Their Role in Studies of Estrogen Formation in Target Tissues. *Cancer Research,* 1982. 42(8): p. 3295-3298.

[66] Wang, M.Y., et al., Lipid peroxidation-induced putative malondialdehyde-DNA adducts in human breast tissues. *Cancer Epidemiology Biomarkers & Prevention*, 1996. 5(9): p. 705-710.

[67] Boyd, N.F. and V. Mcguire, Evidence of Lipid-Peroxidation in Premenopausal Women with Mammographic Dysplasia. *Cancer Letters,* 1990. 50(1): p. 31-37.

[68] Martin, F.L., et al., DNA damage in breast epithelial cells: detection by the single-cell gel (comet) assay and induction by human mammary lipid extracts. *Carcinogenesis*, 1997. 18(12): p. 2299-2305.

[69] Malins, D.C., N.L. Polissar, and S.J. Gunselman, Progression of human breast cancers to the metastatic state is linked to hydroxyl radical-induced DNA damage. *Proceedings of the National Academy of Sciences of the United States of America,* 1996. 93(6): p. 2557-2563.

[70] Martucci, C.P. and J. Fishman, P450 Enzymes of Estrogen Metabolism. *Pharmacology & Therapeutics*, 1993. 57(2-3): p. 237-257.

[71] Welsch, C.W., et al., Influence of Dietary-Fat Levels on Development and Hormone Responsiveness of the Mouse Mammary-Gland. *Cancer Research,* 1985. 45(12): p. 6147-6154.

[72] Nishizuka, Y., Turnover of Inositol Phospholipids and Signal Transduction. *Science*, 1984. 225(4668): p. 1365-1370.

[73] Davis, D.L., et al., Medical Hypothesis - Xenoestrogens as Preventable Causes of Breast-Cancer. *Environmental Health Perspectives,* 1993. 101(5): p. 372-377.

[74] Zhu, B.T. and A.H. Conney, Functional role of estrogen metabolism in target cells: review and perspectives. *Carcinogenesis*, 1998. 19(1): p. 1-27.

[75] Liehr, J.G. and M.J. Ricci, 4-hydroxylation of estrogens as marker of human mammary tumors. *Proceedings of the National Academy of Sciences of the United States of America,* 1996. 93(8): p. 3294-3296.

[76] Cancer, I.A.f.R.o. Colorectal Cancer Incidence, Mortality and Prevalence Worldwide in 2008 Summary 2008 [cited 2012 March 6]; Available from: *http://globocan.iarc.fr/.*

[77] Zock, P.L. and M.B. Katan, Linoleic acid intake and cancer risk: a review and meta-analysis. . *The American Journal of Clinical Nutrition,* 1998.\. 68: p. 142-153.

[78] Davidson, L.A., et al., Carcinogen and dietary lipid regulate ras expression and localization in rat colon without affecting farnesylation kinetics. . *Carcinogenesis*, 1999. 20: p. 785-791.

[79] Dommels, Y.E., et al., Dietary n-6 and n-3 polyunsaturated fatty acids and colorectal carcinogenesis: results from cultured colon cells, animal models and human studies. *Environmetal Toxicology and Pharmacology,* 2002. 12: p. 233–244.

[80] Rao, C.V. and B.S. Reddy, Modulating effect of amount and types of dietary fat on ornithine decarboxylase, tyrosine protein kinase and prostaglandins production during colon carcinogenesis in male F344 rats. . *Carcinogenesis*, 1993. 14: p. 1327-1333.

[81] Reddy, B.S., C. Burill, and J. Rigotty, Effect of diets high in omega-3 and omega-6 fatty acids on initiation and postinitiation stages of colon carcinogenesis. . *Cancer Research,* 1991. 51 p. 487-491.

[82] Whelan, J. and M.F. McEntee, Dietary (n-6) PUFA and intestinal tumorigenesis. *The Journal of Nutrition,* 2004. 134: p. 3421S-3426S.

[83] Tuyns, A.J., M. Haelterman, and R. Kaaks, Colorectal cancer and the intake of nutrients: oligosaccharides are a risk factor. . *Nutrition and Cancer,* 1987. 10: p. 181-196.

[84] Hietanen, E., et al., Diet and oxidative stress in breast, colon and prostate cancer patients: a case–control study. . *European Journal of Clinical Nutrition,* 1994. 48: p. 575-586.

[85] Slattery, M.L., et al., Dietary fats and colon cancer: assessment of risk associated with specific fatty acids. *International Journal of Cancer,* 1997. 73: p. 670-677.

[86] Terry, P., et al., No association between fat and fatty acids intake and risk of colorectal cancer. *Cancer Epidemiology Biomarkers and Prevention,* 2001. 10: p. 913-914.

[87] Koh, W.P., et al., Interaction between cyclooxygenase-2 gene polymorphism and dietary n-6 polyunsaturated fatty acids on colon cancer risk: the Singapore Chinese Health Study. *British Journal of Cancer,* 2004. 90: p. 1760-1764.

[88] Cancer, I.A.f.R.o. Prostate Cancer Incidence, Mortality and Prevalence Worldwide in 2008 Summary 2008 [cited 2012 March 6]; Available from: *http://globocan.iarc.fr/.*

[89] Godley, P.A., et al., Biomarkers of essential fatty acid consumption and risk of prostatic carcinoma. *Cancer Epidemiology Biomarkers and Prevention*, 1996. 5: p. 889-895.

[90] Harvei, S., et al., Prediagnostic level of fatty acids in serum phospholipids: omega-3 and omega-6 fatty acids and the risk of prostate cancer. *International Journal of Cancer,* 1997. 71(4): p. 545-551.

[91] Clinton, S.K., et al., Growth of Dunning transplantable prostate adenocarcinomas in rats fed diets with various fat contents. . *The Journal of Nutrition,* 1988. 118: p. 908-914.

[92] Wang, Y., et al., Decreased growth of established human prostate LNCaP tumors in nude mice fed a low-fat diet. *Journal of the National Cancer Institute*, 1995 87(19): p. 1456-1462.

[93] Rose, D.P. and J.M. Connolly, Effects of fatty acids and eicosanoid synthesis inhibitors on the growth of two human prostate cancer cell lines. . *Prostate* 1991. 18: p. 243-254.

[94] Pandalai, P.K., et al., The effects of omega-3 and omega-6 fatty acids on in vitro prostate cancer growth. *Anticancer Research*, 1996. 16: p. 815-820.

[95] Maggiora, M., et al., An overview of the effect of linoleic and conjugated-linoleic acids on the growth of several human tumor cell lines. *International Journal of Cancer,* 2004. 112: p. 909-919.

[96] Newcomer, L.M., et al., The association of fatty acids with prostate cancer risk. *Prostate* 2001. 47: p. 262-268.
[97] Cunnane, S.C. and M.J. Anderson, Pure linoleate deficiency in the rat: Influence on growth, accumulation of n-6 polyunsaturates, and [1-C-14]linoleate oxidation. *Journal of Lipid Research,* 1997. 38(4): p. 805-812.
[98] Simopoulos, A.P., The omega-6/omega-3 fatty acid ratio, genetic variation, and cardiovascular disease. *Asia Pacific Journal of Clinical Nutrition*, 2008. 17: p. 131-134.
[99] Fischer, S.M., et al., Differential-Effects of Dietary Linoleic-Acid on Mouse Skin-Tumor Promotion and Mammary Carcinogenesis. *Cancer Research*, 1992. 52(7): p. S2049-S2054.
[100] Yasuda, M., et al., Linoleic acid metabolite suppresses skin inflammation and tumor promotion in mice: possible roles of programmed cell death 4 induction. *Carcinogenesis*, 2009. 30(7): p. 1209-1216.
[101] Hariharan, D., A. Saied, and H.M. Kocher, Analysis of mortality rates for pancreatic cancer across the world. *Hpb*, 2008. 10(1): p. 58-62.
[102] Society, A.C., in Cancer Facts & Figures 2010. 2010: *Atlanta: American Cancer Society*. p. 19.
[103] Wicha, M.S., L.A. Liotta, and W.R. Kidwell, Effects of Free Fatty-Acids on the Growth of Normal and Neoplastic Rat Mammary Epithelial-Cells. *Cancer Research,* 1979. 39(2): p. 426-435.
[104] Dippenaar, N., et al., The Reversibility of Cancer - Evidence That Malignancy in Melanoma-Cells Is Gamma-Linolenic Acid Deficiency-Dependent. *South African Medical Journal,* 1982. 62(15): p. 505-509.
[105] Fugiwara, F.T., S.; Imashuku, S., Anti-tumour effect of gamma-linolenic acid on cultured human neuroblastoma cells. *Prostaglandins Leukotrienes Med,* 1983. 23: p. 311-320.
[106] Begin, M.E., et al., Selective Killing of Human Cancer-Cells by Poly-Unsaturated Fatty-Acids. *Prostaglandins Leukotrienes and Medicine,* 1985. 19(2): p. 177-186.
[107] Begin, M.E., et al., Differential Killing of Human Carcinoma-Cells Supplemented with N-3 and N-6 Polyunsaturated Fatty-Acids. *Journal of the National Cancer Institute*, 1986. 77(5): p. 1053-1062.
[108] Falconer, J.S., et al., Effect of Eicosapentaenoic Acid and Other Fatty-Acids on the Growth in-Vitro of Human Pancreatic-Cancer Cell-Lines. *British Journal of Cancer*, 1994. 69(5): p. 826-832.
[109] Merendino, N., et al., Induction of apoptosis in human pancreatic cancer cells by docosahexaenoic acid. *Apoptosis: From Signaling Pathways to Therapeutic Tools,* 2003. 1010: p. 361-364.
[110] Roebuck, B.D., et al., Promotion by Unsaturated Fat of Azaserine-Induced Pancreatic Carcinogenesis in the Rat. *Cancer Research,* 1981. 41(10): p. 3961-3966.
[111] Birt, D.F., S. Salmasi, and P.M. Pour, Enhancement of Experimental Pancreatic-Cancer in Syrian Golden-Hamsters by Dietary-Fat. *Journal of the National Cancer Institute*, 1981. 67(6): p. 1327-1332.
[112] Birt, D.F., The Influence of Dietary-Fat on Carcinogenesis - Lessons from Experimental-Models. *Nutrition Reviews,* 1990. 48(1): p. 1-5.
[113] Ip, C., C.A. Carter, and M.M. Ip, Requirement of Essential Fatty-Acid for Mammary Tumorigenesis in the Rat. *Cancer Research,* 1985. 45(5): p. 1997-2001.

[114] Ip, C., Fat and Essential Fatty-Acid in Mammary Carcinogenesis. *American Journal of Clinical Nutrition*, 1987. 45(1): p. 218-224.

[115] Appel, M.J., A. Vangarderenhoetmer, and R.A. Woutersen, Effects of Dietary Linoleic-Acid on Pancreatic Carcinogenesis in Rats and Hamsters. *Cancer Research*, 1994. 54(8): p. 2113-2120.

[116] Farrow, D.C. and S. Davis, Diet and the Risk of Pancreatic-Cancer in Men. *American Journal of Epidemiology*, 1990. 132(3): p. 423-431.

[117] Howe, G.R., M. Jain, and A.B. Miller, Dietary Factors and Risk of Pancreatic-Cancer - Results of a Canadian Population-Based Case-Control Study. *International Journal of Cancer,* 1990. 45(4): p. 604-608.

[118] Baghurst, P.A., et al., A Case-Control Study of Diet and Cancer of the Pancreas. *American Journal of Epidemiology,* 1991. 134(2): p. 167-179.

[119] Olsen, G.W., et al., Nutrients and Pancreatic-Cancer - a Population-Based Case-Control Study. *Cancer Causes & Control,* 1991. 2(5): p. 291-297.

[120] Zatonski, W., et al., Nutritional Factors and Pancreatic-Cancer - a Case-Control Study from South-West Poland. *International Journal of Cancer,* 1991. 48(3): p. 390-394.

[121] Stolzenberg-Solomon, R.Z., et al., Prospective study of diet and pancreatic cancer in male smokers. *American Journal of Epidemiology,* 2002. 155(9): p. 783-792.

[122] Michaud, D.S., et al., Dietary meat, dairy products, fat, and cholesterol and pancreatic cancer risk in a prospective study. *American Journal of Epidemiology,* 2003. 157(12): p. 1115-1125.

[123] Thiebaut, A.C.M., et al., Dietary Fatty Acids and Pancreatic Cancer in the NIH-AARP Diet and Health Study. *Journal of the National Cancer Institute*, 2009. 101(14): p. 1001-1011.

[124] Clerc, P., et al., Lipid-Dependent Proliferation of Pancreatic-Cancer Cell-Lines. *Cancer Research,* 1991. 51(14): p. 3633-3638.

[125] Poston, G.J., J. Gillespie, and P.J. Guillou, Biology of Pancreatic-Cancer. *Gut*, 1991. 32(7): p. 800-812.

[126] Matsuoka, T., et al., Elevated dietary linoleic acid increases gastric carcinoma cell invasion and metastasis in mice. *British Journal of Cancer,* 2010. 103(8): p. 1182-1191.

[127] Rose, D.P., et al., Effect of Diets Containing Different Levels of Linoleic-Acid on Human Breast-Cancer Growth and Lung Metastasis in Nude-Mice. *Cancer Research*, 1993. 53(19): p. 4686-4690.

[128] Carroll, K.K., Experimental-Evidence of Dietary Factors and Hormone-Dependent Cancers. *Cancer Research*, 1975. 35(11): p. 3374-3383.

[129] Reddy, B.S., Dietary-Fat and Colon Cancer - Animal-Model Studies. *Lipids*, 1992. 27(10): p. 807-813.

[130] Welsch, C.W., Enhancement of Mammary Tumorigenesis by Dietary-Fat - Review of Potential Mechanisms. *American Journal of Clinical Nutrition,* 1987. 45(1): p. 192-202.

[131] Karmali, R.A., Prostaglandins and Cancer. *Ca-a Cancer Journal for Clinicians,* 1983. 33(6): p. 322-332.

[132] Karniali, R.A., Lipid nutrition,prostaglandins, and cancer. *Prostaglandins Leucotrienes Cancer,* 1985. 1: p. 203-212.

[133] Karmali, R.A., Fatty-Acids - Inhibition. *American Journal of Clinical Nutrition*, 1987. 45(1): p. 225-229.

[134] Mccormick, D.L. and A.M. Wilson, Combination Chemoprevention of Rat Mammary Carcinogenesis by Indomethacin and Butylated Hydroxytoluene. *Cancer Research*, 1986. 46(8): p. 3907-3911.

[135] Oconnor, T.P., et al., Effect of Dietary Omega-3 and Omega-6 Fatty-Acids on Development of Azaserine-Induced Preneoplastic Lesions in Rat Pancreas. *Journal of the National Cancer Institute*, 1989. 81(11): p. 858-863.

[136] Karmali, R.A., Omega-3 fatty acids and cancer: a review, in Polyunsaturated Fatty Acids and Eicosanoids, W.E.M. Lands, Editor. 1987, *American Oil Chemists' Society: Champaign*. p. 222-233.

[137] Abouelela, S.H., et al., Eicosanoid Synthesis in 7,12-Dimethylbenz(a)Anthracene-Induced Mammary Carcinomas in Sprague-Dawley Rats Fed Primrose Oil, Menhaden Oil or Corn-Oil Diet. *Lipids*, 1988. 23(10): p. 948-954.

[138] Abraham, S. and L.A. Hillyard, Effect of Dietary Carbon-18 Fatty-Acids on Growth of Transplantable Mammary Adenocarcinomas in Mice. *Journal of the National Cancer Institute*, 1983. 71(3): p. 601-605.

[139] Bull, A.W., et al., Invivo Stimulation of DNA-Synthesis and Induction of Ornithine Decarboxylase in Rat Colon by Fatty-Acid Hydroperoxides, Autoxidation Products of Unsaturated Fatty-Acids. *Cancer Research,* 1984. 44(11): p. 4924-4928.

[140] Berlin, E., E.J. Matusik, and C. Young, Effect of Dietary-Fat on the Fluidity of Platelet Membranes. *Lipids*, 1980. 15(8): p. 604-608.

[141] Lai, C.S., L.E. Hopwood, and H.M. Swartz, Electron-Spin Resonance Studies of Changes in Membrane Fluidity of Chinese-Hamster Ovary Cells during the Cell-Cycle. *Biochimica Et Biophysica Acta*, 1980. 602(1): p. 117-126.

[142] Doi, O., et al., Manipulation of Fatty-Acid Composition of Membrane Phospholipid and Its Effects on Cell-Growth in Mouse Lm Cells. *Biochimica Et Biophysica Acta,* 1978. 509(2): p. 239-250.

[143] Kidwell, W.R.K., R.A.; Vonderhaar, B.K.; Lasonczy, I., E*ffects of unsaturated fatty acids on the development and proliferation of normal and neoplastic breast epithelium, in Molecular interactions of nutrition and cancer,* M.S.V.E. Arnott, J.; Yang, Y., Editor. 1982, Raven Press: New York. p. 219-26.

[144] Zarkower, D.A., et al., Alteration by Prolactin of Surface-Charge and Membrane Fluidity of Rat 13762 Mammary Ascites Tumor-Cells. *Cell Biophysics*, 1984. 6(1): p. 53-66.

[145] Roebuck, B.D., et al., Carcinogen-Induced Lesions in the Rat Pancreas - Effects of Varying Levels of Essential Fatty-Acid. *Cancer Research*, 1985. 45(11): p. 5252-5256.

[146] Gregor, J.I., et al., Does enteral nutrition of dietary polyunsaturated fatty acids promote oxidative stress and tumour growth in ductal pancreatic cancer? *Experimental trial in Syrian Hamster. Prostaglandins Leukotrienes and Essential Fatty Acids*, 2006. 74(1): p. 67-74.

[147] Heukamp, I., et al., Impact of polyunsaturated fatty acids on hepato-pancreatic prostaglandin and leukotriene concentration in ductal pancreatic cancer - Is there a correlation to tumour growth and liver metastasis? *Prostaglandins Leukotrienes and Essential Fatty Acids*, 2006. 74(4): p. 223-233.

[148] Simonsen, N., et al., Adipose tissue omega-3 and omega-6 fatty acid content and breast cancer in the EURAMIC study. European Community Multicenter Study on

Antioxidants, Myocardial Infarction, and Breast Cancer. *Am J Epidemiol,* 1998. 147(4): p. 342-52.

[149] Bartram, H.P., et al., Missing anti-proliferative effect of fish oil on rectal epithelium in healthy volunteers consuming a high-fat diet: potential role of the n-3:n-6 fatty acid ratio. *Eur J Cancer Prev*, 1995. 4(3): p. 231-7.

[150] Simopoulos, A.P., The importance of the ratio of omega-6/omega-3 essential fatty acids. *Biomed Pharmacother*, 2002. 56(8): p. 365-79.

[151] Kris-Etherton, P.M., W.S. Harris, and L.J. Appel, Fish consumption, fish oil, omega-3 fatty acids, and cardiovascular disease. *Circulation*, 2002. 106(21): p. 2747-57.

[152] Organization, W.H., Interim Summary of Conclusions and Dietary Recommendations on Total Fat & Fatty Acids, -.N. *From the Joint FAO/WHO Expert Consultation on Fats and Fatty Acids in Human Nutrition*, 2008, Editor: Geneva.

[153] Cohen, L.A., et al., Effect of varying proportions of dietary menhaden and corn oil on experimental rat mammary tumor promotion. *Lipids*, 1993. 28(5): p. 449-56.

[154] Karmali, R.A., et al., Effect of n-3 fatty acids on mammary tumorigenesis. *Adv Prostaglandin Thromboxane Leukot Res*, 1987. 17B: p. 886-9.

[155] Maillard, V., et al., N-3 and N-6 fatty acids in breast adipose tissue and relative risk of breast cancer in a case-control study in Tours, France. *Int J Cancer,* 2002. 98(1): p. 78-83.

[156] Goodstine, S.L., et al., Dietary (n-3)/(n-6) fatty acid ratio: possible relationship to premenopausal but not postmenopausal breast cancer risk in U.S. women. *J Nutr*, 2003. 133(5): p. 1409-14.

[157] Rose, D.P. and J.M. Connolly, Omega-3 fatty acids as cancer chemopreventive agents. *Pharmacol Ther*, 1999. 83(3): p. 217-44.

[158] Chajes, V. and P. Bougnoux, Omega-6/omega-3 polyunsaturated fatty acid ratio and cancer. *World Rev Nutr Diet,* 2003. 92: p. 133-51.

[159] Leitzmann, M.F., et al., Dietary intake of n-3 and n-6 fatty acids and the risk of prostate cancer. *Am J Clin Nutr*, 2004. 80(1): p. 204-16.

[160] Chajes, V., et al., Plasma phospholipid fatty acid concentrations and risk of gastric adenocarcinomas in the European Prospective Investigation into Cancer and Nutrition (EPIC-EURGAST). *Am J Clin Nutr*, 2011. 94(5): p. 1304-13.

[161] Bougnoux, P., B. Giraudeau, and C. Couet, Diet, cancer, and the lipidome. *Cancer Epidemiol Biomarkers Prev*, 2006. 15(3): p. 416-21.

[162] Bagga, D., et al., Dietary modulation of omega-3/omega-6 polyunsaturated fatty acid ratios in patients with breast cancer. *J Natl Cancer Inst,* 1997. 89(15): p. 1123-31.

[163] Lavecchia, C., et al., Olive Oil, Other Dietary Fats, and the Risk of Breast-Cancer (Italy). *Cancer Causes & Control*, 1995. 6(6): p. 545-550.

[164] Erickson, K.L., Is there a relation between dietary linoleic acid and cancer of the breast, colon, or prostate? *American Journal of Clinical Nutrition*, 1998. 68(1): p. 5-7.

[165] Holmes, M.D., et al., Association of dietary intake of fat and fatty acids with risk of breast cancer. *Jama-Journal of the American Medical Association,* 1999. 281(10): p. 914-920.

[166] Hillyard, L.A. and S. Abraham, Effect of Dietary Poly-Unsaturated Fatty-Acids on Growth of Mammary Adenocarcinomas in Mice and Rats. *Cancer Research*, 1979. 39(11): p. 4430-4437.

[167] Hopkins, G.J.K., T. G.; Carroll, K. K., Polyunsaturated fatty acids as promoters of mammary carcinogenesis induced in Sprague-Dawley rats by 7,12-dimethylbenz[a]anthracene. *J. Natl. Cancer Inst.* , 1981. 66: p. 517-522.

[168] Hopkins, G.J. and K.K. Carroll, Relationship between Amount and Type of Dietary-Fat in Promotion of Mammary Carcinogenesis Induced by 7,12-Dimethylbenz[a]Anthracene. *Journal of the National Cancer Institute*, 1979. 62(4): p. 1009-1012.

[169] Hopkins, G.J. and C.E. West, Effect of Dietary Polyunsaturated Fat on Growth of a Transplantable Adenocarcinoma in C3havyfb Mice. *Journal of the National Cancer Institute,* 1977. 58(3): p. 753-756.

[170] Wetsel, W.C.R., A. E.; Newberne, P. M., Dietary fat and DMBA mammary carcinogenesis in rats. *Cancer Detect. Prev.*, 1981. 4: p. 535-543.

[171] Fay, M.P., et al., Effect of different types and amounts of fat on the development of mammary tumors in rodents: A review. *Cancer Research,* 1997. 57(18): p. 3979-3988.

[172] Greenwald, P., Role of dietary fat in the causation of breast cancer: Point. *Cancer Epidemiology Biomarkers & Prevention*, 1999. 8(1): p. 3-7.

[173] Hunter, D.J., Role of dietary fat in the causation of breast cancer: Counterpoint. *Cancer Epidemiology Biomarkers & Prevention*, 1999. 8(1): p. 9-13.

[174] Matsuba, S., et al., Effect of dietary linoleate/alpha-linolenate balance on experimentally induced gastric injury in rats. *Prostaglandins Leukotrienes and Essential Fatty Acids,* 1998. 59(5): p. 317-323.

[175] Ferretti, A., et al., Moderate Changes in Linoleate Intake Do Not Influence the Systemic Production of E-Prostaglandins. *Lipids*, 1985. 20(5): p. 268-272.

[176] James, M.J., et al., Simple Relationships Exist between Dietary Linoleate and the N-6 Fatty-Acids of Human Neutrophils and Plasma. *American Journal of Clinical Nutrition*, 1993. 58(4): p. 497-500.

Index